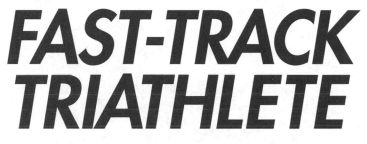

FAST-TRACK TRIATHLETE

**Balancing a big life with big performance
in long-course triathlon**

MATT DIXON

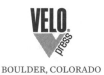

VELO press

BOULDER, COLORADO

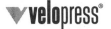

3002 Sterling Circle, Suite 100
Boulder, CO 80301–2338 USA

VeloPress is the leading publisher of books on endurance sports. Focused on cycling, triathlon, running, swimming, and nutrition/diet, VeloPress books help athletes achieve their goals of going faster and farther. Preview books and contact us at velopress.com.

Distributed in the United States and Canada by Ingram Publisher Services

Library of Congress Cataloging-in-Publication Data
Names: Dixon, Matt (Exercise physiologist), author.
Title: Fast-track triathlete : balancing a big life with big performance in
   long-course triathlon / Matt Dixon.
Description: Boulder, Colorado : VeloPress, [2017] | Includes index. |
   Identifiers: LCCN 2017039559 (print) | LCCN 2017039609 (ebook) | ISBN
   9781937716943 (ebook) | ISBN 9781937715748 (pbk. : alk. paper)
Subjects: LCSH: Triathlon—Training. | Triathlon—Physiological aspects.
Classification: LCC GV1060.73 (ebook) | LCC GV1060.73 .D54 2017 (print) | DDC
   796.42/57—dc23
LC record available at https://lccn.loc.gov/2017039559

This paper meets the requirements of ANSI/NISO Z39.48-1992 (Permanence of Paper).

Art direction by Vicki Hopewell
Cover design by Nate Baltikas
Cover and interior photographs by Jeff Clark
Interior design by Anita Koury
Text set in Mercury

17   18   19 / 10   9   8   7   6   5   4   3   2   1

Contents

Introduction

Triathlon is a complex and uniquely challenging sport. It demands a high degree of overall fitness and proficiency in three distinct disciplines that require a lot of sophisticated gear, and it necessitates relentless drive, focus, and many hours of training. Not surprisingly, the sport draws ambitious individuals whose lives are already rich with commitments to their careers and families. Those people seem to have a genuine desire to pursue big goals in Ironman® and Ironman 70.3 races.

Although anyone can enter triathlon at a casual or recreational level, to truly achieve success and continually improve in the sport takes ongoing commitment. You need a focused mindset and pragmatic adaptability to train and race while also performing at a high level at your workplace, within your family and social circles, and in your community. That's often much easier said than done, especially for people who are time starved before they even get started.

The reality is that in many cases, the pursuit of triathlon becomes all-consuming, especially when you are training for an Ironman triathlon. You've probably experienced this firsthand or witnessed it in friends or training partners, individuals who try so hard to achieve their goals in triathlon that the rest of their lives suffer. They become fully invested in the sport; they sign up for a race, buy the gear, and start training only to find themselves overwhelmed and falling behind, both in training and other aspects of their lives. They invest still more time and energy in training, but it only leads to fatigue and anxiety. Suddenly they're not performing as well at work, they're not sleeping or eating well, and they become more susceptible to illness. There might even be added tension with a significant other or family members. Amid this mounting pressure, these athletes continue to push themselves beyond their limits regardless of the detrimental effects.

I found myself in a similar scenario in my athletic pursuits as an elite swimmer and professional triathlete. When I reflect on my career, it is clear that I had a very strong work ethic, and I made it my mission to try to outwork my competition. Although I made the finals of the Olympic Swimming Trials, and I won a couple of professional races over the course of my triathlon career, I underperformed relative to my potential and ultimately burned out. The cause of my underperformance came down to the simple truth that I didn't have a comprehensive approach to training. Despite my educational background in exercise physiology as well as experience coaching collegiate-level swimming, I didn't structure my workouts correctly, and I didn't optimize my endurance training with the essential building blocks of success: strength, conditioning, nutrition, and recovery. I now refer to those four key areas as the pillars of performance because regardless of your experience, you must nurture and develop all of these areas to succeed as an athlete. They have become the baseline educational tools and program framework for all Purple Patch athletes.

I'm here to tell you there is a more realistic, sustainable, and life-affirming path to success. Best of all, it will actually help you overcome challenges in the rest of your life, too. It doesn't require you to maximize the number of hours you spend training during any given week. Instead, it is rooted in optimization of available hours. The goal is to attain the highest amount of quality training you can fit into your week while also maintaining high performance in the other important areas of your life. Your best training recipe might lead you to consistently log fewer hours of training most weeks, but the mission will be for those training hours to be very effective. It is all determined by what works for you.

Having coached multiple professional and age-group world champions and dozens of highly successful amateurs who live extremely busy lives, I've been able to develop a comprehensive framework and methodology that integrate triathlon training and racing into a full life. I wrote *Fast-Track Triathlete* for anyone looking to create and execute a sustainable plan for success. I will show you how to plan proactively, make pragmatic decisions and adjustments over the course of your training, and eliminate or scale workouts when necessary without compromising your key sessions. I've used the same framework and philosophy outlined in this book to help hundreds of athletes achieve their long-distance triathlon goals.

Like my previous book, *The Well-Built Triathlete*, I wrote this book with ambitious, performance-oriented, age-group athletes in mind. However, this book is not just about training for triathlons. Training for a full Ironman or Ironman 70.3 is a metaphor for something much bigger. Yes, this book will help you solve your Ironman challenges, but the intent is to help you do so by creating a sustainable framework for training and racing that also supports your bigger goals in work and life. Ultimately, I wrote this book to help you execute your Ironman goals and everything that goes with them.

Training doesn't have to become a distraction from work, keep you from being present for your family or commitments, or require you to live like a monk for several months. If you are a really busy person, your pursuit of triathlon had better be fun and bring you happiness. Otherwise, what's the point? It's possible for you to train and race in a way that improves your health and feeds your soul, thus giving you something for yourself. You can become a better version of yourself, at which point you will find that you have a greater capacity to focus and think critically at work and be better in your relationships.

Is this a controversial approach? Absolutely. It debunks the prevailing belief that triathlon has to be a selfish, exclusive pursuit that stands between you and your family and friends. Critics of my approach are obsessed, self-punishing types, and they probably aren't training correctly in the first place. They're single-mindedly chasing something unattainable and definitely unsustainable. This mindset can bring down so many triathletes, making their results meaningless in the greater context of life.

The approach we'll explore in this book takes courage. If you choose this journey, you will need to avoid looking over the fence at the athletes accumulating big hours and mileage. You will need to remain focused on your needs (and those of your loved ones) and not fall into the trap of feeling as if you must do more. *Fast-Track Triathlete* doesn't serve a performance-at-all-costs mindset, lining out everything you can possibly do to get faster.

It's more than possible to gain performance with limited training time, and I believe focused training is the best avenue for success. My 14-week race-prep plan will show you how it works, but I hope you will see beyond the training plan and your goals for your upcoming race. Use the same principles in the rest of your life, which is your most important performance pursuit. *Fast-Track Triathlete* demonstrates how to successfully implement an adaptable, pragmatic approach to training in terms of both time management and the habits proven to support performance. By following the principles and operating within the framework outlined in this book, you will make a critical investment in yourself that adds value and performance to every aspect of your life.

CASE STUDY: **EMBRACE THE JOURNEY**

CEO Michael Concannon, founder of three San Francisco–based software businesses, set a goal of completing his first Ironman. Although this aspiration is quite common, Michael was not looking to finish an Ironman as a badge of honor. He is an intelligent, highly motivated individual on a personal quest of sorts, a pursuit to enhance his life.

Michael didn't participate in organized sports when he was younger, but as an adult he occasionally ran and rode a bike. He taught himself to swim after his daughter was born, and six years later he found his way into Olympic-distance triathlons. As his enthusiasm for triathlon training and greater fitness grew, he began looking for a way to balance his many commitments.

When I started working with Michael, we decided to cut his training time back to an average of 12 or 13 hours per week. He could have sacrificed more family or work time, but fewer training hours proved enough to perform well and excel in those areas, too. Michael learned how to scale key training workouts and eliminate some of the supporting sessions as needed. By establishing a sustainable training program rather than consistently dancing on the edge of overtraining, he was able to remain energized on a daily and weekly basis. Coupled with good nutrition and sleep habits, Michael's training kept him fresh throughout the workday and engaged at home with his wife and three young kids.

Michael proactively planned his training, blocking out the time as he would for meetings. This allowed him to be focused during his workouts, which paid off when he returned to the office invigorated. Ultimately, he learned to control what he could control (namely his training) and adapt to the unpredictable nature of entrepreneurial business and the day-to-day life of his busy family. Michael admits that a 5:30 a.m. swim workout is challenging, but he still makes it to the pool two mornings a week. He knows that training block is important to achieving his goals and helps to balance the rest of his day.

If he has a transcontinental trip to New York City for business, he adapts his training before, during, and after he travels. If he's feeling fatigued and knows he needs to skip a certain session so he can finish a work project or attend an event with his family, that's what he does. It no longer makes him anxious. It's a win-win situation for his training, his health, and his daily responsibilities. Furthermore, his wife and children have taken to sport in their own ways, too. They've come to appreciate teamwork, endurance, and mental fortitude, and they understand why Michael's triathlon goals are important. His example benefits the entire family.

PART 1

THE PERFORMANCE JOURNEY

1

Mindset

If your goal is to progress in triathlon, establishing the appropriate mindset is your first order of business. Achieving success in triathlon requires that you maneuver through a complex series of ever-changing challenges. Although triathlon should be approached as a single sport of swim-bike-run, there are three complex disciplines to master against a backdrop of regular stress and fatigue. The sport requires a lot of gear, many hours of purposeful training, and special attention to fueling, hydration, and recovery. The longer the triathlon is, the more challenging the puzzle becomes. There is no simple, formulaic approach to guarantee success in triathlon for the ambitious athlete with a full life and a weekly schedule of work, family, and community commitments. However, if you start with the appropriate mindset built upon a sound work/life balance, pragmatism, and adaptability, your journey enables you to arrive at races optimally prepared for your best performance. It's a rewarding pursuit that renews your motivation to work toward even better results and create an avenue for continued improvement, achievement, and growth in the other important areas of your life.

In your own triathlon journey you have identified some practices that work well for you, and you have achieved some level of success, but no one gets it right all the time. Despite one's best efforts and hundreds of hours of training, the results on race day often yield underperformance and disappointment. Many athletes remain in the dark as to why this is the case, especially after putting in loads of work at the expense of everything else in their lives. Therein lies one of the most glaring missteps that plagues so many triathletes. Underachieving usually can be traced back to being rooted in an unhelpful mindset.

Your mindset is far more important than specific workouts and intervals. I often discuss with athletes the concept of their *potential within the context of the life they lead*. Many triathletes never reach their potential; it's difficult to manage all of the training hours (because of fatigue, poor scheduling, or a training plan at too high a volume), it's not possible to be present and focused enough to train effectively, or the emphasis on training leads to feeling distracted and overwhelmed in other areas of life. Even as athletes try to cram the training into daily and weekly schedules filled with other important commitments, the results become more elusive. That kind of self-pressure puts an athlete on a downward spiral that leads to chronic fatigue, overuse injuries, frustration, disappointment, and burnout.

Ultimately, long-term sustainable success is going to require a clean slate, a new approach that permeates all areas of your busy life. The good news is that if you can take this on, you should not only achieve your triathlon aspirations but also establish a platform for excelling in health, work, and life as a whole.

BALANCING THE SPORT/LIFE EQUATION

In seeking an effective performance model, it's natural to look to those achieving great results. Amateur triathletes as well as many coaches have traditionally turned to top-level pros for inspiration, studied their approach, and mimicked how they train. Although there are certainly many things to learn about training and racing from the professionals, it's a mistake to attempt to emulate a professional approach at the amateur level, especially within the context of a busy life. Professional triathletes train many more hours every week than you can, and they can put more time, effort, and resources toward training and recovery because triathlon *is* essentially their full-time job.

The programs I design for professional athletes are unabashedly built for world-class performance. Many coaches suggest that amateur triathletes try to execute a similar training regimen summarily diluted to accommodate far fewer hours of training every week. However, it's not that simple. In fact, for a busy amateur limited both by athletic ability and by other commitments, a training plan that imitates a pro athlete's preparation develops bad habits rather than performance. If an athlete is never able to effectively execute the requirements of the training plan, it creates a platform for failure, opens the door for many other follow-up mistakes, and ultimately invites overload and exhaustion.

I believe in amateurs pursuing performance in the context of a balanced life. The goal isn't to qualify for Kona, become an age-group Ironman 70.3 podium finisher, or even just improve your time from your previous race *at the expense of life*. Performance should be built on a platform of health. An approach centered on pragmatism and adaptability that takes into account your own life circumstances, physiology, and focus will put you on the path to continued progress and success.

Everyone has a different set of life circumstances, but some basic tenets apply to just about everyone in the sport. It all starts with understanding the context of your life and how triathlon fits into it. That looks entirely different for professionals and aspiring age-group athletes. A professional triathlete doesn't just "fit in" the training; life is anchored by it, and maximizing performance is the highest priority.

In many ways, professional athletes are the barometer for performance. They are our lab subjects for learning how different training stimuli affect the body. The training/adaptation equation is simplified when you isolate the variables in this way. The opportunity to push against an athlete's physical limits in order to gain a positive performance adaptation can be met more easily with an equally appropriate amount of rest and recovery. When we add to this the greater availability of nutritional supplementary therapies for intake, the parameters are widened for continued improvements.

When I coach professional or world-class amateur triathletes, I am looking to suppress all factors that contaminate their sports-life equation. This means reducing their lives to simple components. I'm not aiming for some sort of former Eastern Bloc, machine mentality. I firmly believe professional athletes should be healthy, happy, and able to pursue relationships, but their chosen profession (their job) is world-class triathlon performance. So our collective approach reflects that ambition. I've coached athletes through the transition from amateur to pro. It entails a massive shift in mindset that illustrates why the pro approach isn't a good fit for amateur athletes.

CASE STUDY: **FROM FAST TRACK TO PRO**

When Sarah Piampiano first came to me for coaching, she was a high-achieving, amateur triathlete working long, hard hours as an investment banker on Wall Street. She had a couple of years of triathlon experience under her belt, but she was struggling to fit in the training.

The modest early successes and positive life changes Sarah experienced compelled her to begin training on a regular basis, but what she was doing wasn't sustainable. She was limiting her success in both her high-level job and her aspiring triathlon career. In addition to working the long, Wall Street hours, she was trying to squeeze in 12 to 16 hours of training each week. She didn't have much time for rest and recovery, let alone the ability to focus on proper nutrition, fueling, and hydration. She became more prone to illness and was often fatigued from lack of sleep.

Eventually, Sarah decided to reduce her weekly work commitment to 30 hours per week and focus more on her key training sessions, understanding that the sport-life balance sometimes didn't allow her to execute all of the supporting sessions in her regimen. She immediately started to feel more rested, and performance followed. Sarah achieved such great results that she decided to turn pro in late 2011 and quit her banking job entirely in early 2012 at the age of 31, when most people are becoming more invested in their careers. It was a decision her family, friends, and coworkers didn't all understand, but she knew it would afford her the chance to see how good she could be in triathlon. Shortly thereafter, she won the Ironman 70.3 in New Orleans and later finished 23rd in the Ironman World Championships in Kona.

For Sarah to achieve her performance capacity as a professional, training had to become her absolutely highest priority, and the other aspects of her life had to fit around it. Her weekly schedule grew to include three or four training activities per day. The increased training stimuli highlighted the need for more recovery. Along with putting a premium on appropriate rest and recuperation, Sarah also had to reprioritize nutrition and fueling to facilitate the goals of her training.

It was a tough transition, and Sarah pressured herself because she wanted to justify her decision to quit her high-income job. Early on, she made the mistake of training so hard that she couldn't handle the intensity. Sarah has since found balance and developed a sustainable training regimen. She's collected numerous podium finishes in Ironman and Ironman 70.3 races in recent years, including a 7th-place finish at the Ironman World Championships in 2015 and multiple Ironman championships.

How does that apply to you? Even though some amateur triathletes have more time to train than others do, the majority don't have the opportunity to be relentless in triathlon pursuits. Your approach to the sport starts with a holistic understanding of all of your other time commitments and how they play out on a daily, weekly, monthly, and annual basis. You might have many other performance journeys, be it work, parenting, community volunteering, or leisure pursuits. Of course, you still want to achieve your own version of triathlon excellence. Whether it's winning an amateur world championship, qualifying for Kona, or crossing the finish line in an Ironman 70.3 race for the first time, the common thread is a desire to improve.

So instead of organizing life around sport, you need to pursue rigorous training in the right context so you can give it the appropriate amount of attention. Unlike Sarah's pro situation, which allows for more rigidity and continuity in terms of training, the many variables in your life mean you have a constant need for adaptability and pragmatic decision making. If you're working a full-time job, you might usually have time for only one or, at most, two key sessions per day. You might also have to balance business meetings, presentations, deadlines, work-related travel, and a variety of family, social, and household commitments.

As a coach, I regularly see the same motivation that builds athletes' insatiable appetite for triathlon success applied to the rest of their lives. Most athletes I coach have, to varying degrees, wonderfully big lives that fill their waking hours. They juggle a busy family schedule, social life, holidays, and travel (the list goes on) with highly successful careers, all built upon an unwavering commitment to excellence. I've watched many top-performing business professionals and entrepreneurs carry their athletic success into their families, partnerships, and friendships.

As a coach I recognize and respect the fact that these commitments are critical and unchangeable. After all, you are not *just* a triathlete; you have a livelihood, you have a family, you have a role to play in supporting friends and your greater community. It's important that you thrive in these areas, too. For all of these reasons, from a training-focus perspective, an ambitious, busy triathlete is more or less the opposite of a pro. That is precisely why the training mindset I use with professional athletes is the polar opposite of the mindset I bring to age-group athletes.

INTEGRATE, DON'T ACCUMULATE

The first question I often get from an athlete who approaches me for coaching is, "How many hours a week do I need to train to get ready for this race?" Unfortunately, it's the wrong question. I honestly cannot provide a clear answer as to how many training hours are necessary for this athlete because I don't yet know how many hours are available. I don't have an understanding of the athlete's other life commitments. Furthermore, the question of how much time is required assumes an unlimited supply. In rare cases this might be the case, but it's hardly the norm. Most of the ambitious amateurs have about 10–15 hours per week available, but their time varies greatly from week to week depending on other commitments, travel, and a variety of unexpected contingencies.

The number of hours spent training or how sharp your focus is does not decide the fate of your goals. Establishing the right mindset to maximize the training time you have brings the answer you seek. Let's take a step back and consider what you are aiming to accomplish with training. When we compare pros and amateurs, their priorities and training loads will typically be dramatically different, but the *mission* of training is the same for top-level pros as it is for you. *The mission of training is to arrive at your race ready to perform your best.*

I know it might seem overly simple, but this mission is vital in defining our training mindset. In my experience, too many amateur triathletes make the mistake of setting their barometer of success on the specifics of accumulated training time and mileage. In other words, they're trying to rack up big yardage in the pool, long hours on the bike, and extensive mileage on the run. Instead, they should establish a mindset that considers the context of their entire lives and allows for consistency over many months and pragmatic adaptability on a weekly basis to get them to their races fit, strong, and healthy.

Even that worthy goal comes with a caveat. Too many athletes make it their goal simply to become fitter or stronger, but there are no awards for the athlete who has the highest functional threshold or who has covered the most training miles. If you arrive at the starting line fresh, with the necessary physical and mental capacity and with a clear understanding of how to execute your best swim, your best ride, and your best run on race day, then you are on the path to success.

After you acquire this mindset, you can approach training with a clear intention: Maximize your training load within your realistic amount of training time in a way that achieves a positive life/sport balance in any given week. Resist the temptation to do more for the sake of doing more or because you think you have to or because some of your friends or competitors might be taking that approach. Chasing after amorphous fitness goals will only lead to an unsustainable situation that inserts too much training load into a busy week, making it impossible to maintain an appropriate work/life balance.

Real success is built on the consistent layering of months and months of specific work on a platform of healthy sustainability. Following a realistic approach relative to your specific life circumstances will physically and mentally bolster you to the point that you become less prone to injuries, illness, lingering fatigue, and frustration. This creates the opportunity to arrive at the race healthy, fresh, and energetic with more than enough fitness to execute your best performance.

What you do on a given day, in a given training session, during a given swim, ride, run, or whatever activity (or inactivity, for that matter) will directly affect your physical and mental preparedness at the starting line of your race, but it could also lead to erosion of the harmonious balance of your entire life if not done properly. Going harder is also a relative term, and cramming too much intensity into a program will dilute the quality of positive adaptations because it will not allow you the ability to recover.

The goal is to execute those sessions with intent and balance them with proper recovery to achieve positive adaptations, continually watching for the negative adaptations that can add up to long-term challenges such as chronic fatigue, monotony, increased stress, or anxiousness about other areas of your life. This realization is crucial. That doesn't mean training and its lingering effects should always feel good or that you can't train when you're fatigued, but the goal must always be to achieve positive adaptations from the training load.

Now we hit the real challenge: to achieve our mission in a time-consuming, equipment-heavy, and technique-driven sport given the continual ebb and flow of a full, demanding life. To meet this challenge, I want you to think in terms of *integration*, not *accumulation*. When you successfully integrate an optimal training load into your life, you will achieve your best performance.

In order to improve as an athlete and see different results, you must retain a pragmatic mindset grounded in the realities of your life. You might draw inspiration from the best athletes in triathlon, but stop there. Now your focus shifts to how you can most effectively realize your specific goals. Ask yourself: *How can I go from where I am now to a state of absolute readiness to perform at my best?*

Performance within the context of a busy life is a liberating concept and opens the door to broader success. An executive I train expressly requested that I prepare him to perform at 90 percent of his capacity. This request demonstrated amazing insight because he knew that to reach 100 percent capacity, he would have to make undesirable sacrifices in some, if not all, of the other parts of his life. His pragmatic and adaptable approach, coupled with his willingness to pursue the optimal over the absolute, meant that his performance yield increased across all areas of his life, not just in his sport, thus exceeding his own expectations.

Meeting this challenge via integration is fast-track triathlon training at its best because it sacrifices nothing essential, maximizes everything you do and have, and achieves positive, long-lasting results. It is by no means a short-term panacea because it develops the consistency and framework for your greatest performance yield in both sport and life, year after year.

TRAIN FOR ONE SPORT, NOT THREE

Triathlon is a sophisticated sport that captures the imagination with the distinct possibility of personal achievement. All of the gear and metrics come with an aura of challenge and potential. Long-distance triathlons represent enormous physical and mental tasks and require a significant time commitment, and this is why competing in an Ironman is seen as a badge of honor. The demanding nature of the sport has always attracted driven individuals.

Triathlon is a relatively young sport, with an ever-developing identity. Some of the prevalent training methods are left over from the mindset made popular at the sport's inception in the 1970s. The "more is better" manifesto was adopted by triathlon pioneers who fought for bragging rights with their capacity to log massive numbers of miles and do endless sit-ups in saunas on a bet. The iconic triathletes from the early days of the sport including the big four of Dave Scott, Mark Allen, Scott Tinley, and Scott Molina as well as forerunners Gordon Haller, Tom Warren, "Cowman" Ken Shirk, and early women's champions

Paula Newby-Fraser, Erin Baker, and Sylvain and Patricia Puntous became legendary for their relentless training pursuits.

To the mainstream sporting world, triathlon was a spectacle back then, and these athletes were as interested in pushing the very limits of human endurance as they were in the emerging sport of swim-bike-run. There was not a well-defined training protocol for Ironman in the early to mid-1980s (and certainly few coaches) and that meant aspiring pros as well as ambitious amateurs intrigued enough to want to participate were gleaning whatever training they could from the elite professionals. They were the only role models, and there was little logical sense, scientific understanding, or evidential backing for most of the training at the time. The predominant school of thought was that whoever did the most extreme training leading up to the race would inevitably rule the day. There was an obsession with being excessive, a formula that never served anyone well.

In the ensuing years, triathlon captured the imagination of traditional endurance athletes (swimmers, road cyclists, and middle- to long-distance track and road runners) with abilities and expertise well suited to their disciplines. As participation in triathlon grew, each discipline brought the specialized knowledge and effectively created a circus with three ringmasters under one big-top tent and little chance for cohesiveness. The notion of working on your weaknesses while maintaining your strengths (for example, a good runner might have to put considerably more time into swimming and/or cycling) was formed with good intent, but it didn't consider the relationship of competing in all three disciplines successively.

Triathlon has since evolved into a stand-alone industry with an influential stake in the world of endurance sports. Training has evolved because of better science, better coaching, and of course a broader base of knowledge and experience on the part of the athletes themselves. More and more, professional triathletes rise from pupils of the triathlon, not necessarily from other endurance sports. Triathlon became more mainstream when it was accepted into the Olympics in 2000 and gained increased media exposure, which resulted in monumental growth, especially in Ironman, Ironman 70.3, and other long-course events. Triathlon coaching services, training websites, and enterprising media conglomerates boomed. Despite all of this progress, many amateur triathletes still rely on training advice from the individual disciplines or deconstruct their performance and training into those three disciplines.

Each of triathlon's stages has its own methodology with regard to technique, training, and racing as a single event. Pool swimming technique and training involves big volume and intensity in preparation for events lasting 20 seconds to 15 minutes in a controlled environment. Cycling instruction is largely focused on classics and tour riding, where athletes ride road bikes in pack formation. Classic training approaches to road and track running show no consideration of the aftereffects of swimming and cycling. These methodologies fall short of preparing you for long-course triathlon races. You are first required to have aptitude in open-water swimming, with its dynamic environment and influence of being shoulder to shoulder with many of your competitors. We then begin a time-trial on our bikes, with the need to focus on sufficient nutrition and hydration for the next effort. We start the run in a state of substantial fatigue, dehydration, and nutritional deficit, and performance is dramatically affected by how the previous two disciplines played out. Triathlon must be understood as swim-bike-run; one sport with three disciplines that are not mutually exclusive. As you will come to find out, for the busy amateur, this concept provides both a challenge and an opportunity.

Think of where you most commonly experience a performance decline in a race. For most of us, this is on the run. Fatigue, cramps, and frustration all come bubbling to the surface. When this happens in a race, athletes resolve to focus on the run during the next training cycle in the hope of improving their ability to run through the fatigue next time around. Perhaps this approach will lead to modest gains, but it is a classic example of isolating the disciplines and suffering as a result. Most triathletes fail to recognize that their run performance is influenced by their swimming preparation and ability, their cycling position and pacing, and their nutrition and fueling. It's all well and good to consult knowledgeable swim coaches, bike coaches, and run coaches, but you still have to sift their advice through the triathlon filter.

A poor performance in the run doesn't necessarily mean you have poor running ability. If you come out of T2 fatigued because of inadequate training, overexertion in the swim or on the bike, or dehydration and deficient fueling, it's quite possible that you haven't been given the opportunity to demonstrate your running ability at all. If you want to succeed, start thinking of triathlon as *one* sport.

AVOID THE UNDERPERFORMANCE CONDITION

As a whole, the triathlon community is made up of smart, intuitive people well aware that in signing up for a half-Ironman or Ironman, they are already pushing their limits. Few of us live at 60 percent of our capacity. We strive to make good use of all of our time and energy. This is the hallmark of anyone highly motivated and successful, and it's part of what attracts us to long-course triathlon despite the fact that our days are full and evenings and weekends are harnessed to other enterprises. We involve ourselves in the things that matter to us most, both professionally and personally: a position on a board of directors at work or at a nonprofit, coaching our child's soccer team, taking time each evening to connect with family on what is happening and what is important to them. These things are vital components of our lives.

We bring that same drive to triathlon, eager to begin a training program that promises the results we seek. Meticulously prepared on colored spreadsheets, training plans are triathletes' beacon of performance success. Although they tell us what to do each day, they don't necessarily provide a clear definition of where we are in the training cycle or what it is we are trying to achieve at any given moment. Workouts are prescribed as a given time or distance, progressing on the assumption that these parameters will be met. The most glaring problem is that most of these training programs are too rigid to conform to our lives.

Highly motivated athletes will make every effort to stick to this training program. Unfortunately, life is not a spreadsheet, and you can't crack the code of triathlon success with data or algorithms. Life is dynamic, even chaotic, with something happening every week, or even every day, that disrupts best-laid plans. When the barometer for training success is the accumulation of training hours and the exact execution of every prescribed workout, you're immediately set up for failure.

Panic sets in. A missed 6 p.m. running session moves to 4 a.m. the following morning to squeeze in the missed mileage. One such early morning catch-up session might be manageable, but thereafter, bad habits can creep in (in this case, sacrificing sleep) and quickly take root. Athletes compromise sleep and neglect nutrition to accommodate training. These crucial elements of preparation are the supporting cast to the three stars of the sport (swim, bike, and run). Left backstage, their absence will be felt. The singular focus of achieving a set amount of swim, bike, and run miles or minutes relegates them to an afterthought.

However, as soon as something unpredictable happens, you are left to make your own decisions, lacking the skills necessary to either prioritize or scale workouts. The disappointment of intervals cut short and sessions skipped makes us susceptible to a failing mindset. You can only see one set of numbers. Anything less than those numbers is time, distance, and most profoundly, confidence lost. This panic places the mission and goal of the training program—to create positive adaptations—in jeopardy. Any grasp on what might constitute training success is lost. Although you might be getting more fit in some ways, you mostly become increasingly fatigued.

Don't buy into the myth that training success depends on precisely adhering to an unrealistic, rigid training schedule, the "more is better" paradigm.

A rigid, data-driven mentality chips away at the foundations of performance, leaving cracks and gaps that begin to be filled with quick fixes for damaged or neglected fundamentals. These Band-Aid solutions are the training equivalent of fad diets: short term, unsustainable, misinformed, and ultimately unhealthy. The end result is that you arrive at your races in a state of fatigued confusion, focused on the training you have missed rather than empowered by the training you have achieved.

The underperformance condition is not necessarily failure, but at the same time, it is certainly not success. Underperformance is often the result of a mismatch of agendas in which unrealistic training is forced into a complex life, with resultant conflict. The only constant is consistently poor performance relative to time investment, consistent injuries, and consistent frustration. Arriving at the underperformance condition, triathletes find that their broader lives suffer from similar neglect, likely with the same results. Underperformance puts them in jeopardy of never realizing their true potential.

Looking back on my own career, first as a collegiate swimmer and later as a professional triathlete, I can see that I was first a pupil and then a master of the underperformance condition. In college, my training was primarily focused on pure swimming. I spent about 25 hours a week in the water. I included two hard, nonspecific gym sessions just prior to the afternoon swim session for those days. Time in the water and, to a lesser extent, time in the gym, were the two factors that governed my swimming program.

There was little education about proper nutrition, fueling, and hydration. Water bottles were not allowed on the pool deck during training, even when I was swimming nearly four hours a day. I ate poorly like many university students. Sunday was the only day off from training, and naturally I would go out on Saturday night until the early hours of Sunday morning. I was training very hard, yet I was ignorant of the roles recovery, nutrition, and hydration played in my performance.

When I moved into triathlon, I was in the process of completing my master's degree. My increasingly busy life restricted training time. Though I performed well as an amateur, my move into professional racing led me to where I am today. With the help of a coach, I transferred my world-class swimming mindset and work ethic into the ranks of professional triathlon. I became world-class at triathlon training.

Driven as I was by the culture of triathlon training at the time, anything outside of actual swim, bike, and run training was deemed irrelevant or, especially with regard to recovery, a sign of weakness. Every day was a grind, and every day was big. Ultimately my capacity to handle the training stress, in conjunction with an absence of the supporting cast of sleep, nutrition, and fueling, resulted in a form of chronic fatigue. The only way out of such a condition was to withdraw from training and racing.

This forced removal provided me an opportunity for reflection, learning, and growth. It gave me a new perspective on the landscape of triathlon training at that time and shaped my philosophy and methodology for triathlon and endurance training as a coach. Armed with a master's degree in exercise physiology and collegiate swim coaching experience, I was determined to develop a better approach to training that would combat the underperformance condition.

I am continually learning as a coach (to do otherwise is surely the death of a coach), but the philosophy behind my coaching methodology is fundamentally the same today as it was when I established Purple Patch. Out of my own experiences with overtraining and physical breakdown came a better approach to achieving optimal performance.

A BETTER APPROACH TO TRAINING

One of my priorities as a coach is to successfully educate athletes. I want all athletes with whom I work, whether pro or amateur, to be able to navigate the complexities of triathlon and discern what is most important.

In developing a new approach, I want busy amateur athletes to develop a mindset that could be applied to every aspect of their performance journey, from planning and prescription to evaluation and execution. I want to keep them from falling into a pattern of focusing almost exclusively on swim, bike, and run, so I developed the four Purple Patch pillars of performance.

The pillars of performance include not only *endurance training* but also *functional strength*, *nutrition and fueling*, and *recovery*. At the most basic level, when we view these pillars as equally important, it changes our thinking entirely. For starters, there is just one pillar for three disciplines because we now think of triathlon as swim-bike-run. The other three pillars now bear a higher degree of importance. If any one of those pillars is deficient or absent, the whole is adversely affected.

If we think about what we're trying to accomplish, positive adaptations to training stimuli, it follows that our endurance training should adhere to these important principles:

1. It must enable and maintain the element of *consistency*.
2. It must be *specific* to the needs of the individual athlete.
3. It must allow for continued, smart, short-term *progress* throughout the course of the season and long-term progress season after season.
4. It must be built on a firm understanding that true performance, through both short and long-term progression, requires *patience*.
5. The athlete must be fundamentally *healthy*.

So now we have an understanding that an overall program that delivers training success requires equal respect for its four constituents. It has to allow for consistent, specific training that progresses over time. To develop positive adaptations to training stimuli, there must be a platform of health from which to operate. How, then, do you obtain the greatest return from your time investment? How can you realize your greatest performance yield from a program that meets these complementary criteria?

Ultimately, our goal is to understand individual athletes' life circumstances, research their background and history in the sport, and determine how many hours they have available to train. We then deliver a program built upon key sessions and supporting sessions for all three disciplines. We arm you with the tools to make smart, pragmatic decisions by yourself. Those skills can be applied to various parts of the training approach, but they can also be transferred to other aspects of your life to achieve success.

Before you even consider types of intervals, specific modes of delivery, and training loads, you need to execute the basics well. In doing so, you maintain control of the things you can control: the exercise prescription, equipment choices, nutrition, sleep, and recovery. Definitively, you must also be in control of your mindset; you must understand and embrace the pillars of performance and the keys to success. Harmoniously integrate these things into your life and you have achieved the performance mindset.

CASE STUDY: **LESSONS FROM SAMI THE BULL**

Sami Inkinen came to me just as he was in the thick of launching his San Francisco–based, real-estate search company, Trulia. Although his triathlon experience was limited, he had some solid results under his belt. However, his ambitions were set significantly higher than his modest results. The biggest obstacle to his triathlon ambitions was his work life, a typical story for age-group athletes, particularly those with limited time.

Figuring out how to optimize an athlete's training workload is different for everyone based on physiology, athletic background, work/life balance, and other unique variables. Fortunately, Sami is always diligent in tracking his nutrition, fueling, and sleep in conjunction with his training. We began not by questioning how much training he could do but by deciding upon areas in which he was unwilling to compromise. Atop the list were such items as proper nutrition and fueling, high-quality sleep, and the most specific swim, bike, and run sessions that could be executed well.

Taking these parameters into account left him with 10 to 12 hours for training each week. On paper, this might appear too few hours to truly train successfully as an elite, age-group triathlete. However, the key to maximizing the available hours was in how they were used. As Sami's coach, I was responsible for planning sessions that allowed stimulus for improvement that could be matched with recovery. These would progress with consistency throughout the season to help Sami arrive at key races ready to perform at his best. Aside from a few opportunities to attend a weekend training camp, he never exceeded the

12-hours-of-training-per-week rule. In fact, on several occasions, to uphold consistency, health, and energy, he did less.

Sami's task was to apply the plan intelligently and to make decisions based on logic, not emotion. By planning ahead, Sami was able to counter lost training time and rest resulting from a meeting that required travel time by cutting intensity and duration and delaying key sessions until time allowed. He supported his training with excellent nutrition and fueling and high-quality sleep. His pragmatic approach to training and his insistence on executing sessions well paid off. Sami was able to achieve multiple overall Ironman and Ironman 70.3 wins, overall championships at Alcatraz and Wildflower, an Ironman 70.3 amateur world championship, and his sub-nine-hour time in the Hawaii Ironman.

The beauty of Sami's training approach and results lies in the realization of his physical attributes and incredible work ethic, but it never would have happened without his correct mindset. He knew from the start that he needed to maximize his key training sessions within his limited window of training opportunity. Training just 10 to 12 hours a week for Ironman racing was risky but nowhere near as counterintuitive as attempting to squeeze 13–17 hours of training into each week when his schedule just couldn't accommodate it. This would have resulted in him being very fit but very fatigued. He certainly wouldn't have been in a position to deliver his best on race day or to be effective as a business leader. He approached his training with confidence and an open mind, simply doing all he could do within the constraints of his life, and he did it very well. Although his example is exceptional and his variables are unique to him, all ambitious amateurs living full lives face their own sets of challenges and demands along with the same opportunity to take a new approach to training.

2

Setting the Lens

The right mindset provides a foundation for great performance that extends well beyond triathlon. A myopic focus will not lead to balanced success; you must be able to correctly set the lens to see what effective training looks like in the context of all variables in your life.

It's a learned ability to be continually aware of and organize all of the activities, commitments, and intricate realities in life and the corresponding demands and stresses each one creates. You must recognize the hierarchy of priorities on a daily basis. If you put yourself through hours of training every week without considering how everything in your life fluidly fits together, you will either end up fumbling through the sport and not progressing or, worse yet, floundering in aspects of training, work, or family life. Setting the lens is about foreseeing the successful integration of training into your busy life.

Only as you adopt and understand that realistic focus can you craft a pragmatic approach to your overarching time commitments and how they relate to your training. Although that can be a complex task, it ultimately comes down to developing consistency within chaos. Your ever-changing schedule of events and all the unknown variables that appear every week (an unexpected challenge at work, a sick child at home, a thunderstorm that precludes your track session) represent the chaos. Your pragmatic mindset will stabilize you in the turbulence of daily life, allowing you to maintain a realistic view of your training and adapt it when necessary.

We will establish a framework via the lens of your life that prepares you to have your best performance on race days, and you will learn to manage the chaos and create sustainability for your journey through this training cycle and beyond.

PLAYING THE GAME OF STRESS

There's an undeniable relationship between stress and adaptation. All sorts of stressors can solicit a physiological reaction from your body. Your body's adaptive response to training, the link between stress and performance, can be either positive or negative. This response is influenced by the amount of training stress as well as the influence, or contamination, of other types of stressors you encounter at the same time. It is important to take a step back and view your collective stressors to understand how to manipulate specific training stressors that engender positive adaptations. Your best performance emerges from consistent training that creates positive adaptations, not overly hard training that leads to negative adaptations.

Consider stress a game. Our bodies are amazing adaptation machines that will respond and adapt to any kind of stress without discrimination. It's not a question of whether we are adapting, because we are in a state of constant adaptation. Endurance athletes win the game by facilitating a positive response when they control their stressors as much as possible. Stress, of course, comes in many different forms, and it's really important for us to take stock of the stressors we're managing if we want to continue layering positive adaptations to achieve performance success.

There are two important rules to live by: (1) You simply can't, nor should you even try to, turn your back on the reality of your life and the many stressful situations it entails; and (2) You can't beat your physiology. To develop and improve, you ultimately have to work within the realm of these two ideas. Regarding the first rule, turning your back on life stress while simultaneously manipulating your body with training stress creates an imbalance that isn't sustainable. It's far better to embrace all stressors in your life because, in doing so, you can begin to differentiate between the types of stress and seek harmony between them.

By being pragmatic and adaptable, you can modify negative, stressful situations to maximize positive training stress adaptations.

As for the second rule, physiology is your toughest opponent. Try to circumnavigate the way physiology operates, cheat, or take shortcuts, and you will ultimately lose every time. When you push egregiously past your physical limits, you jeopardize the consistency and quality of your regular training sessions over the long term. Here are some examples of how athletes violate this rule: pushing through a workout despite a sharp pain in the hip; getting up at 3 a.m. to ride on the trainer, going to work, and then not getting to bed until 11 p.m.; or trying to cram in all of the key sessions and supporting sessions in a week that requires work-related travel to a city where there is no access to a bike or pool. Taking each of these foolhardy risks ignores the many additional stressors present, and the buildup of stress could easily flip the switch to the negative adaptations that result in frustration, illness, injury, and chronic fatigue. Disregarding the needs of your body will not get you ahead; it will only get you a loss.

Training Stress

Triathlon training is your specific performance stressor. It's the stress you apply to achieve the positive adaptations you need to be prepared for race day. The majority of training is swim, bike, and run workouts, but it also includes strength training and anything else that adds to the sum of specific stressors, or training stimuli.

Training stress is measured in terms of *frequency*, or how often you train; *duration or volume*, the time spent doing each workout; and the *intensity* with which you execute your training. The accumulation of work across all disciplines (swim, bike, run, strength) gives you the overall training stress load. If we get the recipe for your overall, specific training stress right (or mostly right), then over time you will progress toward your mission of arriving at a race ready to perform optimally. The more specific the training is to your individual needs, events, and particular physiology, the better prepared you will be.

Professional triathletes are generally better equipped to continue to refine their training stress without other stressors becoming obstacles because professionals are unapologetically focused on world-class performance. They can train more or less frequently, increase or decrease duration, play around with higher or lower intensities, and rest more, all with the goal of increased performance.

However, this flexibility is not a reality for most amateur triathletes, especially for those who have important business, family, and social commitments that invariably cause stress, too. Life often gets in the way for the amateur triathlete (and so do bad training plans), continually threatening inconsistency. Whether the athlete is a first-time competitor or an advanced age-grouper, the challenge always entails more than simply adjusting training variables.

Unfortunately, most amateur triathletes obsess over that elusive combination of training stressors and disregard all of the other factors in life that lead to a global accumulation of stress. Even with some smart changes, that formula doesn't offer much long-term, positive change because the equation is constantly shifting. It's an oversimplification to quarantine training from the realities of life. When we focus on one part of a multifaceted story, it's a shortsighted approach to improving performance.

Life Stress

Before we can begin a conversation about the optimal training recipe for you, the specifics of your life must be brought to the fore. Life gets in the way of training because each of the many important elements in your life presents a rich source of stress, and life stressors are typically more difficult to control. Work is one such largely uncontrollable stressor and causes an array of physical effects. Perhaps, for instance, your job is a physically demanding, manual job, or, equally stressful, involves sitting at a desk for a sustained period. Then there are mental stressors such as deadlines to meet, a team to manage, dealing with coworkers, and public speaking, to name a few. Also, regardless of profession, work is associated with financial stress manifested in many different ways.

Furthermore, we each have our own forms of self-stress, such as negative body image, lack of confidence in our abilities, or confusion as to where we are headed in the future. Relationships with husbands, wives, partners, children, in-laws, friends, and so forth, although enriching, can often engender stress, as can social obligations. Many athletes need to manage travel, which often entails genuine physical stress as well as an emotional impact.

All stressors act upon the body at a hormonal level, and although we differentiate between "good" stress and "bad" stress, the body manages all of it in more or less the same way. When we experience stress in other areas of our lives, it becomes part of our overall stress load. These stressors, especially uncontrollable stressors outside of training stress, tend to shift the balance of adaptation from positive toward negative. The good news about training stress is that it's a variable we can control. It is the best tool in our tool kit for adjusting our overall stress load, and we need to use it wisely.

A TOOL KIT FOR MANAGING STRESS

As athletes and coaches, it is our responsibility to create a flexible and dynamic training program that can ebb and flow along with your body's reaction to that training (for example, noting if you are overly fatigued from a workout) as well as what is happening in other areas of your life. You need to approach training in a pragmatic, integrated manner to create a system that facilitates consistency and retains your own specific training stimuli relative to the unpredictable nature of your life. Such a system also should promote the positive habits of *sleep, nutrition, and fueling*, the other essential tools in your tool kit.

If you allow yourself the capacity to focus on proper sleep, nutrition, and fueling, you can offset the burden of other life stressors and increase the yield from training stress. You can even intentionally increase training stress to further maximize yield through promoting better recovery. If used poorly, however, these tools only add to your life-stress bucket. In other words, if you don't refuel immediately after a workout, if you regularly sacrifice sleep (for any reason), or if you tend to have poor eating habits, you are allowing these tools to become negative stressors. I cannot overstate the importance of prioritizing these factors and using these tools to your benefit.

Well-intentioned triathletes and coaches make several stress-induced mistakes regularly. Although radical quick-fix or short-term approaches are rarely sustainable, fine-tuning, habit-changing behaviors that can avoid these mistakes quickly result in measurable performance gains that *are* sustainable. Such performance gains occur not only over the short term but also multiply over the long-term.

You can often make these changes simply by becoming more conscious of where limiting factors can and do arise. Positive adaptations to training come about more quickly and are more significant when implemented with this heightened understanding. In a sense, it's a case of keeping your friends close and your enemies closer, because to optimize your training, you need to know not only what makes you stronger and faster but also what slows you down and makes you weaker.

Adapt Training to Your Stressors

The goal is to set the lens to see what training success looks like. When stress control is removed from your routine through either poor management or misinformation, so is your ability to perform at your best. With regard to your training, control is interrupted or removed when your training plan is rigid. Your approach to training must take into account real outside forces that can throw even the best plans into a tailspin. You might swim every Tuesday and Thursday morning, and you might ride every Friday and Sunday, and you might fit in your key runs on Wednesday and Saturday, but trying to follow that plan precisely without considering the stressors from other parts of your life or how your body is feeling and performing in a given week only leads to disaster. What happens when you have a business trip from a Tuesday through a Friday, and you have no access to a pool or a good bike or treadmill? What happens when your Saturday long run gets postponed because of a thunderstorm? What happens when a school function, a sick child, a traveling spouse, or a stressful project at work gets in the way of your training, sleep, and good nutrition habits? You need to be able to adapt.

Simply executing the plan does not automatically guarantee success. When athletes come to me confused by their lack of success despite completing everything set out on their plans, I immediately suspect an imbalance of stress. A busy athlete can't adhere to a rigid Ironman or Ironman 70.3 training plan without the bucket of life stress overflowing at some point. I can appreciate that people like routine and often feel in control if they are sticking to that regimen, but life can't always match up with their routines. A schedule easily executed one week could be grossly mismatched on a number of levels during another.

Implementing a flexible training schedule will keep your training lens in focus. At the beginning of each week (and even each day), you need to focus on a number of criteria before you execute the plan. What is your *intention* for the week ahead? You need to focus on your intended training goals for the coming week relative to your current physiological state, which will affect the duration or training load for that week. You need to do it *all within the context of your life and your anticipated stressors for that week*. I encourage the athletes I coach to follow a routine in which Sunday planning helps set the tone and structure for the week ahead.

If you tried to replicate a previously successful week while on vacation with a week filled with work commitments that included a long flight for a meeting, rearrangement of school drop-offs and pickups (and the family friction that can result), can you realistically expect the same training adaptations from the same intentional training stress? Absolutely not. It would also be harder to dig into your tool kit to respond accordingly.

Here's where mistakes are made. While your body is trying to manage time-zone shifts, stress on the home front, and interrupted sleep from travel and work deadlines simultaneously with the training stress, the overall stress input is far greater, and the hormonal response from your body will reflect the increased load. Your adaptation to the net sum of those stressors, therefore, will not be the same as it was during the relaxed vacation week.

Execute on Intent

Even with a well-designed program, athletes often fall into a pattern of poor execution relative to the intent of the training. The athletes see limited results because the prescribed training was performed at the wrong intensity. More often than not, this means going too hard in a session designed to be at lower intensity. (We do not often see the opposite problem because of the triathlete's penchant for overachieving. When I do encounter lazy long-distance triathletes, there's usually another underlying cause.) The effect of poor execution is twofold: It reduces the necessary polarization of training intensities and often results in insufficient recovery.

First, when you push too hard during an easy session, you miss the intention of the easy session (to exercise aerobically, work on a technical aspect of form, or promote recovery). The by-product is that your capacity to perform at a harder intensity during what might be a key session, possibly on the same day or the following day, is reduced or diluted. Poor execution can then lead to a state in which the gap between "hard" and "easy" is less well defined and, more importantly, not as easily recognized by your body. Here, you are entering a state of *monotony*: a highly stressful situation to which your body finds it difficult to adapt because there is a lack of differentiation between training intensities and corresponding stresses. If you bring the bottom (or your easy sessions) up, you wind up with a blend of moderately hard. It's hormonally corrosive because you are carrying more fatigue, which makes it difficult to be emotionally engaged during your hard sessions.

Increasing intensity in easier workouts also means you are not getting the desired recovery from sessions designed for that purpose. This renders your body susceptible to increased structural stress on your muscles, tendons, ligaments, and even bones. You are also putting into jeopardy your ability to recover hormonally. Both can add to the risk of injury and to the accumulation of stress during the course of the week. Furthermore, going too hard on the easy days often leads you down the "accumulation path," where success depends on racking up training miles or hours.

Once again, the effect of overtraining moves you away from layered positive adaptations, and therefore renders you less prepared for their races. Decreased recovery leads to not only the inability to perform with the proper intent and intensity in key sessions but also an increase in the overall stress hormone. Your body, because of what quickly becomes a chronic condition, starts to enter a maladaptive state. This is where you commonly see secondary symptoms of increased overall stress and under-recovery. Sleep is disturbed, and your body craves certain foods (often sweets or other empty carbs), causing compromised eating habits. Now you see physical underperformance, and the pillars of performance begin to erode. Rather than supporting performance, they work as stressors. You must retain a high degree of variability in training intensity throughout a given week to avoid the dangerous state of monotony.

When a program is designed with too much intensity, there are similar effects: not enough recovery between intense sessions, lack of variety leading to monotony, and increased risk of injury and physical exhaustion. In my coaching experience this problem is particularly prevalent among older athletes and female athletes. In both cases, not only do they take longer to recover at a hormonal level but also they fail to recover adequately before putting in more high-intensity training.

The same can be said of too much volume or duration of training, particularly on top of a busy life. The implications are obvious: potential monotony, stifled variability, and reduced recovery. Here you also encounter the detrimental effects of reduced down time. The time you take for yourself is a valuable commodity, in a space where the usual suspects that cause stress aren't present. The absence of down time not only takes away rest and recovery but also adds emotional stress, counteracting your energy level and your ability to prioritize. It's easy to become overscheduled and overprogrammed. Meanwhile, the supporting cast of sleep, nutrition, and fueling fades into the background as the attention and focus training requires is all but impossible.

Safeguard Sleep and Recovery

When stress control is lost, athletes feel forced to compromise by shifting the shortfall from one area of life to another. One of the first casualties is sleep. It's a common reaction to a value proposition: Training is important, so is family, and so is the deadline at work, so we give up sleep to make it all happen.

The value of sleep is measured not only in the number of hours but also in the quality of those hours, much as training is. Some people need six hours per night, but others need eight or even nine hours on a regular basis. Quality is the non-negotiable commodity, and it is affected by nutrition, the amount of "screen time" in the evening, whether your bedroom is cool and dark enough, and your state of mind.

Most of us will subtract sleeping hours to fit in more training. After you've put in a full day of work, driven your kids around, and attended to other family or personal matters, what is left to sacrifice? Only your time to sleep. You end up justifying poor sleep habits for the wrong means. The effects are wide ranging, but even in the short term, there's an adverse reaction in your ability to make positive physiological adaptations.

The reduced neurological function and coordination that come with sleep deprivation affects economy; that is, your ability to train or race at a specific level while expending the least amount of energy. Economy is an essential component to Ironman and Ironman 70.3 performance. Training in a sleep-deprived state will translate to poor execution on race day, especially if it becomes chronic, at which point it can have similar effects to alcohol. The difference is that when you feel the effects of alcohol, you know what is happening; with sleep deprivation, you often don't recognize you're suffering from it, and that leads to other problems.

Lack of proper sleep also typically compromises your ability to adhere to good nutrition and fueling habits. Your capability to focus and make sound decisions is reduced as are your resistance to poor food choices and portion control. Your susceptibility to cravings increases. Digestion and synthesis of macronutrients affect your overall health profile, and a suboptimal digestive process can result in increased fat retention.

When an athlete has body composition issues despite training hard and focusing on a healthy diet, I know to look beyond diet alone. Sleep and training load have dramatic effects on body composition, which is especially susceptible to stressors. If diet is in fact the underlying cause, it's usually a case of the athlete not eating and fueling enough to cover the body's caloric and nutritional requirements.

Sleep is vital to performance in both triathlon and life. Chronically sleep-deprived athletes enter a suboptimal state of being. They might not comprehend what a well-rested state is; their definition of "normal" requires resetting. An athlete's training, nutrition, fueling, and sleep habits are inextricably linked. However, rather than try to fix these components all at once, I go after the sleep disturbance. I'd often much prefer that overstressed athletes reduce their overall weekly training time from 16 hours to 12 hours a week to get more quality sleep.

Prioritize Nutrition and Fueling

Your nutrition habits have the potential for mistakes despite your best intentions. This is not just in relation to how sleep deprivation affects eating. At a baseline level, you need to build a platform of health rich by eating wholesome, not overly processed, quality foods throughout the day. This is where you get your major supply of proteins, vitamins, minerals, and fats for cellular function. If these are lacking, your body starts to run on less-preferred fuels, even before the supply-and-demand complications training brings.

Taking in calories during exercise can be important, but postexercise fueling is critical. I tell athletes to eat real food including protein, fats, and carbohydrates immediately after a workout. A few hundred calories will go a long way toward kick-starting the recovery process. Undertaken correctly, this simple habit serves the interest of any athlete in training. If calories are not consumed within one to two hours after exercise, the athlete moves into a state I call *athletic starvation*. As you exercise, the level of cortisol (your most prominent stress hormone) rises to help you perform. However, when you stop exercising, you want those levels to decrease to a baseline level as fast as possible. This reduction mechanism is greatly impaired with inadequate or no fueling after workouts, which means stress hormones are likely to remain elevated longer than they need to be.

Protein resynthesis and the restocking of glycogen in the muscles and liver are impaired without adequate postexercise fueling, which prolongs or shortchanges the recovery process. If the predominant fuels you use during training (carbohydrates and fats) aren't replaced, your body will detect the shortfall and react with cravings later in the day. Typically, athletes encounter cravings for sugar or starchy carbohydrates; some crave ice cream, chocolate, and cakes, and others crave pasta, pizza, and rice. These cravings challenge good food choices and portion control in athletically starved triathletes.

Finally, hydration, although fundamental and widely understood, can become problematic for athletes. Failure to hydrate adequately is inexcusable in serious triathletes. Most athletes do a reasonable job at keeping themselves hydrated during their regular days. The biggest mistake, and the one that causes the most stress, is failure at *postexercise hydration*.

Even if you do a good job of taking in fluids during training, you are always going to finish in a state of dehydration. After exercise, your objective is to return to a fully hydrated state as soon as possible. Hydration maximizes your cellular function and immune system health. Water is fundamental to cellular rebuilding in your muscles. When you don't drink enough after exercise and throughout the day, your recovery is impaired. Also, poor cellular function compromises your immune system, reducing resistance to infection. Dehydration also causes energy levels to vary, which will prevent you from bringing your most focused self to life.

I classify these issues regarding training, sleep, nutrition and fueling, and hydration as mistakes because they are controllable. They lie at the heart of good performance, and you can better prepare for race-day performance simply by focusing your lens on their importance.

Optimal performance depends on the integration of controllable stress into life. This is only possible when you actively manage this stress. When you work with life (not in ignorance or defiance of it), you can promote a strong health profile that brings more balance and productive energy to all aspects of your life. The greatest effect is that as your energy increases, you can more readily absorb specific training stress, and now you have synergy. This harmony between life and sport surpasses the individual benefits of controlled stress and positive training adaptations.

When you know the stressors that can drag you down, it's a lot easier to control them and avoid their pitfalls. This information also increases your understanding of how the mechanisms for improvement work so you can turn your attention to the key training elements that lead to greater performance.

MASTERING POSITIVE ADAPTATION

Training success depends on metering out enough stress to produce the physiological responses that will create positive adaptations. Your ace in the hole is the principle of efficiency: *It is far better to perform less training well than it is to perform more training poorly.* This does not translate to "less is more"; you can do more *if you can adapt to it positively.* However, your goal should be to generate the most positive adaptations with the least training stress. Achieving this success requires that you remain flexible in your planning and pragmatic about adjusting frequency, intensity, and duration to your greatest benefit. Consider training a tool to achieve that goal, and make sure all of the training you undertake is *effective* training.

Consistency drives success, specifically when it's attained amid the chaos of everyday life. Nailing every session week after week is neither realistic nor sustainable over the long term. When you are able to arrive at an approach that more or less guarantees you can always train consistently within the context of your busy life, you have the ability to produce long-term performance improvements.

Know Your Tipping Point

I want to highlight once again that it is better to train below the tipping point of your capacity. Keeping your training below capacity facilitates flexibility. You can't expect to remain at 100 percent capacity, 100 percent of the time. You are human, and you naturally think about other aspects of your life and carry with you other physical stressors during training. If you are having an emotionally stressful day or a physically stressful week at work, you are more at risk of pushing yourself beyond the threshold when adaptations begin to turn negative. It is certainly easier to maintain focus at 80 percent of capacity, and if you can achieve this, if you are skillful in controlling the stress, you will begin your training on a firm foundation.

This "capacity buffer" allows your workouts to be a release. Not only are you getting the training stimulus that brings about positive adaptation but also you experience opportunities to temporarily escape your other commitments. The focus you bring to your training creates a chance for mindfulness, or even meditation. The ability to be present allows you to detach from the chaos of life.

The Real Value Proposition

If, on a week-to-week, day-to-day, or task-to-task basis, you focus on training that feeds your soul and promotes self-improvement, you will bring yourself many benefits and even happiness. It's important that you have an escape and a place for mindfulness, purely for you. Even if you are passionate about your job, it does not necessarily serve this purpose. The same goes for your family and social life because you are often still making sacrifices in these areas.

Not all training can achieve this ideal; in fact, some athletes never rise above a state of physical struggle, particularly if they haven't learned to be present during their workouts. However, if you can break that code that enables you to be truly mindful, you will reap benefits even beyond the layering of positive adaptations. You will experience an immensely positive, soul-enriching, energy-feeding, spiritual component to training that will benefit your overall health, reduce stress, and help you become whole as a person.

As effective training becomes habitual, the training itself (even the hard interval training) can become recharging. Such opportunities to recapture personal energy are rare for busy people, but in striving to become intentional athletes, you can improve athletically and use your athletic pursuits to benefit your broader busy life. You can transform this renewed energy into greater focus and banish those typical mistakes made through stress mismanagement.

When the right mindset is employed to habitually practice effective training, the overall life yield is so great. This approach to training is grossly understated as a value proposition. If you retain a fear-based mindset focused on gauging your success via accumulation of mileage, volume, or duration, you will enter a black hole of performance predictability and never reap this success on a broader scale.

PLANNING AND INTEGRATION

Knowing the lay of the land in your complex life is essential to planning and integrating training. This is a multistep process in which you aim to achieve a firm understanding of your life landscape. You first need an honest assessment of your true time available for training. What's the purpose of creating a 16-hour weekly program when you really only have 12–13 hours to train each week? When you do know your available hours, you can start to build the scaffolding for your integrated training program. This is essentially a challenge of optimization of your time.

You first require healthy doses of realistic assessment, pragmatism, and personal introspection. It is rare for ambitious triathletes to step off the treadmill of life long enough to perform such a mental exercise, but it is very valuable because it provides clarity and context. Athletes often discover that it is easier to establish realistic goals within the context of life than it is to start with idealistic hopes and dreams. It might mean that the Ironman you signed up for last week on a whim isn't realistic right now, and within the context of your life and your experience in the sport, you might be better off training until next season. It is better to acknowledge limitations now rather than have them become painfully obvious down the road after months of frustration.

Seeing Your Life Landscape

To begin this process, review every area you manage in your life. Athletes often operate day to day or week to week, knocking out each task on autopilot. You must step outside that detailed perspective to truly see what your life entails. A great triathlete naturally inhabits the bigger picture and can be invaluable in getting the most out of this task. However, even with a coach's involvement, athletes need to see their life landscapes for themselves. When athletes possess this clarity, they are much more likely to be pragmatic in their decision-making, better adhere to a program they helped build, and ultimately have the ability to manage the process.

Start with a typical week and put together an exhaustive picture of how it is you live every day. This includes work commitments, commuting time, family responsibilities (both in and out of the home), and typical social or community events. Even mealtimes, eating habits, down time, and sleeping habits count. A wearable tracking device can be useful in this exercise. Particularly where perception can differ from reality, having some quantifiable data can provide real insight, especially with regard to sleep. When you note even the smallest things (when you drink alcohol, how often you have dessert, when you grab snacks on the go rather than eating a proper meal, etc.), your picture will become more clear. This process of examining your daily and weekly life routines can produce some harsh realities, but it can also reveal areas in which to improve as you get into your training program.

Allowing for Contingencies

After you have gained this clarity, look into common contingencies that have introduced chaos into your day-to-day lifestyle. Travel for business or pleasure is a good example of this, or a child's sports tournament or dance competition to which you must commit for several days in a row. Illness, a seasonally changing work schedule, and even adverse weather conditions where you live are factors to take into account. What has created roadblocks in your life landscape? You might have experienced situations that throw you out of whack for a day or a week, and most are unpredictable. However, being able to predict any eventualities that occur more often than not is helpful (for example, how often does traffic cut hours out of your day that you were expecting to spend on other activities?) Any such expectations you can build into your planning will help you remain flexible about training.

Learning from Your Past

In the third step, look back at some of the obstacles you have encountered in previous attempts to achieve your triathlon goals in establishing a baseline of fitness, in executing specific training, or in racing. Have you struggled with injuries? Have you made costly compromises to fit in your training? Did you deal with frequent illness or have trouble overcoming even a common cold? Did you suffer a lack of confidence in your abilities because of missed sessions? Did you feel excessively fatigued or burned out after completing every part of a training program? After you see how past attempts have been stymied, the symptoms of those overprogrammed, overcommitted, and less-than-successful attempts become more obvious.

Integrating Training Time

Now, hold on to this baseline picture of your life as your begin to think about integrating your training into it. *Within your life landscape,*

- When can you (*nearly*) *always* train?
- When can you *typically* train?
- When can you *perhaps/potentially* train?

These questions help you shape a prioritized timeline of when you can train during any given week.

For example, perhaps you always have Tuesday and Thursday evenings free, along with Saturday mornings. Sunday mornings are mostly free, unless your family attends church or your children have sports commitments. Monday evenings you have board meetings, but not every week, so they hold potential, and on Wednesday mornings, it is possible to start work a little later because your company's headquarters is several time zones away. Friday evenings are reserved for family time, and weekday mornings are always about getting the kids ready for work and school and then commuting. It's different for everyone, but you might recognize some of those situations in your own life landscape.

Before you can map some definitive training times into your weekly schedule, you need to look at some other important factors. The biggest one is when you sleep, mostly because, as stated earlier, the quality of your sleep (or lack thereof) can and will affect everything else you do. You need to look closely at your week as it is now and ask whether there is adequate time available for sleep.

Many athletes believe they can fit in regular training during the early hours of their days, so they seek to train as often as possible in the morning. However, your new map of your life landscape with your perceived available hours for training might reveal a shortage of sleep hours. If that board meeting on Monday evening tends to go overtime, getting up early on Tuesday to train might rob you of sleep hours. You might be willing to sacrifice sleep on a Friday morning, but does that mean it will affect your family time that evening because you're too tired to go out to dinner and a movie? Where are you are reserving your down time? Has personal time been reallocated to training? True down time is often overlooked because it can't be defined easily, but it must not be missed. Adjust your training time accordingly.

It is important to be courageous: From your first attempt at integrated mapping, you must have the gumption to trim your availability. *It is easier to grow into more training than it is to retreat when contingencies get in the way.*

Whenever athletes have to downscale training time, they have a potential sense of failure. Start with realistic and reasonable expectations. Remember, the total hours of training in a given week will not necessarily help you improve; only through maximizing effective training will you find consistency amid the chaos of life and be able to facilitate those positive adaptations.

All of this leads back to that pesky question: How many hours do I have to train? Now that you've gone through this exercise, you realize why I always respond to an athlete who asks that question that I have no idea. It is only through this customized, personal process that you can determine how many hours you can actually train.

Optimizing your available hours is the secret to a sustainable training program.

If you have performed this optimization exercise correctly, the total number of hours you have available for training will likely be fewer hours than you thought, or at least fewer than you might have hoped. For some, this exercise might reveal 12–14 hours of availability, or perhaps more. However, for many it will be fewer, maybe as few as 10 hours. You now have a picture of your life landscape, your availability, and your priorities, the final adjustment in setting your lens. The mission from here is to take those truly available hours and maximize their effectiveness. You need to remember that the mission is *not* how to fit in more training hours.

Now that you understand why your approach to training (which really means your approach to all of life) is so important, you can start to actually plan your training to avoid unnecessary sacrifice, setbacks, and poor performance. This puts you in a position to succeed both sustainably and beneficially to all aspects of your life. The resulting training plan (the workouts contained within; the volume, duration, and intensity of the workouts; and the available time in which those workouts are executed) should specifically cater to you and the unique way you live.

The Athlete-Coach Relationship

Working with a coach can be a smart and beneficial step to help you achieve success in triathlon. However, you must understand that the coach is not the catalyst for your success. A good coach can guide you on the path to success, but you determine if you'll achieve success. If you get into Harvard, it's still what you bring to Harvard (work ethic, smarts, curiosity, ambition) that determines what you'll get out of that experience.

If you're looking for a coach, consider what you need to be successful and what type of person will help you the most. Just as you should do your research and shop around before you make a big investment, you will want to talk to several coaches. If pro athletes come to me about coaching, I insist that they also talk to two or three other coaches to help them find the best fit for them, instead of me simply selling my guidance and services. If they find a better fit, super; if I am still the best fit for them, then the relationship begins with clarity and commitment.

Look for someone with whom you can build a solid relationship. You don't want to be just an addition to a stable of athletes. A coach's reputation is often built on the results of a single great athlete. Does the coach you are considering have a history of developing athletes? Have the athletes stayed with that coach for a while? Does the coach have a wide range of athletes, with many at the same level as you? Does the coach have consistent results with athletes at your ability level or at the level you want to reach? Just because a coach has helped an athlete win a world championship doesn't mean he or she can help you reach the finish line of your first Ironman.

Every coach offers something different. If you're fairly new to triathlon, it would be smart to look for a local coach known for working with new triathletes and first-time 70.3 or Ironman competitors. In getting to know a coach's personality and background, you might find out a certain coach is known for making great runners but not as proficient in helping athletes improve on the bike. If you're a good runner and a weak cyclist, that might not be the best coach for you.

The essence of working with a coach is building a relationship. As with any relationship, you want it to evolve over time. There are many great examples of athletes who remained patient and committed to a program: They bought in, did their homework, and over time they achieved great success. One of the best examples is Brent McMahon, who worked with coach Lance Watson for 22 years. In that journey Brent became junior world champion, competed in the Olympics, finished an Ironman in under eight hours, and successfully raced in several Ironman World Championships. That's an impressive evolution, and the athlete-coach relationship deserves some of the credit. On the contrary, when athletes change their coach from one season to the next, it diminishes their ability to build toward ongoing success. Instead, they're stuck in a pattern of adapting to new training philosophies, new workouts, and new relationships.

I've been fortunate to work with many great athletes: Meredith Kessler, Jesse Thomas, Sarah Piampiano, and Tim Reed, among others. When they made the decision to work with me they bought into the program, and every year they reinvest in the program and begin building on what we did the previous year. Their continued progression is built upon a successful, ever-evolving relationship.

3

Planning Your Training

Now that you have a real understanding of your life landscape, it's time to put the concept into action and actually plan your training. Consider how to optimize your training within your available hours. This involves more than simply planning your swim, bike, run, and strength workouts; you are creating a personalized road map that integrates training into the broad scope of your life. You began with a bit of introspection, a healthy dose of reality, and a pragmatic mindset applied whenever necessary. The real picture of your life, especially your availability, will keep you on track and allow you to execute practical steps that lead to improved performance.

Take charge and own this process. Even if you are working with a coach, you need to be at the controls and steer yourself to a true and honest look at your life. This is your passion, so you need to understand precisely why, how, and when your training will take place.

PLAN YOUR SEASON

Before making your weekly and daily workout plans, pull back to get a bird's eye view of your entire year. The best way to approach your training is to examine the timing of your goal races. Even if you intend to work toward just one major race (or A race), you'll want to schedule other races along the way and quite possibly another A race. For example, you might plan a couple of Ironman 70.3 races before the Ironman Arizona in mid-November, your A race, or you might compete in two full Ironman races in a year, even though Ironman Arizona is your key goal.

There are many reasons to choose certain events as goal races: Perhaps you've always had your heart set on a certain race, your training partners are doing that race, or you want to take your family on a vacation to that region. Think about what you wish to accomplish with that race and how it fits into the rest of your year. Choose your races carefully to allow for the most sustainable training; avoid events scheduled during or after major life events.

For example, don't choose Ironman Lake Placid in late July if you know your kids are out of school and you will be traveling a lot with them. This means you won't really have time to train in the months leading up to the Ironman. Similarly, if you're an accountant, don't sign up for Ironman Texas in late April, just after your big tax season. If you are an executive at a company that reports quarterly earnings or is preparing for an IPO, avoid choosing a race that would interfere with those protracted busy periods.

Ultimately, the plan for your year should put you in a position to be optimally ready for your goal race. You should also have a secondary goal of evolving your fitness and skills year after year, which is only possible with a holistic perspective and sustainable habits. Although it might seem daunting to plan multiple races that lead up to an Ironman, it's a smart maneuver because it places strategic training blocks and performance peaks in your year. It will also keep the focus off of your goal race until it is time to begin training specifically for that event.

It won't serve you well to sign up for an Ironman goal race, such as Ironman Arizona in November, and then focus on that starting in December of the previous year, especially if you're shooting for a lifetime dream of finishing your first Ironman. You want to arrive prepared for the race and emotionally and physically fresh to give your best effort on race day, but it's counterproductive to focus on one event for such a long time. It doesn't matter who you are or what kind of experience you have as an athlete; it will become mentally and emotionally burdensome and eventually drag you down over the course of the year. It most likely won't be a sustainable or successful training process because at some point you'll begin to feel like you're just trying to get that monkey off your back. A two-pronged approach to your training makes it easier to maintain your effort, enthusiasm, and consistency as you methodically build toward your big goal, improving your abilities progressively.

Ultimately you're aiming for sustainability in training, performance, and lifestyle so that however time starved you might be, you will not be training at 100 percent of your capacity for the majority of the year. Only in the few months leading up to a key race will you be edging up toward maximum capacity. At times during the year you will need rejuvenation, so you'll need to back off the training intensity and adjust your focus accordingly.

Striving for consistency and specificity in training requires unyielding dedication and focus. However, you also need to progress, and you cannot progress if you are always maxed out. Progression develops through training and racing spurts connected by breaks for rest and recovery. By approaching your training with a pragmatic mindset, you are empowered to make smart decisions about how you feel and what you need to do on an ongoing basis. If you sense you're overly fatigued or repeatedly skipping workouts, it might make sense to retool your training program so you can fit more sleep, active recovery workouts, or down time into the rhythm of your work, life, and training.

Planning the Buildup to Your Goal Race

Only for the 14 or so weeks leading up to your A race will you be in full-on Ironman training mode. I like athletes to place a mark on the calendar that denotes that emotional shift so that they can maximize focus in that period. The rest of the year is governed by pragmatism; you rein yourself in, train sustainably for other goal races or tune-up races, and develop your skills and athleticism.

During your race-prep cycle, you will hone in on that race in particular in the context of the rest of your life.

The race-prep period will include some bigger training days that might involve multiple workouts and as many as six to eight hours of total training. These big days are key building blocks for developing your physical, mental, and emotional strength and endurance for race day. I ask amateur athletes to identify a few opportunities for bigger training days or weekends during the final 12–14 weeks leading up to their goal race, whether on weekends or even via a three- to five-day personal training camp where it is possible to be fully immersed in training.

Using Ironman Arizona in mid-November as an example, you might look at your calendar and decide that you have time and space for big days on September 7, September 25, the weekend of October 1–2, and October 12. You'll have to make sure that these dates work within the rest of your life; you might have to negotiate with your boss or your family to get the buy-in you need from the people around you. There is a direct correlation between their support and your success. If you plan ahead, you can reduce distractions and have more ability to focus on the intention of and rhythm of your workouts. Mark those on your calendar as cornerstones of your training schedule and avoid any conflicts on those dates. If one of your big days is interrupted by a conference call for work or stress over what your family is doing that day, it will be challenging to achieve your workout goals.

These big-day training sessions bring the Ironman-distance race within reach. You can successfully race Ironman 70.3 events without them, but the long-course distance will be particularly challenging. For most athletes, missing these bigger workouts is a deal breaker. After you have those bigger days on your calendar, you'll also want to plan ahead for moderate- to big-mileage days on weekends. This looks different for everyone because it is based on the context of your life. For some athletes, it's possible to commit to big mileage every Saturday. They train from 6 a.m. to 3 p.m. and tell the people in their lives that they are completely unavailable during this window.

Success Starts Here

Too many athletes lack an understanding of what they need to be successful, which leads them to merely train hard without commensurate performance gains. In working with top pros and aspiring amateur athletes, I regularly see these four factors as a precursor to success at any level.

A SMART TRAINING PLAN. This is obvious, but it's also more than just having a good training plan. It's about having a smart plan that fits an athlete's specific needs and work/life schedule. You can't just follow the fast-track program or the plan your coach devised for you; you have to execute it with the proper intent and rhythm. Behind every successful athlete is a smart, well-executed plan that allows or encourages flexibility and pragmatism.

ACCOUNTABILITY. After arming yourself with a smart training plan, adding accountability facilitates your progress. Although triathletes are highly motivated individuals, we all tend to do better with accountability from a coach, a training partner, a mentor, or a training group. It might even come through a tune-up race, as race results tend to give an authentic measure of where you are in your training.

FEEDBACK AND SUPPORT. A support network provides perspective and encouragement for even the savviest of athletes by helping you make smart decisions, keeping you motivated, and grounding you in real life. Honest feedback and support serve as personal checks and balances. If you are hoping to do an Ironman-distance race, this support is essential.

COMMUNITY. People thrive in a community setting, especially in sports. It brings a sense of belonging, and even the most challenging situations are more fun and enjoyable when shared with others. Local or regional training groups are invaluable for this reason. Although the dynamic is different, you can still benefit from the shared passion and commitment of an online club or forum. At Purple Patch, we have a group swim session twice a week at 5:30 a.m., and it's always sold out. People aren't just coming for the training; they're coming because it makes their lives richer.

This is not a practical or sustainable option for many people because of family dynamics and a variety of commitments on weekends. In those cases, the timing of your weekend training sessions will vary based on some give-and-take and pragmatic thinking. It might mean that one weekend you're free to do a six-hour ride outside, but the next weekend you have time for only a two-hour bike session indoors with a two-hour run the next day. It might mean that you carve out time for a two-hour run on Saturday morning but then are involved with family responsibilities for the rest of the day and have to play it by ear for Sunday.

Planning Other Races

After you have your Ironman buildup mapped into your year, you can start to plan additional races. Again, if your ultimate goal is Ironman Arizona in November, you might add an Ironman 70.3 race in early May and another by the end of June or in early July. Sometimes you can cluster races, even on back-to-back weekends, but you should select each race based on everything you have going on. The Ironman 70.3 race in Santa Rosa, California, held in mid-May, might fit into the bigger context of your life, but then again, maybe it's the same day as your daughter's dance recital, your son's big soccer tournament, or just a week before your busiest season at work. Find a race that both fits into your season and works for your business and family endeavors, too.

Just because you plan races leading up to your goal race later in the year, your B races are no less important and merit no less focus on performance. Instead, those B races form a progression for your season and help you structure your training for specific cycles. Your A race (in this case Ironman Arizona) is where you're targeting your final training so that you'll be optimally ready to race to your fullest potential. Your B races serve as important stepping stones and as test races in which you build your skills, fitness, and experience. Even so, you will show up and race to the best of your abilities, which might lead to a breakout performance.

THE PHASES OF TRAINING

Now that you have settled on some races, let's consider how the season takes shape. Two important phases, postseason and preseason, allow for athletic development and set up the success of the season (see Figure 3.1).

FIGURE 3.1
Outline of a Typical, 2-Cycle Season

POSTSEASON
Oct. 23
Oct. 30
Nov. 6
Nov. 13
Nov. 20
Nov. 27
Dec. 4
Dec. 11
Dec. 18
Dec. 25

PRESEASON #1
Jan. 1
Jan. 8
Jan. 15
Jan. 22
Jan. 29
Feb. 5
Feb. 12
Feb. 19
Feb. 26
Mar. 5

EVENT-SPECIFIC #1	
Mar. 12	
Mar. 19	
Mar. 26	Local Olympic Race
Apr. 2	
Apr. 9	
Apr. 16	
Apr. 23	
Apr. 30	Ironman 70.3, B Race
May 7	
May 14	
May 21	
May 28	Local Olympic Race
Jun. 4	
Jun. 11	Ironman 70.3, A Race

TWO WEEK BREAK
Jun. 18
Jun. 25

PRESEASON #2
Jul. 2
Jul. 9
Jul. 16
Jul. 23
Jul. 30
Aug. 6

EVENT-SPECIFIC #2	
Aug. 13	
Aug. 20	
Aug. 27	
Sep. 3	
Sep. 10	
Sep. 17	Ironman 70.3, B Race
Sep. 24	
Oct. 1	
Oct. 8	
Oct. 15	
Oct. 22	
Oct. 29	
Nov. 5	
Nov. 12	Ironman, A Race

TWO WEEK BREAK
Nov. 19
Nov. 26

POSTSEASON
Dec. 3
Dec. 10
Dec. 17

Postseason Phase

This critical phase starts with a complete break from structured training following the final race of your season. I recommend that athletes take two full weeks off to relax, do some low-impact active recovery exercise, and don't even think about triathlon. Many triathletes remain active after a goal race with a variety of exercise, including yoga, hiking, mountain biking, and relatively unstructured swimming and cycling. Few pro triathletes detrain in the same fashion professional runners or cyclists do, but it is important for all athletes to engage in a postseason phase before the start of their next season of racing. If recovery isn't your focus, you are likely to miss the desired effect. The postseason phase might last 2–6 weeks for pro triathletes and 5–10 weeks for amateurs depending on their experience and when the next racing season begins in earnest. For many triathletes in North America, the postseason typically ends with the calendar year, allowing a clean break at the end of December and beginning anew in January. After this break, the postseason should include a block of training with low physical stress during the least physically taxing period of the year.

Although some coaches and athletes might consider this "base training," I avoid that term because it creates the impression that you'll be accumulating miles at slower paces, and this is not the focus I recommend. The majority of Ironman training is endurance oriented, which by definition is base training. In fact, over the course of the season triathletes need to be training with more speed and power to increase their cardiovascular capacity.

To optimize this off-season preparation, the postseason phase should contain a good amount of high-intensity training, plenty of neurological timing work, and some stimulation of form and technique (see Figure 3.2). Think about strengthening your tendons and ligaments to absorb the running you'll be doing later in the season, along with developing coordination, synchronization, and agility. This is a good phase for trail running both because it's less structured than the road- and track-running sessions you'll do later and because the uneven surfaces and lateral movements tend to correct the natural gait issues with which some athletes can be afflicted by the end of racing season.

FIGURE 3.2
Typical Postseason Training Week

	M	T	W	TH	F	SA	SU
S1	Supporting Swim or Bike or Run	KEY SWIM Technical ·	KEY BIKE + RUN End-of-Range	KEY SWIM Endurance	KEY RUN Technical	KEY BIKE or Outside Fun Ride Replacement	Supporting Swim Endurance
S2	Core & Light Strength	KEY RUN Technical	Strength & Conditioning			Strength & Conditioning	KEY RUN Endurance

By the time you are building up to your Ironman or Ironman 70.3 race, you will be well accustomed to heavy work and low cadence on the bike and plenty of strength-based hill running. The building blocks of work, as we call them, begin in the postseason. Your key bike sessions might be a seven-minute interval of moderate effort in which you dip from moderately low to very low rpm. The goal is not only to help you refine posture and pedal stroke but also introduce your muscles, tendons, and ligaments to overload and strength-endurance work. Don't hope for massive fitness gains or power jumps, but prepare the body to absorb the heavy upcoming work over the next few months and establish a platform of great form and posture.

The ultimate goal of the postseason phase is to transition from your previous race season into the preseason of your next year healthy and rested, with some consistent training and good habits under your belt. It's really a preparation phase that will help you get ready to absorb harder work in upcoming phases.

Preseason Phase

The preseason phase is a transition to a period in which an athlete needs to develop big muscular resilience. It involves concerted foundational efforts that will help maximize the yield of the specific training later in the year. Because your A race(s) are not yet on the horizon, you have the license and capacity to train less specifically to the demands of longer-distance racing. There's no need to worry about Ironman-specific race pace this early. Instead, this is a time to focus on sprint- or Olympic-distance, high-power training to increase your cardiovascular capacity and muscular strength and refine your form and technique.

The preseason phase is also a good time to integrate hill running and low-cadence strength and endurance training on the bike. In contrast to the preparatory and introductory, low-cadence work described for the postseason, the focus here is overload intervals at a strong effort with similar low cadence. This work differs from an Ironman run or ride, but it builds power, strength, and resilience that will benefit you later in the season. You will also want to do some high-intensity training. Try a main-set swim session of really fast 50s; for example, 10 × 50 yards at "best effort" on the minute. This is nothing like an Ironman swim, but it improves your ability to hold and move water with great force. When you layer endurance on top of this preparation, you'll be even more effective at swimming the 1.2 miles in an Ironman 70.3 or the 2.4 miles in an Ironman.

Another example of a preseason workout is a 10 × 30 second hill-running workout that has you close to maximum effort on each rep. That's a long way from what it's like to run 26.2 miles off the bike in an Ironman, but you're developing athletic awareness, timing, power, and leg turnover. In addition to building a foundation of fitness, the types of workouts you'll do in the preseason can also help you overcome weaknesses by emphasizing proper form and building good habits for later in the season (see Figure 3.3).

The preseason phase typically lasts about 10–14 weeks (roughly from January through March for North American triathletes), but it depends on how early in the year your first race might be. For example, you could plan an abbreviated preseason phase and make a spring vacation out of an Ironman 70.3 in New Zealand, Puerto Rico, South Africa, or one of the many other races held late in the North American winter. Following a short break after that race, you would then plan another preseason phase leading up to the 12-week buildup to your next scheduled Ironman 70.3 in May (likely one of your A races).

As you go through the year, the preseason cycle becomes familiar and energizing because you've already experienced it once or twice. It's a great way to

FIGURE 3.3

Typical Preseason Training, Week 1

	M	T	W	TH	F	SA	SU
S1	Supporting Bike	KEY SWIM Endurance	KEY BIKE + RUN Strength-Endurance	KEY SWIM Endurance, Speed, and Power	Supporting Swim	KEY RUN Strength	Supporting Swim
S2	Core & Light Strength	KEY RUN Technical	Strength & Conditioning	Supporting Run Endurance		Strength & Conditioning	KEY BIKE Endurance

Week 2

	M	T	W	TH	F	SA	SU
S1	Supporting Bike	KEY SWIM Endurance	KEY BIKE + RUN Strength-Endurance	Supporting Swim	Supporting Swim	KEY BIKE + RUN Strength-Endurance	KEY SWIM Endurance
S2	Core & Light Strength	KEY RUN Technical	Strength & Conditioning	KEY RUN Strength		Strength & Conditioning	KEY RUN Trail/Endurance

reinvigorate yourself for the next race cycle and keep from getting stale during the middle of your season, with your ultimate goal race still many months away.

Race Cycle Phase

The race cycle is the essential training to build up to your goal race. Many athletes fall into the trap of forgetting the elements that have worked in their evolution up to this point of the season, and they make a massive shift to weeks of training focused on event-specific intensity. For Ironman-distance athletes, this means repeating session after session of steady and smooth endurance training, a divergence from the high-value training that entailed working across the range of intensities. I've created a modular approach to the final block of work leading into the race with a clear weekly focus. You will notice similar variation in the training to what you have done in the postseason and preseason. The modular format also allows you to shift the weeks around to better accommodate travel, life obligations, or other races, which we'll explorein the case studies in Part 2 (pp. 226–228).

BUILD

To avoid getting stale, I have athletes execute some high-volume running and riding early in a race-prep phase. You return to banking the miles in some key sessions closer to race day, but this approach facilitates confidence in doing the distance and avoids the need to "go long" every weekend.

STRENGTH ENDURANCE

Following the initial build, you have about two weeks of heavy strength-endurance work. Otherwise known as the "special sauce," this is where you get your magical strength endurance. "End-of-range" biking and running are retained throughout the event-specific phase. It has proven to be effective in developing invaluable tools and resilience for athletes.

TRANSITION

You want to avoid lingering heavy legs from that strength-endurance work, so shift the focus, remove a little stress, and transition to a week focusing on speed to refresh and remind yourself of the range of intensities you can hit. The typical transition week will carry more overall training load than race week, but the rhythm and intent of the work will be similar. Don't think of these as recovery weeks; they hold high value in the training progression.

EVENT SPECIFIC

Aim to hit two weeks of event-specific training load before freshening up and sharpening with a shift in focus. For an Ironman buildup, this means a return to miles with plenty of race simulation (including specific run-off-the-bike sessions) and over-distance work, but now with greater intensity. A few weeks before your key race (or for a B race, in a case where you are doing more than one race-prep phase in a season) is a super time to do a shorter tune-up race

FIGURE 3.4
Typical Training Progression for Race-Specific Phase

CYCLE 1, BUILDUP TO 70.3		CYCLE 2, BUILDUP TO IRONMAN	
Mar. 12	Endurance	Aug. 13	Build
Mar. 19	Endurance	Aug. 20	Endurance
Mar. 26	Transition, Local Olympic Race	Aug.27	Strength-Endurance
Apr. 2	Transition	Sep. 3	Strength-Endurance
Apr. 9	Strength-Endurance	Sep. 10	Transition
Apr. 16	Strength-Endurance	Sep. 17	Race Week, Ironman 70.3, B Race
Apr. 23	Transition	Sep. 24	Transition
Apr. 30	Race Week, Ironman 70.3, B Race	Oct. 1	Event-Specific
May 7	Transition	Oct. 8	Event-Specific
May 14	Event-Specific	Oct. 15	Transition
May 21	Event-Specific	Oct. 22	Event-Specific
May 28	Transition, Local Olympic Race	Oct. 29	Event-Specific
Jun. 4	Transition	Nov. 5	Transition
Jun. 11	Race Week, Ironman 70.3, A Race	Nov. 12	Race Week, Ironman, A Race

to remind your body of the race effort and act as the final catalyst for race-day fitness. Also practice race day fueling and hydration. To prevent slow-cadence riding, you also do a mix of both low rpm work and high-rpm challenges during this two- to three-week period.

PREPARATION (RACE WEEK)

With the hard work behind you, push toward race day with two weeks of feel-good training, choosing your best type of training. Avoid aiming to get more fit because you can't get any fitter at this point in your buildup.

After you've been through one or two race cycles that culminate in Ironman 70.3 races, you will likely start to approach your prep for a full Ironman. After an early to midsummer Ironman 70.3, you'll take one to two weeks off, then perhaps do preseason work until your actual Ironman race cycle begins. As you begin that race cycle, you will learn from your previous race cycles and evolve as an athlete. What worked? What didn't? This familiarity allows you to focus on execution, make adjustments that work for you, and achieve greater predictability in your race performance. Figure 3.4 shows how the race cycle progresses over the course of the season.

For pros and elite age-groupers, that usually means a 12- to 14-week cycle in July, August, and September in preparation for the Ironman World Championships during the first week of October. Other athletes who might be focusing on Louisville, Kentucky, in mid-October or Panama City or Arizona in November can take a slightly longer preseason before beginning in August to ramp up to the fall Ironman.

PLANNING YOUR WEEKLY TRAINING

In Chapter 2 we defined the landscape of your life on a weekly and daily basis; now it's time to start mapping your workouts. Revisit the weekly schedule that you roughed out in Chapter 2. Create slots for morning, midday (or lunchtime), and evening workouts, and use different colors to highlight the times when you are always available to train, typically available to train, or sometimes available to train. Define a realistic time frame for each of those slots: Are you available for 2 hours or only 45–60 minutes? These become your weekly training opportunities (see Figure 3.5).

You will place the four key activities of triathlon training (swimming, biking, running, and strength and conditioning) into your available slots. Anchor your week with two swim sessions, two bike workouts, and two runs. Strength and conditioning (described in more detail in Chapter 4) is an important component of performance. Plan for two sessions a week, each lasting 15–40 minutes, but don't allow these workouts to detract from the bull's-eye of swim, bike, and run training. Keep in mind that you are a triathlete first and foremost. Those key swim, bike, and run workouts can fit into your schedule differently in any given week, but you should have this template going into the Sunday planning session that kicks off each week.

Always Available

First, plan for your "always available" time slots. These are good opportunities for key sessions because they're predictable and repeatable. The particulars of each session are irrelevant at this stage. Your key workouts will not always be extraordinarily difficult. Of those six key workouts, you might have two or three sessions dedicated to your bigger, harder workouts because you know you'll have time, energy, and focus to approach those sessions with proper intent and rhythm. If you have been honest about your true availability, these key sessions should fit harmoniously into your life landscape.

As you plan, allow enough time in these availability windows to complete your workouts properly. Each session will have a warm-up, a pre–main set, a main set, an optional extra set, and a cooldown. This framework shouldn't keep you from being adaptable and taking the license to make well-informed decisions. Without knowing the specifics of the workouts yet, you'll likely want a 1.5- to 2-hour window, but some sessions can be as short as 45 minutes.

It's not as simple as planning your key sessions here, here, here, and here, and *bada-bing*, you're done. Although the key sessions are typically high-yield workouts, training this way exclusively does not constitute a successful program. It might work for a particularly busy week at some point during the season, but it's not a good strategic plan overall. You will also need to layer in secondary sessions and optional supporting sessions that might include active recovery work, additional endurance training, and technique work. Find the amount of extra training hours that are both sustainable relative to your life and conducive to positive adaptations. These workouts balance out the key sessions and give your body time to recover and absorb the training.

Consider some standing sessions that take place at a specific time and place: masters swim sessions, indoor cycling classes, group track workouts, or Saturday group rides. Group training is viable if it can be integrated into your week without interrupting your plan. Even though these workouts can detract from specificity, much can be gained from them. If you struggle to show up for early morning sessions, accountability to a class or group can help you be more consistent. These sessions can offer healthy competition, social interaction, and food for your soul in a way solo training cannot. Consider yourself lucky to have the opportunity and to show up to what might be a harder workout than you expected. As long as your standing sessions fit into your life landscape in "always available" slots, plan to participate in them on a regular basis.

Typically Available

After you've filled the slots when you're always available to train, consider those when you can typically train. These are secondary in your hierarchy, meaning sometimes it will take a bit of negotiating to make them work. This is where you should put your recommended sessions, workouts you want to get in if you have time or sessions that allow you to train more in a specific discipline. It's a lower tier of importance, but it's based on what you need. For example, if you already have two key bike sessions in your schedule but feel like you need a third one, place it in one of these slots. It might mean you lose an extra swim, but so be it. Let your priorities arise according to where you need to build fitness, enhance your skills, or improve on a weakness.

These "typically available" time slots might be the first to go when important work or family obligations conflict with them. Maybe you sometimes have an important work meeting on Tuesday morning, or perhaps in the winter you drive to a ski resort for the weekends, eliminating Thursday or Friday evenings and forcing you to consider how you might get in a recovery run or easy spin bike ride the next morning.

Sometimes Available

Last, consider the time slots when you can sometimes train. During any given week you might be able to pencil in supporting sessions or optimal sessions. Active recovery, general endurance, and technical proficiency are the best activities for these slots. If you don't get them in, don't feel like the sky is falling or give in to frustration or disappointment. These sessions are helpful, but

FIGURE 3.5
Weekly Trianing Template

	M	T	W	TH	F	SA	SU
5 A	Additional sleep	KEY SWIM 1 hr.	KEY BIKE 2 hr.	Additional sleep	Additional sleep	Additional sleep	
6 A		Additional time		KEY SWIM 90 min.	Supporting session 2 hr.		KEY BIKE 3 hr.
7 A		Breakfast	BRICK RUN			KEY RUN 2 hr.	
			Breakfast	Breakfast			
8 A							
9 A							Breakfast
10 A	Work	Work	Work	Work	Work		
11 A						Family	
12 P							
1 P	Supporting session	Meditation 15 min.	Meditation 15 min.	Meditation 15 min.			Family
2 P					Optional workout	Nap	
3 P						Family	
4 P	Work	Work	Work	Work	Work		
5 P						Strength	Optional workout
6 P		KEY RUN		Optional workout	Dinner and rest	Social	Work
7 P	Dinner	Additional time	Strength	Additional time	Social		
8 P	Work	Dinner and rest	Dinner and rest	Dinner and rest			Dinner and rest
9 P	Rest	Rest	Work	Rest	Bed	Bed	Bed
10 P	Bed	Bed	Bed	Bed			

■ ALWAYS AVAILABLE   ▨ TYPICALLY AVAILABLE   ▢ SOMETIMES AVAILABLE they're not the meat and potatoes of your week, and perhaps there is another slot when you'll fit in the work.

Maintaining the Mindset

After you get your week mapped initially, step back and take a deep breath. Between work and training sessions, you still have to identify your sleep time and down time, along with time to spend with family. If your initial view of the week has you getting up at 4:30 a.m. four days a week to make it to a particular group workout, now is the time to think about whether that is sustainable given the other commitments in your life.

Generally speaking, most people (and particularly amateur triathletes balancing work and family life) are quite overscheduled. If you have created a weekly schedule that puts you at maximum capacity, open up some of the potentially available time slots for contingencies. Everyone benefits from having time in the week when there is nothing scheduled (and then it somehow disappears). Remember, training has to integrate into your entire life. To make training work on a consistent basis, you need to be really brave but not foolish.

It's easy to become overzealously aspirational about your training schedule. Genuinely ask yourself, "This is the reality of my life right now, so where and when am I best able to train?" Compromising other parts of your life to fit in more workout sessions isn't sustainable. You are better off to be cautious and conservative from the outset so you'll be able to achieve your goals on a regular basis. You want to evolve and grow, not be burdened by training.

Build a regular template for your life so that it all works and is enjoyable for you. Busy people generally do better with a regularly structured schedule or at least a template with several regular features. They know they swim on this day at this time or run on another day at that time. If your life is more flexible, you can adjust as you go along. Most of us struggle with a more scattered approach. Having a replicable schedule can boost your confidence, energy, and even your soul.

For example, starting your week with a strong early Monday morning run can set the tone for both your training and your work week. Perhaps you anchor your week with Tuesday/Thursday morning swims and a Wednesday morning bike/run with a group. Maybe you enjoy your Saturday endurance rides with your buddies, and you prefer to spend Sundays with your family after a swim and run in the morning.

As you outline your weeks during your Sunday planning sessions, build your training around your key sessions. Then consider what it will take to feel good during those sessions and recover from those sessions. Fine-tune it with optional sessions that will enhance your overall approach. How many hours of training you are getting in is the last thing on my mind as a coach, and it should be the same for you. On the contrary, if you find out you have only 10 hours of training planned, you might be able to add more.

Even for athletes who have fewer time commitments and less life stress, the training schedule is not based on accumulating a set number of hours. Start building the week with the key sessions and determine the workload from there. This planning exercise might seem simple or even obvious, yet it's a wonder so few athletes can do it from the start. This process can enrich your whole life experience, not just your triathlon training. You have the luxury to customize an optimal, flexible training program that fits within your life. Planning is a golden opportunity to streamline your life, which can be a catalyst to greater success at work, relationships with family, and of course training and racing.

This lens enables you to deal with the inevitable changes, compromises, and sacrifices required on a weekly and daily basis. No doubt you'll have to skip or postpone workouts, scale workouts, or perhaps reorganize certain sessions in different time slots. That's where the pragmatic mindset will help you adjust. However, if you start by setting up your framework with the ability to execute two key sessions each of swimming, biking, and running per week, you will have a strong basis of training upon which other supporting training sessions can be layered in the time available.

PLANNING INDIVIDUAL WORKOUTS

As you venture into developing and executing your training approach, you will do a blend of workouts within each block of training to create the desired training stimuli and response. On an ongoing basis your training might be influenced by outside stress factors, and how you manage and juggle the plan will create your success. This is why I want you to understand the why and how of the program. Your best outcome won't likely arrive from following the program verbatim. I have done the job of detailing the building blocks and key sessions of the training in a sensible and dynamic manner. Your task is to plan each week, integrate the key sessions when most appropriate, and support them with the optional sessions. Remember, life is not a static spreadsheet, so you cannot expect your training approach to be so either.

In Part 2, The Performance Plan, you will find weekly templates and key workouts for the postseason and preseason phases of training as well as a 14-week race-prep plan that details every session of the event-specific phase. As you compare these with your own weekly schedule (especially in the race-prep program), you will need to shift workouts to shape the upcoming week of training. There are some general rules that will help your week go more smoothly and effectively. For example, it's often optimal for your key swim to be the first workout of the day. With two key sessions back to back, it's typically better to do high-intensity workouts before endurance workouts. So, if you're doing the hilly loop for your hard run, do that on a Saturday and then do an endurance ride Sunday morning or even later in the afternoon on Sunday. Conversely, if you have bike intervals on a Saturday, do your endurance run on Sunday. This works well because it tends to amplify the effectiveness of the endurance work. If you attempt to go on a four-hour endurance ride on a Saturday morning and then do a hard, hilly run session later that day or early the next morning, you're going to carry fatigue into the workout and jeopardize your ability to meet the intention and rhythm of that workout. If you have a ride on Friday for muscular stimulation, then do the hilly run workout on Saturday and an endurance ride on Sunday, you're likely to have tired legs on Sunday, but that can actually be good preparation for an Ironman or Ironman 70.3.

The bottom line is that I can't create a utopian, one-size-fits-all plan that's 12–15 hours a week and say, "Good luck, now you're on your own!" You develop the concept, and you then see it into action through the landscape of your life. We'll develop rules in Chapter 4 on how to manage training with a pragmatic mindset and how to effectively scale a workout when your training availability is reduced or when you're overly fatigued from training or less sleep because of a business trip, late-night meeting, or any number of unexpected eventualities. The scaling rules offer a couple of options so that if your original training time slot is reduced from 75 to 45 minutes, you can still effectively achieve the original intention and rhythm of the workout instead of postponing it in panic, haphazardly truncating it, or skipping it entirely. Although I might seem to be giving you an out here, it's important that you see how adaptability works. Whether time or fatigue is your limiter, this adaptability is essential for a successful triathlete.

You understand now more than ever the need for consistency in creating positive training adaptations. The yield from your available time is far greater if you work with focus from an intentional framework in which training synergistically fits into the rest of your life on a weekly and daily basis. You also understand the need to be vigilant about controlling life stress. Now you can customize your specific progression to facilitate consistency and performance.

4

Executing Your Training

Now that you've developed a new mindset, set your lens on your available training time, and learned how to plan your overall season and weekly workouts, it's time to execute your training. This chapter will explain how to structure your training. Specific workouts and more information for each phase of the season are in Part 2, The Performance Plan.

At this point you understand that your goal is to optimize your training within the scope of your busy life and maximize its yield. To do that, you have to actively participate in your own process. No matter whether you're guided by a coach or an online training program, you cannot just follow prescribed workouts, power levels, or heart rate zones from a spreadsheet. You can learn and you can be guided, but if you're wholly relying on someone else to manage your process on a daily or weekly basis, without any of your own self-management, you'll not likely reach your fullest potential. It's your sport, and to get the most out of it, you have to take ownership of your training and be responsible for it on a daily basis. Investing in this process is the way to achieve the race results you want and continue to improve in triathlon.

NON-NEGOTIABLES
Know the Intent of Each Session

To execute your training properly, you need to know the intent and rhythm of each workout and the goal you are trying to achieve in each session. It takes more than pure endurance to prepare for long-distance triathlon. The workouts in the Fast-Track program are organized by the different adaptations they bring about.

TECHNICAL

Low-stress sessions that emphasize form, recovery, and skill acquisition. They are often used as preparation for an upcoming race or tougher session. Run sessions are focused on easy endurance, including hops, bounds, and even walking with great form.

ENDURANCE

Focused on improving muscular and cardiovascular endurance and conditioning. Endurance sessions are not easy, especially endurance rides, but the steady-state work is the bedrock of preparation in long-distance triathlon and a key to building resilience as an athlete.

INTERVALS

Typically higher-intensity, short-interval sessions that vary speed and effort to increase maximal steady-state pace. Although effort is increased, the importance of retaining good form remains unchanged.

END-OF-RANGE

Specific to cycling, these workouts are the "special sauce" of Purple Patch training. Each session includes a mix of very-low-cadence and very-high-cadence work that develops resilience, pacing, and better management of the terrain on the bike.

EVENT-SPECIFIC

As the name suggests, these sessions serve as preparation for the demands of racing. Workouts target the specific pace, effort, or power appropriate to race goals and simulate typical race situations to allow practice at execution.

An educated athlete is much better equipped to adapt to the vicissitudes of life, never losing sight of the focus and purpose of training. Part 2 includes a workout glossary describing the different training stimuli within each of these categories (see Figure 4.1 for an overview) and road maps for each phase of training. With these tools in hand, you will know specifically how to execute the key sessions, and why that work will produce the intended outcome. Likewise, you can include supporting sessions with full understanding of their purpose. For example, if you schedule a technical run, you should know it promotes general resilience, active recovery, and an opportunity to work on form. You can expect the overall stress level to be low so that you can adhere to the intent and focus of that workout and have the capacity to focus on form. Contrast this with an interval session that includes 6 × 5-minute intervals at very strong effort;

FIGURE 4.1
Workout Types

WORKOUTS	SWIM	BIKE	RUN
Technical	Recovery Form Speed and power Prep	Recovery Prep Activation	Recovery Prep Activation
Endurance	Short intervals Over-distance Building	Over-distance General endurance	Over-distance General endurance
Intervals/ End-of-Range	High-intensity Building	Strength endurance Building High cadence (rpm)	Strength Tempo Speed
Event-Specific	Pyramid Threshold Race simulation Open water	Building Intervals Race simulation	Building Intervals Race simulation Run off the bike (brick)

output and intensity will be high. In each scenario, you are mindful of what's come before that day's workout and what's coming next, and you understand how it all fits into the bigger picture of your week. This allows you to be present and ready to execute both the work and the recovery process that will bring about both consistent training and positive adaptations. It also helps you make smart decisions when life events or fatigue create the need to scale or prioritize workouts.

By placing that workout within the larger montage of your week, both in terms of training and the rest of your commitments, you can set yourself up physically, mentally, and emotionally with proper sleep, hydration, nutrition, and recovery and manage job responsibilities and family matters. It might mean you pay more attention to your hydration the night before the morning of a hard workout. Or it might mean you finish a report for work so you can have a clear mind when you show up for your workout. It could even mean that you allow an extra 15–20 minutes of time in the car on your way to the track so you can drop the kids off at school and not feel pressed for time when heading to your challenging session. The bottom line is that you want to have all of your physical, mental, and emotional resources available as you begin the session, especially if it's a key workout that requires intense focus and presence.

The actions that set you up for success are entirely individual and relative to your fitness, your capacity for training, your experience as an athlete, and numerous variables in your own life. Athletes who are 25 years old, working less demanding jobs, and are more physically and mentally resilient can manage a considerable training load; in fact, even if their preparation lacks precise focus or effectiveness, they're likely to improve. However, as athletes get older they are typically more restricted by their schedules and life stress. The appropriate amount of weekly training time is bound to decrease, which only increases the demand for acute focus to get the maximum yield out of training. Less opportunity (fewer swimming strokes, fewer pedal strokes on the bike, fewer running strides) means you need to make the available opportunities as effective as possible. As life becomes more complicated, the requirement for training optimization increases in parallel.

Bring Your Best Self

Another key to executing effective training is to have all resources (or energy) available to put forth strong efforts in key sessions. Remember, training is not about cramming in hours, simply "punching the clock." You need to perform with focused intent despite the fact that the physical and mental capacity you bring to a session will fluctuate from day to day and session to session. No matter what energy level you bring (whether your legs feel heavy or your shoulders are tight, whether fresh or fatigued), you must bring the best of yourself to each session. Physical training is just one part of this equation. Athletes also need to detach themselves mentally and emotionally from outside stressors for the duration of the training session. Not every day will hold spectacular results, but if you can draw upon all of the resources available to you that day, you will get the most out of that session. Practicing this mindset will serve you well on race day, when the goal is to always maximize your resources. When you develop the capacity to be consistently present and focused, it means your program is sustainable. It also shows that you have successfully integrated your training program into your life.

For any given workout, you need to have presence, understand the purpose of the workout, have your resources and energy available, and make a habit of executing the intentions of that workout.

Let's consider how these resources are put to the test in training. If you're training for an Ironman and you have a 4-hour ride on your agenda that includes 6 × 5-minute hard intervals in the middle of the ride followed by two additional hours of endurance riding, each aspect of that workout has a different purpose. The 2-hour effort at the end is not meant to be a leisurely ride or a long cool-down. To continue riding with good form you will need to actively manage the physical and mental fatigue that creep in after a few hours. In other words, it's not about holding 200 watts the entire way but about continuing to ride the bike well with great posture and pedaling dynamics even when you are tired.

When you are mentally and physically fatigued, you are prone to stop sitting on the bike in good position and stop navigating the terrain of the course in best fashion. Look at athletes in the initial miles of the bike leg of an Ironman. They typically have great form and posture on the bike, they're riding powerfully and efficiently, and they're attacking the course in a smart and logical way. However, by Mile 90, those same athletes often aren't maintaining the same power or speed. The first place athletes and coaches tend to look is simply at output, blaming fitness for being the performance limiter. However, form is noticeably compromised: posture has morphed into a rounded back and hands are choked back on the aero bars, creating poor aero position, and efficiency and output have dropped. If you didn't know better you might think the athletes stopped halfway through the race to change their bike fit to a terribly uncomfortable position.

These athletes lack the postural fitness to retain the aero position, but also they've suffered a loss of focus. It isn't just how the athletes sit on the bikes. Instead of riding through a roller and pedaling strong at the crest of the hill, the athletes began moderately riding up the inclines and then coasting out of them a bit, reducing their speed relative to their input of effort, dragging down their average power and speed. Being present and understanding the intent of the workout is crucial to building habits that prepare you for race situations like these. If you know the last 2 hours of a 4-hour ride are about endurance, you still need to maximize your effort with great focus, not by riding hard but by riding smart, with the appropriate effort, good posture, and precise focus on how you're navigating the features of the course.

Many times in a training cycle, you'll have lingering fatigue when you go into a workout. Whether or not the fatigue is apparent when you begin, when you recognize it you need to have the presence of mind to understand that it might lower your output but not to get discouraged. For example, let's say your prescribed running workout is 5 × 1 mile on the track at a 7:30 pace, but because of hard sessions you did earlier in the week and a bigger training load the previous weekend, you're only able to hit the first two 1-mile intervals of that workout at about 7:40 pace. It would be easy to see this as failure, evidence that your training is not progressing and maybe even going backward. These are logical conclusions when metrics are taken out of context. Instead, you need to remain present and understand that running that workout at 7:40 pace is acceptable. Acknowledge that you have lingering fatigue and that maybe your physical resources aren't quite as good as they were three weeks ago when you did the same workout. Leap at the opportunity to retain running with great form and focused intent, maximizing the resources you do have on that day. With this subtle shift the day quickly evolves from failure to high value.

There could be many other factors, too, including carryover of emotional fatigue from life stress. Maybe your sleep was compromised from a busy week at work or a business trip, maybe you have been dealing with a stressful family situation, or maybe you've been trying to fend off a head cold. Some women's monthly cycles can significantly affect resources available from one week to the next. Don't let fatigue compromise your workout or metrics change your outlook as you approach your next session. It might sound trite, but part of being present and executing a workout with intent is simply swimming, riding, or running well despite the variables of any given day.

Bringing your best self requires focus, and even when you are not feeling fatigued, the longer sessions that build endurance will put that focus to the test. These sessions are best broken down into more manageable increments. If you set out to do a swim workout that includes a main set of 20 × 200, don't let yourself become daunted by the 20 intervals. Focus on executing 5 intervals at a time, and pick off each of those intervals with strong intent. After you finish a set of 5 intervals, move on to the next project.

The same mindset applies to racing. We don't think about racing 26.2 miles. Instead, we break down the marathon into logical intervals we know we can execute. You might choose to use literal mile markers or less formal milestones on the racecourse: the turn up ahead, the lollipop loop, the next major intersection. This is what I call making every day a masterpiece. It's the ability to hold yourself accountable to get the best out of that session you can. If that attitude becomes habitual, you'll maximize the effectiveness of your training on a daily and weekly basis.

Focus on the Process, Not the Outcome

The optimization challenge requires you to shift your focus away from your desired outcome and instead become process-driven. It doesn't matter if your goal is qualifying for the Ironman World Championships or finishing your first Ironman, if you are thinking about that outcome every day of the week, you're not thinking about what you can control on a daily basis or even in a specific moment of a workout or a race. What you set out to do in training is to maximize positive adaptations so we can perform optimally on race day. The fitness you develop in training is only a portion of what you need to reach your goals. Performing well in an Ironman or Ironman 70.3 is all about economy and resilience: you have to maintain efficiency from start to finish, think pragmatically, and problem-solve. These are habits to develop in training.

To be process-focused, you need to regularly check in with yourself regarding how you're feeling and how you're performing relative to the intent of the workout. The three key questions are:

- How am I feeling?
- How am I pacing?
- How is my form?

However, you also need to ask: How is my focus? How is my mental energy? How is my physical energy? How is my fueling? Am I bonking? Am I thirsty? Training is an opportunity to refine your ability to discern what's going on internally and make the necessary adjustments, even when you feel fatigued or stressed. Cultivate the ability to remain present and aware in workouts so you can use that skill on race day. You can't let the perception of how your session is going, positive or negative, have an effect on what you're doing at that moment or what you have left to do. Focus on what you can control in the present.

Form retention is pivotal to performance, and it is something you can control. As you perform each discipline in training, continually check in and think about whether your swim strokes are effective, how you are sitting on the bike, and if you are maintaining your running form. Part of this involves a technical check-in: What is the angle of your arm as it enters the water or the angle of your foot as it hits the ground? The other part is about rhythm: What is your pedaling cadence or your running cadence? Are you in a state of flow? You can't engineer all of these aspects of efficiency all of the time, but they are extremely important considerations as you train. As you train, so shall you race. Make these actions more automatic through the training process. By race day your posture, form, and flow within each discipline should become almost more intuitive, only requiring periodic check-ins.

Ultimately, your success will be based upon how well you achieve your race goals, but it's less about your final Ironman or 70.3 time (that's just a number). More importantly, how well did you carry out your race plan and navigate the challenges within each discipline? Both in training and in racing, good execution requires that you remain focused on the process.

Detach to Gain Awareness

It is extremely important to be detached from everything else when you are training, especially during key sessions. We all know people (friends, colleagues, teammates, training partners) who constantly check their phones immediately before and even during workouts. Some people leave their phones on the pool deck and check them after a warm-up session or between intervals. Some even try to respond to text messages while riding. These behaviors are sheer madness and should be eliminated. Not only do they cause you to lose mental focus but also they add emotional and physical stress to your workout.

I can't be more serious: Leave your phone behind when you head into a workout (unless you are bringing it along for safety reasons). I work with some of the busiest and most in-demand executives of major companies, and I haven't met one who has to be absolutely accessible all of the time. We are prone to continually checking our phones, but there are ways to detach and communicate with people about when you can be reached. For example, if you have pressing family or work matters, take the extra step of explaining where you will be and precisely how long you'll be out of touch. If the situation merits it, tell a few people that if there is an emergency during that 60- to 90-minute span, they can call you. Leave your ringer on so you can see who is calling without repeatedly checking your phone.

Leaving your phone out of your workouts isn't the only type of detachment that leads to success. You also need time to be untethered from metrics and monitoring devices so you can embrace the simple joys of the sport. You want to enter every workout session with a clear, alert mind so that you can achieve the intent of the workout and remain aware of opportunities to enjoy this kind of freedom. If you're out on an easy evening trail run with friends or training partners, don't let yourself worry about your running pace or splits or inadvertently start one-upping the group just because you think you should be running at a certain speed. Instead, enjoy the run and the flow of the session. Focus on your running form as well as the social aspect of being part of a like-minded community. Similarly, when you're out riding with a friend, don't let your metrics from a power meter dominate every pedal stroke you take. You are allowed to have fun, engage in conversation, and immerse yourself in the experience. Know when to be absolutely focused and task-driven and when to enjoy the simple pleasures of the sport.

Having the ability to shut out distractions and be present in your training fosters a sixth sense of awareness. For example, if you are running or riding your bike through the city, you can look around and observe and react without thinking much at all. You can anticipate a car that might turn into your path well before it happens. In your mind, you'll be anticipating what that car is doing and whether the driver might decide to wait for you to pass or to sneak out in front of you. The same goes for when you're running on trails. The more you can calm your mind, the less you think about specific obstacles on the trail such as rocks or roots, which minimizes stress and the likelihood of tripping and spraining an ankle. It's a learned sense based on the habit you develop of being present.

This state of awareness also has implications for your technical riding. If you're out on your bike and riding with a clear mind, presence, and focus, you'll better be able to gauge your pedaling mechanics, how well you are cornering, and how well you are descending and ascending. You'll be able to better manage your effort and execution relative to other aspects of riding, such as wind direction, terrain, and whether you need to stand up out of the saddle to get over the next roller. In a race you will be in a better position to deploy your resources against your competition. Although this aspect of racing mostly applies to professional athletes, having this sense of awareness can help every athlete execute the intervals of a workout or finish a race strong.

Without this presence, training or racing can go wrong in a hurry. Let's return to the same scenario of riding or running on city streets: if you're stressed about work and worried that you haven't checked your phone to respond to an important text, you won't have the capacity to be alert and embrace your surroundings, let alone keep yourself safe amid the many moving elements of traffic. That's when you're bound to run into a turning car at an intersection, hit a curb, or misjudge a traffic light.

Riding or running in traffic is an obvious example, but awareness plays a role in any workout setting. I could share countless real-life examples from the Purple Patch training camps. Because the training rides cause nervous energy in many newer riders, they sometimes experience lack of focus, self-management, and control in the early stages of the rides. An athlete's focus is often driven by the group environment, and all consideration of proper riding mechanics, pacing, and fueling or hydration is replaced by a mindset of keeping up with better athletes or proving self-worth within the group of athletes. By the middle of the ride, some athletes find themselves in deep fatigue, underperforming, and slogging home with a bewildering lack of energy. They suffer not because of poor fitness or inexperience but as a result of poor pacing. This was such a challenge for us in the early years of hosting these training camps that we now take steps to reduce the opportunities for new riders to make these mistakes. Naturally, if this behavior occurs in a training camp, it's even more likely amid the stress, excitement, and challenge of competition.

Distraction about life commitments and expectations could hold you back from reaching the next level. Or, if you buy into the program and all that it represents, then triathlon training can become a form of meditation that will feed your soul. Being present and engaged in an activity so narrow in focus connects you with your body. Myriad other things happening in your life are irrelevant to the task at hand, so set them aside. Believe me, those family, work, and other life obligations are extremely important, but they also carry emotional baggage and anxiety. Develop the ability to train with focus and presence, and triathlon becomes a genuine escape, holding a powerful, stress-reducing role in your life.

THE ELEMENTS OF A WORKOUT

To achieve the goals of your workouts, you need to understand how they are organized. Every session is organized around the main set, which reflects the intent and focus of that individual workout. To prepare you for that work, every session has a warm-up and a pre-main set leading into the main set. Some workouts will have additional elements after the main set and before the cool-down to work on physiological aspects of training such as speed or technical acuity. The main set typically makes up at least 50 percent of the total time for the workout. Those additional sets and even the cool-down might become optional or expendable if a lack of time or overwhelming fatigue inhibits your ability to complete a workout or execute the main set with purposeful intent. We'll look more closely at the details of scaling workouts later in this chapter.

Warm-Up

In this phase you're simply moving your body with easy effort to activate the muscles and increase blood flow, but it is a critical part of every workout. An attempt to do mild- to high-intensity work without warming up can have detrimental effects, such as your inability to achieve the goals of the main set. The only exception to this is specific race simulations in preparation for a competition that you know will allow minimal opportunity for warming up.

The low-stress effort is the key to a good warm-up. In terms of form, you just want to make sure you're moving with the same mechanics you'll use throughout the workout. Most time-starved, amateur athletes go too hard in their warm-up sessions. In some of the early morning swim sessions I coach, we've got the pro athletes in Lane 1 and the slowest group of age-groupers in Lane 8. During a workout, pros can do 100-yard intervals in around 1 minute, whereas the slower age-groupers typically can do those intervals in 1:45 to 2:10. During the warm-up, the pros will typically be going at an easy 1:30 pace, and the slower age-groupers will be cruising at a 1:49 pace or something very close to their real time. The pros tend to know the intent of the warm-up and execute it properly, but the amateurs fail to do the same out of misunderstood intent, misplaced competitiveness, or anxiety about keeping up with the other swimmers. Regardless of whether you're doing a swim, bike, run, or strength workout, the warm-up portion should be about moving blood, not seeking fitness gains, so be sure it is a very low effort.

Pre-Main Set

The pre-main set usually has one or two purposes aligned with the main set: developing a technical skill and/or getting your body prepared to be optimally effective. During a running workout on the track where you'll do hard 6 × 1-kilometer intervals as your main set, you might do a mile or two of easy running as a warm-up, followed by a series of 50-meter buildups or strides at a hard effort, and then maybe 3 × 200-meter sets at 80 percent effort to really get your motor primed. By increasing your heart rate and executing the explosive strides and contained sprints while also paying attention to technique and form, you'll be positioned for the best yield possible from your main set. If you're time-starved, you can skip some or all of this work. Without the pre-main set you can still achieve the goals of the 6 × 1 km interval session, but it will be tougher to perform consistently in pace, rhythm, and form in the initial intervals.

Some Training Is Better than No Training

High-value training comes from following the rhythm and intent of the prescribed sessions, but you are sure to stumble upon days when you just aren't feeling it. Don't fall into the habit of pulling the pin or just going easy every time you begin a session feeling lethargic. There is often a massive difference between your actual physical resources and your perception of your resources, so it pays to give yourself a shot at the workout.

On days when you aren't feeling it, I suggest you still begin a session. If your system opens up and you start to feel good, finish the workout as intended. If you continue to feel lethargic, remove the intensity or main work of the day. Retreat from the work, focus on executing good form, but with less physical stress. You should aim to go home feeling revived from an easier, more therapeutic session.

In a busy life there will be days when you need to shift the focus of a workout, but this doesn't signify failure.

Main Set

The main set is the gold in the treasure chest. You'll want to treat the main set of key sessions accordingly, both in your focus and execution of the intent. It is most important to preserve the integrity of these sessions in the event that you need to restructure your week or even scale down your workouts because of fatigue, illness, or time conflicts. Whether it's a swimming, biking, or running workout, the main set is aimed at building a specific aspect of your fitness or developing race readiness. The main set of any workout is the piece that is most closely guarded if and when a workout must be scaled.

Cool-Down

One of the most overrated pieces of triathlon training is the cool down, especially for the time-starved athlete for whom every minute of training counts. Because triathlon is an endurance sport, with few sessions of very high intensity, the physiological necessity for a cool down is limited. If you are forced to scale a workout, keep as much warm-up as possible, which prepares you for the main set, and be willing to trim or skip the cool down.

The one value of a cool down is to emotionally and physically return you to homeostasis, and many athletes enjoy finishing with some easy work to settle out of the rigor of training. There is nothing wrong with this, so feel free to include cool downs when there is time, but don't skip or trim the main set because you feel you must have cool down. What should be a non-negotiable is your recovery process following, particularly postworkout fueling and restoring your hydration status back to baseline.

Recovery

Although specific workouts don't have a recovery phase built into them, taking the time and steps to ensure proper recovery after hard sessions is extremely important. Oftentimes that can include a prescribed active recovery session on your training schedule, such as an easy run or an endurance ride. However, the most important recovery effort you make is to develop the habits that support performance. Primary among those habits is eating a snack or small meal as soon as possible after your workout. Maintain good hydration and eat balanced, nutritious meals throughout the day. Be sure to get good, quality sleep at night. Chapter 5 will address the supporting habits in detail, but consider these behaviors part of the recovery from every workout you do.

TRAINING INTENSITY AND METRICS

To execute each workout as intended, you need to understand the different levels of training intensity and the use of metrics. In addition to managing your awareness and your form, during training you navigate the data-driven framework of power, pace, training zones, and other measurements. Too many athletes chase an exact intensity, heart rate, or pace for every session. When combined with various life stressors, management of the physiological response to training load is a messy undertaking. It's very tough, if not impossible, to mathematically frame an exact power output at which to ride to achieve a desired response. Human physiology is highly variable, and responses to stressors only increase that variability, so one has to acknowledge how every workout fits into the bigger picture. A thinking athlete can train with intent within a framework of metrics considered both in the context of each session and as part of the bigger picture. With this mindset, the athlete can make informed, pragmatic decisions about the intensity of workouts.

Training Zones

When it comes to training intensity, many athletes establish training zones via benchmark assessments or lab-based tests and then apply a "set it and forget it" approach. No matter how the training session is going, nor their level of fatigue, athletes chase their preset power zones or heart rate zones. They are led by the power meter and heart rate watch. Although nearly every Purple Patch athlete uses devices such as power meters, GPS watches, and heart rate monitors, I don't generally like metrics to drive training intensity. I much prefer to lean into the intent of the training prescription and have athletes develop a feeling of the effort prescribed. Then they can use the information from the devices as an objective measurement of their output to review their training *after the fact*.

I view training zones as indicators of several factors: power/pace, heart rate, perceived effort, and intended intensity. When I coach individual athletes, I prescribe training in terms of easy (Z1), smooth (Z2), strong (Z3), very strong (Z4), and hard (Z5).

The majority of work falls into these categories, and individually coached athletes quickly gain an understanding of how each zone feels. In working with athletes, we align our expectations for the power, pace, and heart rates that accompany these efforts. You will see these descriptors in the workouts used in this book.

Some of the event-specific sessions target specific outputs in terms of pace or power. Imagine that an athlete has run a 1:33 half-marathon off the bike, but we set a goal to break the 1:30 barrier. In order to run under 90 minutes off the bike, the athlete must become comfortable at a sub-6:50-mile pace off the bike. Rather than ask the athlete to run "strong to very strong" off the bike, I would include specific sessions that train the athlete to retain form and become familiar with running at goal pace and faster. In this example, I might prescribe an off-the-bike run session that develops the ability to "get to pace" quickly, then train at and above that goal pace:

RUN OFF THE BIKE
5 min. build to 6:45-mile pace Just faster than goal pace
2 min. form-based smooth running Not easy, but steady endurance running with a chance to recapture form
3 min. at 6:45-mile pace Just faster than goal pace
2 min. form Reset posture and form
2 min. at 6:40-mile pace Training leg speed at faster than goal pace
2 min. form Reset posture and form
1 min. at 6:35-mile pace Shorter interval length as pace increases to above goal pace again
2 min. form Reset posture and form
2 min. at 6:40-mile pace Returning to more realistic sustained pace
2 min. form Reset posture and form
3 min. at 6:45-mile pace Back to about race effort
2 min. form Reset posture and form

This adds up to 28 minutes, but we now go back to *feeling* because it is a critical piece of race-day running. I want you to be able to feel race pace and establish form at the pace required. This is vastly different than simply locking into a pace and allowing the mind to wander. With this goal in mind, I might have the athlete finish the session with an 8-minute interval at race-goal effort without looking at the watch. The mission is to lock into sustainable and fluid running with good form. I often see race pace or faster from the athlete here, but it has to be accompanied by great form.

Less-established runners might aspire to run as much of the run portion of the race as possible. We apply a similar approach, but with a run-walk strategy:

And so on. The run session retains the purpose.

Balancing Perceived Effort and Metrics

To help you establish a framework of pacing and power in the event-specific training, especially in sessions that ask for *race pace* or *race effort*, use Figure 4.2 as a guide to help you gauge output and metrics for how the work feels. If you prefer to keep things simple, just follow the descriptions of perceived effort outlined in the zones.

You'll notice that I am not asking you to go through a benchmark assessment to establish a framework of specific zones for heart rate, power, and pace. In my experience working with athletes, this classic approach has proven problematic. As you can tell by now, I strongly advocate a focus on the art of "doing." I want

FIGURE 4.2
Training Zones

Z1	Z2	Z3	Z4	Z5
Easy	**Smooth**	**Strong**	**Very Strong**	**Hard**
Blood is moving without big effort. Used in warm-up and recovery sessions; well below the effort typically deployed in racing.	An endurance effort that can be sustained for extended periods without accumulation of fatigue or residual effects the following day (e.g., soreness). Many athletes maintain an Ironman race pace at the upper range of this effort.	This effort is sustainable for extended periods with strong focus. This requires steady effort, but not to the point of being breathless.	This is the maximum amount of work that can be sustained over a set duration, combining the athlete's current fitness and good form but without force. The result is an uncomfortable effort that requires dedicated focus to maintain.	Force is added to form and fitness to achieve a high-intensity effort for a short period of time. This effort will put athletes into duress and cause residual effects if too much time is accumulated in this zone.

my athletes to remain focused on the task at hand and develop a feel for training intensity, which I call *minding the internal clock*. In my experience, when you provide athletes rigid power, pace, and heart rate zones, the athletes become shackled to the metrics rather than riding or running well. I wouldn't say you should dismiss a coaching style that adheres to a more rigid, metrics-based approach; it just isn't my style. In my own coaching experience, when I prescribe strict training zones based on an assessment, athletes become confused about how to execute the training. My prescription doesn't fit neatly with the data, which confuses the intent of the session and often leads to flawed execution.

Let's take a closer look at how this phenomenon plays out in training. John completed a classic 20-minute time trial to establish his training zones, riding his bike on a trainer as strongly as he could sustain for the duration while maintaining a self-selected cadence of 85 rpm. From this single assessment John established a series of training zones from Z1 to Z5. His metrics for Zone 3 were:

ZONE 3 METRICS

Power 210–245W
Heart rate 147–159 bpm
Perceived effort 7 out of 10

John is feeling confident about these numbers and ready to conquer specific training. Unfortunately, when he begins his End-of-Range strength-endurance training he encounters some problems.

5 × 5 min. Z3, at < 60 rpm

John sets his trainer at 230 watts, right in the heart of Z3, but he doesn't have any experience doing strength-endurance work at a lower cadence (rpm). He finds the work very challenging, and his legs ache, but he cannot get his heart rate up to Zone 3; it remains at 143–145 beats per minute. He wants to know what he is doing wrong, but the truth is that he isn't doing anything wrong; his body is responding as as anticipated. The session is designed to stress the muscular system, and the corresponding heart rate stress will be lower with this type of work. Having the ability to generate good power at lower cadence can be used in racing, especially on climbs, if John wants to vary the type of global load or lower the heart rate associated with higher cadences across most efforts. The development of this tool in John's tool kit will bring a lot of value. If John remains focused on hitting the specific power zones, he will miss out on this training tool. Imagine John's frustration when he is then asked to execute a session that demands both ends of the cadence range.

6 × 6 min. Z3 on a 4% grade hill:

Odd intervals at <60 rpm, even intervals at >90 rpm

The data from John's ride shows a massive cardiovascular response from the high-cadence pedaling as John struggles to keep his heart rate in Z3 when he climbs at high cadence. The cost is great, and similar power does not equate to a normal heart rate response.

ODD INTERVALS	EVEN INTERVALS
Power 250W	**Power** 245W
Heart rate 145-149 bpm	**Heart rate** 162 bpm
Cadence 50 rpm	**Cadence** 95 rpm

This same problem plays out in many of the workouts specified in this book, and it's possible to learn from each scenario and make adaptations. It is far easier to execute the sessions based on the intended feeling and the description of the effort and then review the different output metrics and physiological responses relative to effort. Used in this context, the metrics become a better tool to apply in the real world of training and racing.

SCALING WORKOUTS

Inevitably contingencies will challenge your ability to execute workouts as they are prescribed. There will be times you will need to scale down a workout or truncate part of your training week, either because you have less time to train or because your body is excessively fatigued, overstressed, and run down.

Scaling Workouts for Time Constraints

Changes in your daily work schedule, business travel, and life with family and kids are bound to encroach on your training. For example, you might have set aside time to do your 90-minute swim workout only to have a work meeting run late, and suddenly you have time for only a 45-minute workout. Although this can be frustrating, if you consistently bring a pragmatic mindset to planning and executing your week, you make smart adjustments and scale the workout as needed. This accomplishes your primary mission of maximizing training time with positive adaptations and still doing at least a portion of your key workout. Here is a protocol for scaling your workouts according to value of each set within your session.

1. Eliminate the extra segments after the main set.
2. Reduce or eliminate the cool-down.
3. Trim or reduce the pre-main set.
4. Trim a small portion of the warm-up.
5. Trim the length of the main set. (This is the least-preferred option.)

For example, let's say you have a 90-minute swim workout that includes 10 minutes of easy warm-up and 15 minutes of a pre-main set, a 50-minute main set, and 10 minutes of speed work at the end followed by a 5-minute, easy cool-down. However, your day goes sideways, and you only have 45 minutes. Following the scaling protocol, you could do a 5-minute, easy warm-up followed by a 10-minute pre-main set, scale down the main set to 30 minutes, and skip the final speed session and cool-down.

SCHEDULED WORKOUT	SCALED WORKOUT
Warm-up 10 min.	**Warm-up** 5 min.
Pre-main set 8 × 100 with fins and paddles, building every two intervals	**Pre-main set** 6 × 100 with fins and paddles, building every two intervals
Main set 8 × 300 on 5 min. 16 × 25 speed work	**Main set** 5 × 300 on 5 min.
Cool-down 2 min.	(Speed work and cool-down are eliminated.)

Whenever you scale workouts, the time you spend on the main set will increase proportionally; in this case, it went from 50 percent to 66 percent of the total time. This preserves the intent and focus of that all-important set. After you complete the workout, you'll be happy to know that you achieved a high-level workout in a condensed amount of time.

Scaling Workouts for Fatigue

As another example, imagine you've had a really hard couple of days at the office while preparing for a big presentation. You have been a bit scattered all week, you didn't sleep well on back-to-back nights, and you are feeling fatigued as you head to the track for your prescribed interval workout session of 5 × 1 km at hard effort. Are you physically or emotionally ready and able to run hard with presence and achieve the intent of the workout? Probably not, but what should you do?

First, you have to do a check-in to get a relative assessment of where you are. You might tell yourself you feel lousy and really don't want to do the workout because you think you will tank the intervals and perform awfully based on how sluggish you feel. (It's important to note that this scenario assumes you're not dealing with injuries or sickness, only life and training fatigue.)

In this situation, you have to pull back from the myopic lens of "if I don't complete this workout, I'm a failure" and always keep an eye on the larger land-scape (the mosaic of the training week and of what's happening in your life) and start to connect the dots. Remember that *some* training is nearly always better than none. Even if you're not feeling great (whether because of fatigue, a busy day, or lack of sleep), you should never pull the pin on a workout or reduce your intensity until you at least try it.

Your perceived energy is often different from your real energy. You can't be your own judge and executioner before you have even started the workout. Don't set yourself up for failure by declaring you're bound to have a bad session because you're feeling some level of emotional or physical fatigue. Give your body the opportunity to showcase its actual physical resources.

Start with the intent of getting through the workout. Do the warm-up session without any emotional judgment, and prepare for the pre–main set and main set. If you believe training stress is the main cause of your fatigue (more so than life stress), try extending your warm-up slightly. As your blood begins flowing faster, the neurological synergy of the movement can actually make you feel better, and you might be surprised by your ability to execute the workout.

From there, hold on to that good intent and go through the pre-main set (which might be two or three repeating sets of 60 seconds at a moderate pace, followed by 30 seconds at an easy pace), and then continue to the first interval. There's a chance you might run that first 1 km interval pretty well, even if just slightly slower than the prescribed goal time. If that's the case, check in with yourself again to see if you feel well enough to continue with the second interval. However, if you run that initial 1 km interval, and it is clear that you still feel emotionally or physically fatigued, and your body is unable to respond, or if you are experiencing a higher rate of exertion than usual, then it's time to scale the workout.

Here are some additional clear indications that you should make adjustments to the workout:

- You can't stay mentally present
- Your performance is poor
- You are running with bad form
- Your perceived effort is high, but your heart rate remains low

- Your pronounced muscle soreness doesn't dissipate post–warm-up
- You just don't want to be there

In these situations, instead of punishing yourself and feeling guilty, remove the hard work from the session. This might mean that you turn the workout into an easier endurance run for the remainder of the time (e.g., finishing with 45 minutes of easy running) or perhaps running a few more 1 km intervals as moderate efforts that build more gradually. The best-case result might just be that you have increased your heart rate and had a therapeutic session for the soul and the body. Ultimately it comes down to being pragmatic and understanding precisely how you feel.

After the workout is done, you'll need to determine what caused you the fatigue and what you can do to recover from it. Determine whether you need more rest days, whether you should move your key running session to later in the week, or whether you just need to move on and put it behind you. It will depend on your week, what else you have going on, and how much time it will take to recover. However, generally speaking, if you're that fatigued, your best option is to put it in the rearview mirror and continue to focus on facilitating better recovery.

It's easier to do this without guilt or worry if this is a rare occurrence. If it is happening frequently (at least once or twice a week), you probably have some other issues to look at, such as insufficient sleep, poor nutrition, or fueling mistakes, all of which are possible indications of overtraining. Start troubleshooting to find the real issue and reexamine your work/life balance and weekly schedule as well as your sleep, nutrition, and hydration habits.

Scaling Workouts for Illness

No matter how smart and careful your approach is, you will inevitably have bouts of illness to navigate over the course of any training cycle and likely more than one over the course of an entire season. Although we hope to avoid those situations and remain healthy, when mapping the seasonal plan, you need a cold contingency plan. Illness is part of life, and the point is that performance readiness is a result of many weeks and months of consistent training. It takes five full days of inactivity before the effects of detraining begin to occur. Your contingency plan is an important buffer for the common head cold and short bouts of the flu. Although it is emotionally tough to be slowed by sickness, you have some wiggle room before the positive adaptations and fitness from previous hard work are compromised.

So how do you manage training with a cold or minor illness? Focus on positive adaptations. When your body's immune system is under attack from a virus, its capacity to make physiological gains from stressful training is greatly compromised. Furthermore, maintaining a normal schedule of endurance training is likely to extend the duration of the virus. I've seen this play out, and I'm sure you have as well. Two athletes become sick, and the first athlete responds by getting a good amount of sleep and rest with no training or other activity and drinking many fluids for 48 hours. The second athlete stubbornly refuses to give up the heavy training and remains immersed in work commitments and other demands. The first athlete recovers from the cold in a few days, but the second athlete is still dealing with symptoms 10 days later. It's no coincidence. When athletes practice patience and commit to rest, they mitigate the loss of valuable training time.

Here is a cold contingency plan to keep you from getting derailed for long periods and dealing with lingering fatigue, at which point it is difficult to fully recover. In general, there are a few tips to follow:

- *If you don't feel well above the neck line, keep moving:* If you have the classic head cold symptoms, without fever or a chesty cough, you can keep moving but avoid hard training. Try to keep your training to 60 minutes or less per session at Zone 2 or under. Respect what your mind and body tell you to do.

- *If you're not feeling well below the neck line, complete rest is in order:* If you have any body aches, fever, chesty cough, and so forth, at least 72 hours of rest is optimal before resuming training, and only resume training when these symptoms have improved.

- *Sleep and rest to accelerate recuperation:* Get as much sleep as possible, especially when you're not feeling 100 percent.

- *Hydrate the immune system:* Drink plenty of fluids, including teas, soups, and water, optimal supporters of both your cellular health and your immune system.

- *Don't let cold medicines mask logic:* There is nothing wrong with taking (legal) supplements to help diminish the effects of a cold. However, don't let the diminished symptoms lead you to make poor decisions about training. Just because your sinus headache dissipates by midday doesn't mean you'll suddenly have all of your resources to properly execute a track workout or interval bike trainer session. Even if you can get through it, you'll run the risk of not feeling well later in the day.

After your symptoms diminish, you can begin ramping up to train. The first day is purely about moving blood, so stick to short durations and low-stress efforts. The second day should be endurance focused, with normal duration of training and willingness to back off if you're not feeling good. Assuming you're feeling closer to 100 percent, the third day is when you can resume regular training with typical intervals. If you feel worse following any of the days, then add another low-stress or endurance day before resuming intervals.

It's important to note that ongoing illness can be a symptom of other problems. If a cold lingers much longer than for most other athletes or much longer than normal for you, or if you begin getting colds frequently (more than two per year), then it is likely worth reflecting on your training load, key supporting habits such as sleep and fueling, and other factors such as scheduling.

In 2016 Tim Reed won the Ironman 70.3 World Championships following a nasty cold about 10 days before the race. He didn't let the cold affect him mentally on race day, and you shouldn't allow that to happen, either. Forced rest can sometimes help eager athletes and coaches. Remember that performance isn't built on hitting every single prescribed session. It is built on consistent training and arriving at race day healthy, fresh, and eager to embrace the day.

New Bike, Same Old Engine

Obviously, triathlon is a very gear-intensive sport. Not only do you have three separate disciplines that have very specific types of equipment, but also there are hundreds of options to consider when you're acquiring gear. I don't have any direct relationships with companies in which I have to promote a certain brand of bikes, wetsuits, or running shoes, but even if I did, I wouldn't want to suggest a specific brand or model to an athlete because it might not be the right thing for that individual. Because of the marketing efforts behind products, it's easy for athletes to want to be drawn to the most expensive gear, the most aerodynamic gear, or the lightest gear. However, that's not always the best choice for a particular athlete's needs. There is a blizzard of equipment choices out there, but there are a few basic rules and details for athletes to keep in mind when they're considering gear purchases. Whatever equipment you choose, remember it will only be as good as you are on race day.

WETSUIT. The best wetsuit for you is one that fits your individual physique well. At Purple Patch, we've done a lot of wetsuit testing, and we've seen a wide discrepancy in the performance from suit to suit and from athlete to athlete. A specific model could be a great wetsuit in someone's wear-test review, but if it doesn't fit you it's not going to put you in position to swim your best during a race.

After you find a wetsuit that fits you properly, you need to put it on correctly so as not to alter that great fit. You really have to snug up the lower half of the suit so you can have maximum flexibility and range of motion in the shoulders. For weaker swimmers, the mid-range and low-end wetsuits of a brand's line are often preferable to the highly flexible, high-end wetsuit. In truth, the more restrictive lower-end suits tend to help the swimmer maintain better posture in the water. Although it sounds a bit counterintuitive that a restrictive wetsuit could aid muscular movement, support and buoyancy have proven more effective for many amateur athletes.

GOGGLES. Outside of training and preparation, the biggest predictor of a good open-water swim performance is your ability to swim in a straight line. It's startlingly simple, but it's true. That means you'll need to practice sighting when you swim, even when you're training in a pool. On race day, you'll want to choose equipment well suited to the conditions of the race. If it's dark or gray outside, you'll want to wear goggles with rose-colored lenses. On contrary, if it's bright and sunny, you'll be better off with goggles that have dark or mirrored lenses. Be prepared for either situation with two different pairs of comfortably fitting goggles.

TIME-TRIAL BIKE. The superbike, priced from $10,000 to $15,000, is a bit like a Formula One race car; it is very fast, but I would not recommend that you go out and buy one unless you have superior mechanical skills or consistent access to an excellent mechanic. Because many races involve taking your bike apart, packing it up, shipping it, and then rebuilding it, the unbelievable difficulties that occur with these overengineered bikes are maddening. We have more athletes who waste energy manically running around the day before a race trying to get their bikes serviced because they're too complicated for anyone but a reliable mechanic. If you go one step down from the high-end bike, it tends to have less integrated components and only negligibly less aerodynamic advantage. These bikes are much easier to disassemble and work on, and they have more sensible designs that facilitate getting into a comfortable, sustainable position. Because of all of those things they'll bring you much less stress. Just because your favorite professional athletes are riding high-end bikes, it's not necessarily the best choice of a bike for an amateur athlete. We have a saying at Purple Patch for this: "New bike, same old engine." What's important is learning to ride your bike well in a sustainable position that will allow you to run your best in a completely uninhibited manner.

WHEELSETS. Unless you really like your toys and you have a massive expendable income, you'll want to choose a wheelset that can be used for all types of courses and conditions, one that allows you to ride with confidence to the best of your ability. I typically recommend getting a wheelset that includes a more shallow front wheel. The front wheel is most affected by crosswinds. In windy conditions, the front wheel is moving the bike all over the road, disconcerting for athletes who are not great at riding in the wind. The rear wheel is less susceptible to wind and all about aerodynamics, so it can be a slightly deeper wheel.

ELECTRONIC SHIFTING. If you are considering a bike with electronic shifting, make sure you have the ability to change gears at the base bar and not just out front on the tip of the aerobars. This will allow you to shift gears in variable terrain; for example, when you're climbing or going over rollers and find yourself standing out of the saddle. You'll want to be able to shift gears easily from any position, and you can't do that on most time-trial bikes. It's not just about having a bike with fancy electronic shifting; it's about having maximum functionality.

RUNNING SHOES. Fortunately, running requires minimal equipment, welcome news when it comes on the heels of swimming and cycling. Don't be tempted to invest in racing flats. Only elite runners have refined their form to the point where they can turn a lighter shoe into a faster time.

5

Developing Habits to Support Performance

We've been taking steps to create a sustainable training framework that will allow you to achieve triathlon success. Many commitments are involved in that structure, including starting from the right mindset, properly setting the lens on your available training time, and executing your training consistently. Within each of those major steps, dozens of small actions lead to your optimal performance.

Don't worry: however complex this might seem, much of it boils down to simple habits and behaviors conducive to your success. I am primarily talking about how sleep, nutrition, fueling, and hydration affect your performance in work, life, and triathlon. The key to achieving sustainability in optimizing these behaviors is to make some basic but important behaviors as habitual as possible. These habits start as learned behaviors gleaned from being present and pragmatic in your journey through triathlon and the rest of your busy life.

The easiest way to think about this is to view your endurance training as the centerpiece, or star, of your performance endeavors; sleep, nutrition, fueling, and hydration make up what I call *the supporting cast*. They're not in the spotlight, but if they are not properly developed, the whole performance production is bound to fall apart. The importance of sleep, nutrition, fueling, and hydration is backed by science, but information on how best to make good habits of them is less reliable and often highly individualized. Cultivating sustainable habits requires the same level of focus, intention, planning, and smart execution that you put into your training. You can't achieve consistent success in triathlon, or life, without incorporating these behaviors effectively on a regular basis. This is why, when talking to athletes about their training program, I always focus on the whole production. The goal is to retain a view of all elements that go into consistency and success, and this means viewing nutrition, recovery, fueling and sleep as a part of the program. The minute that these become afterthoughts, then neglect and poor decisions occur and challenges lay ahead.

Sleep is one of the pillars of performance, a crucial resource in your training tool kit. Dozens of variables in your daily life can affect sleep, and the science of sleep is still evolving. Similarly, the sciences of performance nutrition and hydration are still in a nascent stage. The different schools of thought can lead to general confusion, not to mention that the philosophy of fueling is radically different now than it was 20 years ago. The same applies to hydration. Should you drink when thirsty, or should you proactively hydrate at specific intervals? You read reports about people becoming hyponatremic (an imbalance of salt and potassium in the blood caused by overhydration) during a race, but underperformance as a result of dehydration is typically more common at longer distance endurance events. Even outside of competition, most people don't understand the broader importance of hydration in daily life, with its effects on cellular health, managing energy levels, and many other factors.

Compounding the confusion is rampant marketing of products to fuel peak performance. Many products in the sports nutrition and hydration marketplace are designed for mass-market consumers (as opposed to well-trained athletes) and often primarily consist of starchy carbohydrates and fat. They might taste good as snacks, but they're not what you need to train, race at a high level for hours on end or recover properly. Also, eating and drinking can involve emotional attachments or negative thought patterns about body composition and body image, which makes it harder to determine true best practices.

These topics are complex and sometimes polarizing, but my goal is to filter the information and focus on the habits that yield the biggest return in your performance. We will look at each of these issues through the lens of current science, what we know works in triathlon, and what specifically works for you. It takes some effort to separate the wheat from the chaff when making and executing decisions about sleep, nutrition, fueling, and hydration. Think and act logically, not emotionally, and always be present, practicing solutions in race-simulation workouts and recovery so you can make pragmatic decisions that work for you.

SLEEP QUANTITY AND QUALITY

Sleep is just one aspect of preparation and recovery, but quite simply, it is your most powerful and effective recovery tool, so we will take the time to explore it. Your ability to perform and improve in the sports of triathlon and life depends as much on your sleep as it does on any hard work you do. Although you train in the pool, on the bike, on the run, and in the gym, your body absorbs that training largely during sleep (and various forms of active and physical recovery). Sleep rejuvenates your muscular, cardiovascular, and skeletal systems and allows you to keep progressing on a weekly, monthly, and yearly basis.

In 2006, Dr. Chris Winter and colleagues, leading sleep experts, published a longitudinal study about Major League Baseball players pertaining to many aspects of the players' lives, physical preparation, and mental approach to the sport. They concluded that sleep habits were the greatest predictor of the longevity of a baseball player's career. Think about that: how long a professional baseball player can expect to remain on the roster depends on the quality of his sleeping habits. If sleep is that important to a professional athlete (regardless of the sport), it must be crucial for a busy, amateur triathlete with considerably less time and fewer resources. The takeaway is clear: Performance improves when you maximize sleep.

In general, your body likes to "regress to the mean," and rest, sleep, and low-stress environments support that restorative state. Of all the things you do in a given 24-hour period, sleep is the critical one in facilitating:

- Positive adaptations to exercise and training,
- Readiness for subsequent training sessions,
- Mitigation of injury risk,
- Optimal energy levels in your day, and
- Focus and critical thinking.

Most of us are overscheduled with work, family, and other commitments, but the fact still remains that we cannot "beat" physiology. It always starts with the question: Are you working hard, or are you working effectively? There is a vast difference. In all arenas (sport, business, or life), working smart must be embraced. This doesn't make things easy, but should make your hard work be effective, and deliver results.

As much as we all realize the importance of sleep, it's typically the first variable compromised by motivated and busy people, especially triathletes. If you're cutting corners when it comes to sleep and not fully resting and recovering after workouts, the restorative process that happens during a good night of quality sleep won't be complete, which means your body won't be ready for additional training. If I asked you how many times this week you got at least seven hours of sleep in a single night, you might realize that even in a good week you end up inadvertently skimping on it a bit to connect the dots during your waking hours.

Getting the right amount of quality sleep is your mission. Although the quantity of sleep is highly individual, the importance of getting quality sleep is not. Some people require seven or more hours, and others function well on six hours, but quality is critical and easily influenced by your environment (noise level, light exposure, temperature, etc.), schedule, diet, and other factors.

For a highly motivated triathlete, the typical day starts with an early morning swim, ride, or running group workout before the workday. Following a long day at the office, there's often another workout, an evening meal, and family time, by which point it's typically 9 p.m. or later. That's a great time to shut down and start calming your body, but that's often when we have habits that cause us to restimulate our brains: watching TV, working on our computers, or answering emails and texts on our phones.

The light emanating from these devices triggers the brain and disrupts the biorhythms and hormone (melatonin) that aid the natural sleep cycle. Using those devices in the hour or so before you plan to sleep seriously disrupts your ability to relax and quiet your mind so you can get quality sleep through the night. Try to spend the hour before you go to bed away from any screens (no TV, no tablet, no phone) and use that time for reflecting on the day and looking ahead to tomorrow. Also, wear loose, comfortable clothes and create an ideal sleep environment: a room that is dark, quiet, and relatively cool.

Sleep isn't sexy, but it is a performance enhancer, and the wise leverage it to their advantage.

The nutrition and hydration choices you make both throughout the day and in the hours leading up to sleep also affect its quality. Proper hydration is important and can facilitate quality sleep at night. It is best to avoid caffeinated beverages for several hours prior to bedtime, especially if you are sensitive to these drinks. Prior to sleep, a small snack is often helpful to trigger best sleep and promote recovery. This could come in the form of some protein, such as yogurt or nuts, or carbohydrate-focused snacks, such as cherries or bananas.

Our electronic devices are merely a symptom of a much bigger problem. Culturally, we are susceptible to the "more is better" attitude, and whether regarding training, work, or other worthwhile commitments, the barometer of success is how much we accomplish and how many hours we invest. Many still view lack of sleep is viewed as a badge of honor and an indicator of commitment; valuing sleep is often viewed as a sign of weakness or laziness. We hear war stories of all-nighters from people with incredible drive, but we seldom hear about the power of quality sleep, rest, and recuperation. You compromise both the quantity and quality of sleep when you are determined to fit in one more thing on your to-do list. It's a corrosive habit that limits the effectiveness of what you can bring to training or work, and it undermines your health.

CASE STUDY: **FIT AND FRESH VS. FIT AND FATIGUED**

The accumulation of training and toughness are considered the greatest rewards of training success, but this method sets up athletes for suffering, not performance. I have no shortage of athletes who have improved their results by prioritizing sleep, but I've seen no athlete benefit more than Jim, a highly ambitious and keen triathlete based just outside of New York City. Jim's life is rich with commitments and opportunities, including a demanding job with plenty of upward mobility and the ambition to qualify for Ironman 70.3 World Championships. Yet he still wants to be present for and supportive of his young family with two children. Factoring in the 45-minute daily commute to his job in the city, Jim could become overloaded with stress. Underpinning this reality is Jim's character, marked by unyielding toughness and commitment. Although he rarely complained, Jim's resilience and force of will was an obstacle to evolving his performance.

The goal was never to seek some form of utopian balance within a highly goal-driven individual; rather, as a coach I needed to ensure that Jim could be effective in his pursuits and maximize his performance gains. As soon as I dug into the details of his weekly schedule, it became clear where the casualties of his equation came into play. With so many commitments and an underlying belief that achieving his triathlon goals would require at least 15 hours of weekly training, Jim simply slept less. Each day started with early morning sessions lasting 90 to 120 minutes. Evenings often included a short session, such as a higher intensity work on the trainer or an additional run. These evening workouts made it tough for Jim to fall asleep despite his underlying fatigue. He claimed a consistent five hours of sleep on weeknights, but it was often broken. Weekends didn't bring much relief, with commitments to family time and kids' sports. His longer rides began at 5 a.m., in order to be back for his family by 8 a.m. or 9 a.m. He often included a second daily session prior to dinner. Sunday was his day to sleep in until 6:30 a.m., providing some respite but not real rejuvenation. I saw scarce time in his schedule for downtime and decompression, which compounded the sleep compromises.

Jim's performance displayed this accumulation of fatigue. He had seen little performance progression over the last few seasons and underwhelming race results. His commitment to the sport wasn't declining, but he looked and felt every one of his 43 years, and he certainly wasn't thriving.

The intervention was simple, but it took massive persuasion. For the second half of his season I had Jim remove all of his evening sessions except for an easy spin on Monday evening, which wouldn't affect his sleep. I removed the Monday morning session to add two more hours of sleep. Every other weekend included a trainer ride of 90 minutes to 2 hours, which he could start at 7:30 a.m., allowing extra time to sleep in. The final piece of the puzzle was to find four weekend days over the course of the season designated for sleeping in and spending the day with his family, also including some down time for himself. In exchange, Jim secured two "bike days" over the course of the season where he could leave at 8 a.m. and have until 2 p.m. in the afternoon to train. These weekends were planned in advance and allowed the family to participate in the process. The end result was a drop to about 12 weekly hours of training, with an extra 4–5 hours of weekly sleep. Jim managed to gain focused time for family and his own training and health.

You can imagine how the rest of the story played out. Jim reported better daily energy, a more manageable schedule with time to think, and, best of all, a net performance gain with fewer training hours. The takeaway is not that less is more. Jim made a strategic plan to secure "more" of what was holding him back: sleep. He ended up making performance gains in sport and life as a result.

NUTRITION, FUELING, AND HYDRATION

There are many books and studies about sports performance nutrition, fueling, and hydration. I am not a dietician or a nutritionist, so my goal here is to give you some sustainable habits you can integrate into your life. We will focus on nutrition, fueling, and hydration habits that help you execute your training and achieve your performance goals within the scope of your life.

First, let's distinguish between fueling and nutrition. Think of fueling as the calories you consume during and immediately following a workout to optimize performance during the session and the physiological adaptation afterward, facilitate recovery, and prepare your body for subsequent training; in other words, fueling affects your energy balance well beyond the training window. When you fail to refuel adequately, you are likely to experience cravings later in the day and have to manage a host of other stress responses. Nutrition, on the contrary, represents the vitamins, minerals, and macronutrients you consume in regular meals throughout the day that provide a platform for good health. The food you eat every day obviously contributes to energy production in a workout and recovery from a workout, but it is easier to view breakfast, lunch, and dinner as your nutritional platform. Fueling, on the contrary, is the calories needed to support performance and recovery, which we approach with a different mind-set. Distinguishing between nutrition and fueling in this way makes sense of the decision to consume a soda or other sugary fuel replacement in the middle of training, whereas you would seldom consume such calories to achieve optimal nutrition in daily life.

Fueling and nutrition that benefit performance also enhance everyday life. We want to maximize the positive adaptations in training, but we also want to minimize the negative, stressful impact training can have on your ability to thrive in life. We are looking to strike a balance. To do this, the approach we take to fueling and nutrition must help us avoid unnecessary spikes in energy and massive crashes of fatigue; we want the ability to retain focus so that we can maintain great critical thinking and decision making.

The ideal scenario is metronome living: you have predictable, consistent energy to maintain your sweet spot of energy both during your work and home lives and during workouts. The functions of life served by fueling and nutrition are quite different, but there is basically one set of habits that carries over into everyday life. The bottom line is these are good habits to develop, no matter your fitness or athletic ability; these habits will help you stay properly fueled, hydrated, and balanced.

Performance Depends on Good Nutrition

In our society, many people regularly consume starchy carbohydrates and processed and packaged foods typically high in sugar, sodium, and other ingredients not particularly conducive to their health. Processed foods are often more quickly accessible, but they don't offer the benefits of real, whole foods. Triathletes are typically self-motivated individuals who strive for success in everything they do, but the effort to maintain a healthy diet is often at odds with their need for convenience.

It's no secret that to achieve your optimal performance, you need to eat well-balanced meals and healthy snacks on a consistent basis. Yes, you could merely limit the number of times you eat dessert, comfort foods, and other guilty pleasures but probably not to the point of counting calories or avoiding those entirely. Interestingly, many people who train for triathlons then undereat relative to the demands of training. Perhaps unsurprisingly, these athletes are also typically overtraining relative to their life demands, which further complicates the nutrition equation.

Good nutrition actually starts with post-workout fueling. You might follow a pretty effective nutritional regimen and do a good job of staying hydrated, but when you don't engage in the habit of eating a purposeful snack or small meal after a training session, this can throw everything else out of balance. Proper fueling, starting with those postworkout calories, satiates your appetite between meals, preventing hunger pains and the physiological starvation mechanisms that come with being underfed for the calories you have burned. Strategic fueling will help you maintain good nutrition and reinforce your ability to control portion size and food choices throughout the day. It will also set up a much-improved balance of alertness and energy outside of training.

The Fueling Window

Fueling can make or break your performance. Executed well, it safeguards your energy during a workout, helps you stay in balance throughout the rest of the day, and facilitates the recovery process in the ensuing hours and days that follow. There are two questions you need to explore regarding performance fueling:

1. Are you taking in enough calories from the appropriate foods immediately after training sessions?
2. Are you consuming the right types of calories at the right times during training sessions and races?

Every athlete should be consuming a smart mix of calories within an hour after finishing a workout, in what I label your *fueling window*. What does that mean from a practical standpoint? As a general rule, the more you can consume real food during that window (including some protein, carbohydrates, and a little bit of fat), the better off you'll be. If you can plan your post-workout snack or meal in advance (even when you're planning your workouts for the week), then you won't have to leave it to chance (which can lead to poor choices) or suffer long gaps that could leave you underfueled and therefore under-recovered and a victim of distressing energy swings.

Failing to consume calories immediately after a workout is a top-of-the-list poor habit that can lead to numerous other problems. When athletes have issues such as frequent injuries, unusual fatigue, or retention of fat, they are likely not consuming enough calories immediately after workouts. Even with athletes who maintain a healthy, well-balanced diet, poor fueling habits can be the root of the problem.

Although I'm a proponent of eating real food, consuming smartly engineered nutrition products is sometimes warranted. For example, if you have a high-intensity session and you know that eating real food is likely to give you a too-full feeling or lead to digestive issues, you might drink a protein shake. These products are a good mix of carbs, protein, and fat that can be processed and absorbed more quickly than chicken and rice or a sandwich. Although sugar is something we typically want to minimize in our diets, the sugar in recovery drinks can be quickly converted to glycogen and burned as fuel when your metabolism is

Change Has to Be Focused to Be Effective

After you figure out your approach to training, there are work/life habits to be addressed, adjustments to be made to nutrition and fueling, and more. It winds up creating a mile-wide puddle. Rather than try to clear it in one giant leap, narrow your focus.

When you change too much too soon, you can miss the greater effects of change. Decide on one or two things that will act as a catalyst for further change. For example, when an athlete is not training consistently, not sleeping well, frequently sick, and repeatedly getting injured, I typically attack postworkout fueling first. Why? Getting into the habit of fueling properly right after a workout will affect several facets of an athlete's health. After four or five days, athletes will feel an uptick in recovery, which means they will be more fresh going into workouts, have better energy balance throughout the day, and show more control over their eating habits. One simple change addresses many issues.

Change also has an emotional effect. When a new habit is forming, it feels good. This helps you buy in further, making incremental changes that support your new habit. One simple change won't create a utopian transformation, but it often turns the tide. In the case of our athletes who started by focusing on postworkout fueling, the knock-on effect was a significant reduction in hunger pangs, which made it easier to eat better and avoid unhealthy snacks and meals. Because the athlete maintained better energy throughout the day, there was less of a need for caffeine in the afternoon, which in turn led to better sleeping.

For busy professionals who get up very early to do a run or a swim and then go on with their day, energy fluctuations can be very disruptive. After I know they have good postworkout fueling habits, I turn to daily hydration. Dehydration leads to some awkward sensations and energy lulls that are often mistaken for hunger or fatigue. I instruct these athletes to regularly drink fluids from the time they arrive at work and continue throughout the day. This habit causes them to move around the office more (because there will be a need for more frequent bathroom breaks), but that's good for energy, too. Good hydration habits help the body's overall function and improve cellular health and recovery.

Evaluate your own situation and hone in on one or two things that will make an impact and naturally lead to other physical and emotional changes.

peaking after a particularly hard effort. However, avoid shakes or smoothies with too many antioxidants immediately after a hard workout. You don't want to interfere with the oxidation process, so it's wise to save foods such as berries, dark chocolate, pecans, artichokes, kidney beans, and cranberries for a different time in the day. If you're going to have some kind of starchy-carbohydrate-based food, after your workout is the best time to indulge in the pasta or pizza you love.

FUELING DURING WORKOUTS

Over the past decade or so, athletes and coaches have paid more attention to fueling during workouts. This coincides with an influx of engineered nutrition products geared toward endurance athletes. Some of the products marketed to the mass population of runners and general fitness enthusiasts might seem good for you because they are made of natural ingredients, but many products will not yield your highest energy return. Don't be a victim of the marketing hype.

First you need to determine whether you even need to fuel during a workout. All decisions around fueling are best made when you are able to remain present and understand what your body needs instead of preemptively devouring a pack of energy chews before you start a morning workout. There are some general rules to follow:

- *If your workout takes less than 60 minutes,* you probably don't need to take in calories during the workout. Your body can use stored glycogen before it needs to convert additional food into energy. An exception to this rule is to *consume calories during a workout if you know you won't have immediate access to a regular meal afterward.* In this situation, an engineered recovery drink that includes protein, carbohydrates, and fat will help maintain your energy and put you on a path to proper recovery.

- *If your workout takes more than 60 minutes* or is extremely high intensity, such as a brick that involves running off the bike, you should ingest some calories to maintain your energy level. This is when engineered foods can be most effective. It generally takes about 10 to 15 minutes to start absorbing calories, so don't wait until you start to crash because you will have difficulty recovering. Oftentimes as your energy stores are depleted, your mind will wander, compromising the focus and rhythm of the session.

- *If your workout is less specific or not a race simulation; for example, a longer-duration session at lower intensity such as a 3- to 4-hour endurance ride*, you don't need to pump yourself full of engineered food. Also, if you go on an easy 90-minute trail run in the off-season, you might not need any calories at all. The food you consume in your daily meals has supplied your body with plenty of glycogen to provide energy for workouts like these.

Real food can play a role in endurance workouts. For example, if you go on a trail run, mountain bike ride, or road ride lasting two hours or more, you might try eating a bit of trail mix, small bites of peanut butter and jelly, a few coconut macaroons, or even hardboiled eggs. A mixture of real food can be good for maintaining your energy level and more appetizing than engineered food. Although real food is more difficult for the body to digest, your gastrointestinal (GI) system is not compromised because the workout takes place over a few hours. Personally, I have no issue with athletes using real food during workouts, but it comes down to what works for each individual. As soon as intensity goes up, absorption rates go down. This is the time to gravitate toward sugar as a fuel source. Engineered foods (gels, blocks, jelly beans) can play a big role in your fueling strategy.

Use these guidelines to experiment with your fueling while training. You also need to practice what works for you during a race. Ultimately, you can fuel during workouts to get through the training session or you can fuel during workouts to simulate race conditions.

During any session that approximates race day, practice with the type of fuel and hydration you intend to use, replicating the timing and amount you intend to consume. On race day, you're looking to essentially "drip feed" consistent shots of calories at specific time increments over the course of each hour and support that caloric intake with proper hydration. Chapter 7 includes an overview of the fueling and hydration protocol for race day, but in training it's important to practice and refine your own approach, so we'll explore this topic in more detail here.

Fueling and Hydration for Racing

Athletes tend to underfuel during training and then when it comes to race day, they're so worried about bonking that they fuel to the point where they experience the negative consequences at the other end of the spectrum. As your stress level increases (your physical stress from racing three sports at the optimal level and your emotional stress from anxiety), your ability to absorb calories is greatly reduced. The physical demands of racing cause you to generate more heat, which means more blood goes to the skin to dissipate that heat. At the same time your muscles demand more oxygen, which blood must deliver to the muscles to create energy. Blood then clears the unwanted by-products of energy production. The competition for blood, both to cool the body and to supply oxygen to the muscles, results in less blood flow to your abdomen, which limits the absorption rate in your gut.

At this point, when their bodies are least efficient at calorie absorption, some athletes are trying to consume 300–400 calories per hour. That often leads to GI problems, most notably stomach cramps or bloating. If you ingest so many calories at once and are likely underhydrating relative to the food consumed, you wind up with an undiluted mass that is hard for your GI system to manage. For this reason, it's better to be slightly underfueled and catch up than it is to be overfueling and suffering from stomach distress.

Although research has shown that an athlete can consume roughly 3 or 4 calories per kilogram of body weight per hour, I recommend that athletes err on the lower side, in the range of 2.5 to 3 calories per kilogram of body weight per hour. As a basic framework for fueling strategy in a race, I tell athletes to consume a small amount of calories (in whatever form works for them) on the bike at 20 minutes, 40 minutes, and 60 minutes into the ride. Those feedings are supported with hydration at 10-minute increments to help absorption in the gut. That means, depending on your size, you'll be taking in roughly 70 to 85 calories at each 20-minute interval, as opposed to taking in much larger amounts of 100–125 calories twice an hour.

The timing and amount of fuel and hydration you take in on race day also depends on the weather. In heat and humidity, it is much easier to consume slightly smaller amounts of calories every 20 minutes. In cooler weather, the challenge is remembering to fuel consistently because athletes have fewer hunger signals in lower temperatures, and they tend to forget or ignore hydration signals under those conditions. Regardless of how you choose to get your calories (whether through blocks, chews, or gels), you need to dilute them with about 6–8 ounces of hydration. You should drink a diluted electrolyte solution to match your body chemistry. For every 100 calories you consume, you need to drink about 12 ounces of water or very diluted sports drink. This is another argument for not fueling with more calories twice an hour. It's very hard to drink 12 ounces of fluid all at once while racing.

The reason you start your fueling at 20 minutes into the bike ride (especially if you have come out of a saltwater swim) is because you go from a prone position for the swim to a quick run into the transition area, which is likely to get your heart rate to its highest point of the entire race. After pulling off your wetsuit and getting on the bike, your body takes a certain amount of time to settle, especially if you have inadvertently swallowed some sea water. If you drink anything, make it plain water to settle your stomach and offset the high osmolality of the saltwater. You'll see plenty of athletes in T1 trying to fuel up by shoving gels or blocks into their mouths before they get on the bike. For a recreational athlete deliberately slowing down to get ready for the bike, this might work, but if you're racing through T1 you are better off waiting to take in any calories until you're on the bike and feeling settled. In an ideal world, your first intake of hydration would precede your first intake of calories. However, if your body isn't yet settled and you miss or forget the first 10-minute drinking session, be sure to drink fluids at 30 and 50 minutes past the hour. From there to the finish, hydration continues at 10, 30, and 50 minutes.

This framework is meant to be a helpful guide, not a definitive rulebook. It simply offers some structure to your race-day fueling strategy. Admittedly, it's something of an art and a science. You have to test it out repeatedly in training, but to stay on top of it during a race, you have to tap into your acute self-awareness. You should always be checking in with yourself, asking questions such as: How's my motivation? How's my fatigue? How's my focus? If your thoughts are wandering and you're losing motivation, it's often a sign that you are calorically deficient, so you ought to start playing catchup on calories. If you're feeling a little sick, you're burping, or you have some GI distress, your gut's ability to absorb those calories might be faulty, so back off the calories and dilute them by drinking more water.

Just as with training, race fueling does not come from a spreadsheet. Managing your fuel intake is seldom mentioned by dieticians and underrepresented in the guidelines given to athletes. Your race-day fueling strategy might represent your best-laid plan, but successful navigation of that plan involves thinking your way through it and adapting on the course. Through self-awareness and pragmatic thinking, you can make adjustments so that challenging situations don't lead to much bigger problems.

For example, you might get to 20 minutes past the hour and take in calories, but then 10 minutes later you still feel weak. If that's the case, you can decide to take in more calories again at 30 minutes past the hour and again at 40 minutes past the hour before getting back on your regular protocol of 20/40/60. On the contrary, if you take in calories at 20 minutes past the hour and by 30 minutes past the hour you are burping, hydrate with water or a diluted electrolyte solution and potentially skip taking in more calories at 40 minutes past the hour. After that feeling goes away, go back to your regular fueling protocol.

How do you find out what works best for you? The key is practicing fueling and hydration in race-simulation sessions. Much strategy starts with trial and error, sampling products, and respecting the process and consistent time intervals. On any type of race-simulatin bike ride, brick workout, or tempo run, start with this framework for fueling and hydrating. You might discover you like fueling every 10–12 minutes. If that's the case, set a timer on your watch for every 12 minutes. It doesn't have to be every 20 minutes, but it shouldn't be 30. If you're taking in calories just twice an hour, by definition you're taking on a gut bomb of calories.

The ultimate goal of hydration while on the bike is to set up your ability to run. You'll continue to shed more fluids on the run, but instead of drinking when thirsty you'll actively hydrate at every aid station. You can slow down and even walk if that's what it takes for you to consume enough calories and stay hydrated. However, success on the run demands a controlled regimen on the bike. That means self-management of strategy, pragmatic decision making, and, obviously, mental presence throughout your race.

If you were doing a 112-mile bike time trial (or a 56-mile time trial for Iron-man 70.3 races), you could afford to be relatively dehydrated (at 3 or 4 percent below normal hydration level) as you reached the finish line. You wouldn't ever get dehydrated enough to experience real performance declines (which research suggests happens at beyond 4 percent dehydration level). However, our challenge is that we're doing a 112-mile bike ride followed by a marathon (or a 56-mile ride followed by a half marathon). Because of that, you want to get off the bike with a closely limited level of dehydration (about 1 percent below normal hydration level) so you're ready for the demands of the run.

When you are running, especially in hot environments such as Hawaii, Texas, or Florida, even if you're consuming fluids at every single aid station, you will be losing body fluids the entire way and you can't completely catch up. In an Iron-man-distance race the dream scenario is to finish the marathon at about 4 percent dehydration, right on the cusp of performance declining. If you get off the bike and start running and you're already at 3 percent dehydration, you will certainly experience performance decline as you continue through the marathon.

One question that always comes up is whether you should be drinking water, consuming whatever sports drink is available on the course, or mixing both. We know that drinking only water is typically not optimal, and recent research has shown that consuming an advanced hydration product rooted in science (such as those developed by Osmo, Nuun, Skratch Labs, or SOS) is optimal. The only challenge is that those specific products might not be offered at the aid stations, so you need to find out what works for you.

That's not to deny the research, science, or pragmatism, but if you can combine water, always freely available on the course, and whatever sports drink is available, you'll have a better chance of maintaining your hydration and fueling and avoiding GI distress. Also, if your bottle containing Skratch Labs hydration formula drops out of your bike cage, you'll better be able and willing to use whatever is offered on the course. One advantage of front-mounted hydration systems is that you can easily create a diluted solution by adding water and Gatorade at a ratio of one part Gatorade to two parts water. Maybe it's not optimal, but it's a start.

Everyday Hydration

Maintaining an optimal state of hydration is integral to all aspects of your life, including your capacity to manage your energy throughout the day. Even if you're hydrating well before, during, and after your workouts, you're still going to exit each workout with some level of dehydration. To optimize recovery from that workout and maintain energy, you'll need to rehydrate and then continue to hydrate throughout the day. The old rule of drinking eight glasses of water a day is not particularly useful, but there are some simple habits you can develop to help maintain optimal hydration.

Start by having a glass of water with every meal: breakfast, lunch, dinner, and snacks. In between meals and snacks, carry a water bottle. If your training is particularly intense or you are feeling depleted, add a pinch of salt and a slice of lime or lemon to your water. If you don't like drinking plain water, flavor your water with a splash of juice or lemonade, other fruits or vegetables, and possibly a small amount of sugar to make the act of hydrating more enticing and habitual. Adequate hydration minimizes energy fluctuations, supports performance, and helps you avoid those between-meal hunger pangs.

Optimal hydration does entail more frequent bathroom breaks. Instead of seeing this as an inconvenience, consider it an opportunity to recharge and refocus. Studies have shown that most of us work better in spurts, and taking short breaks can lead to greater mental clarity and acuity. You could even incorporate some mobility exercises or light stretches into your breaks. Hydration is a simple habit with the potential to optimize your day in many ways and put you in a better condition to tackle your afternoon or evening workout sessions.

CAFFEINE

Caffeine is not as detrimental to endurance athletes as we once thought, depending on your individual sensitivity to it. One study showed that caffeine's role as a diuretic is minor, especially when it is consumed before or during exercise. In fact, some athletes find that caffeine improves their mental acuity and ability to be present during training and racing. If this is your experience, you should keep using it to your advantage. Because caffeine increases your body's absorption of carbohydrates and conversion and storing of glycogen, it can aid the recovery process. Whether you start your day with caffeine, have a caffeinated drink following your workout, or occasionally drink some Coca-Cola at an aid station (or a gas station), it's unlikely that you would be better off caffeine free. The only time caffeine is truly bad for you is if it disrupts your sleep. If you are sensitive to caffeine, it's best to avoid it after 1 p.m. because it can have subtle to serious effects on the quality of sleep you'll get later that night.

For anyone who seeks caffeinated drinks in the afternoon to stay alert for the final two to three hours of work, it's important to understand the bigger picture of what's going on in your body. When you go to sleep your body enters a restorative state in which your core temperature drops slightly. You have a similar circadian rhythm in the afternoon, when your temperature drops and you tend to feel sleepy. Although a coffee or energy drink counteracts these slumps, you can achieve the same result without the spikes or crashes that come with stimulants such as sugar and caffeine. It's the temperature of your midafternoon beverage that matters most because a hot drink helps to offset your internal cooling and reinvigorates you for the final hours of work. Like any Brit, I recommend hot tea, but hot water with a slice of lemon will also suffice. The trouble with drinking caffeine late in the day is that it can cause a vicious cycle because you are less capable of getting quality sleep and become more dependent on caffeine the next day, affecting your sleep for a second night. Ultimately this undermines your body's ability to recover fully.

ALCOHOL

Drinking alcohol is a recreational and social activity that can mix with athleticism in moderation. Seen through the right lens, it is part of the larger picture of life and accompanies many pleasurable rituals and traditions. Consequently, I'm not going to suggest that you can't or shouldn't drink alcohol; this kind of ultimatum doesn't create sustainability in your pursuit of sport and life.

However, there are some effects to consider when consuming alcohol. First, imbibing multiple drinks will disrupt the quality of your sleep that night. Whether you acknowledge it, if you drink three glasses of wine per evening on a consistent basis, it can affect your sleep, training, or your nutrition habits. Yes, sometimes people choose to pay the price. Sometimes you have to punish yourself a bit in the name of having a good time and then realize the need to get back on the course of your underlying framework. If you truly wish to adopt a performance-oriented lifestyle, that's a habit you should curtail.

Depending on how your weekends look (i.e., if there is more time to sleep and less stress), you might consider drinking less during the week. If you work a typical 9:00 to 5:00, Monday-to-Friday week, the nights when sleep is most likely to be compromised are Sunday through Thursday, so eliminating or reducing your alcohol intake then can have a great impact. If you really like it and it's a part of your life, one glass in the evenings is probably fine.

With any of these supporting habits, you need not live like a monk and make extreme sacrifices. However, you have to make sure you're giving your supporting cast the respect it deserves to ensure you can optimize your training and race to your fullest potential.

Nailing the Basics

In this media-driven world, it can be a real challenge for athletes to have clarity on the most important elements of preparation. With all promises of "free speed" and no shortage of advice from media or friends, it's easy to end up focusing on things that yield trivial returns in terms of performance.

At Purple Patch, we always talk about nailing the basics before we think about anything else. Those basics refer to executing the intent and rhythm of the training, practicing proper recovery and fueling, doing the prescribed strength training and mobility work, and making sure you are sleeping and eating well. Before you think about wetsuit brands, wheel depth, power meters, or anything else, be consistent about the pillars of performance. These are the boulders on which you will build your performance castle. If you can get those boulders into place, you can be successful. Even for the most experienced athletes, a back-to-basics approach can pay off. Professional athlete Tim Reed has always been a very smart, pragmatic, and hard-working athlete. Rich in talent, he is also very thoughtful and a wonderful racer. Tim and I worked with each other throughout many of his developmental years as a professional athlete, culminating in his victory at the 2016 Ironman 70.3 World Championships in Maloolaba, Australia. In his journey, Tim has always enjoyed process of learning and ownership of his training, from substantially contributing to his training approach to choosing equipment and seeking ways to incrementally improve. These are wonderful traits, but they can also be challenging if they begin to pollute the baseline development and progression of the key elements of performance.

I felt that, after a few seasons of development, Tim fell into an over-complicated approach and "paralysis of analysis" in the 2015 season, especially in areas of equipment and training. His thoughtful and smart approach was causing each session to be a test, and it deflated some of the passion and joy in the simple journey. He was working harder than ever, but I didn't see him enjoying the journey each day. In 2016, we decided on a mantra I often use with my pros, focused around nailing the basics. We stripped the program down to the fundamental level, decided on equipment early in the season and stuck with it throughout, and we approached racing with a pure joy-of-the-sport mindset. The outcome was an opportunity to race with freedom and get back to a fun attitude, but it also allowed the key elements of performance to be the driver of his performance gains. The results speak for themselves, with the world title, but it proved to be a powerful growth opportunity. Tim now has a backbone of a recipe that he knows works, and he can carefully integrate opportunities to improve and evolve while retaining the recipe that works for him.

6

Travel Protocols for Training and Racing

Many triathletes must manage travel on a monthly or even a weekly basis. Like many aspects of their busy lives, travel is a unique variable they have to properly plan, manage, and execute. It is inescapable that the addition of travel signifies an important uptick in global stress that the athlete must consider within the scope of their week. Whether their trip entails a business presentation or a goal race, to achieve the best results, they want to make travel as easy on themselves as possible.

Although traveling might seem simple and even pleasurable (or perhaps a necessary evil), for triathletes each trip is actually a complex prospect. Traveling involves numerous factors that affect athletes' general well-being, mental state, training, nutrition, fueling, hydration, sleep, and recovery. In essence, it cannot be taken lightly. After we recognize travel as such an undeniable physiological and emotional stressor, we can start to address it.

To mitigate the effects of travel, you can and should prepare for it in advance, whether you will need to adapt to different time zones, climates, or cultural considerations such as mealtimes. You'll find that a small misstep in one or more areas of self-care during travel can have real consequences. My goal is to guide you through the details so that travel is less disruptive to your training and racing. The information, tools, and tricks here are drawn from three main sources: the professional and executive athletes I coach along with key experts around the subject.

The pro athletes in the Purple Patch program travel multiple times per year across the country and around the world in their quest to achieve the best performance possible. Traveling to South Africa, New Zealand, or even Boulder, Colorado, is no easy task, and doing an Ironman race there adds several layers of planning, management, and execution. Although you might be competing at a different level, following the example of professional athletes can pay off in your race readiness.

We can also lean into the insights of CEOs and executives who travel on a regular basis for work. We frequently train athletes who, for weeks on end, sleep no more than one or two consecutive nights in their own beds because of their business travel. As much as they are committed to their careers, they are also dedicated to their pursuit of triathlon. When athletes travel that much, we manage travel as a part of their program and plan ahead for the types of stress it causes. Let's learn how they sustain such a schedule while simultaneously training at a high level.

Dr. Chris Winter, one of the country's foremost sleep experts, has helped to shape the travel protocols we use with Purple Patch athletes. He advises that travel success is all about keeping the body's expectations and rhythms as consistent as possible. Smart, gradual adjustments are good, but drastic changes are not.

MITIGATING TRAVEL STRESS

If you are an ambitious, time-starved athlete, you might not have much capacity to absorb the stress of travel. There's probably little room for adjustment in your daily schedule as it is. You can mitigate some of the physiological and emotional stress of travel by problem solving as you would an important deadline at work, an unexpected illness, or a storm that keeps you from training outdoors. You do this by focusing on the aspects of travel you can control.

Some issues are beyond your control; for example, delayed flights, lost luggage, or even a piece of equipment you accidentally left at home. You'll need to deal with those contingencies as they happen. However, there are four primary factors you can diligently manage: planning your travel with serious attention to detail; maintaining good nutrition and hydration; managing your environment; and executing functional movement and specific exercise before, during, and after traveling. Implementation of those four strategies will make the physical and emotional process of traveling go much more smoothly.

Planning Your Travel

Your departure and arrival times will significantly affect your ability to acclimate (or intentionally not acclimate) to your destination. Book your flights or plan your driving time to strike a balance between getting rest and being productive; that is, sort out the best flights and fares based on the scope of your busy life. This might seem painfully basic, but it's common for time-starved people to rush through the planning process and thus miss arranging details to their advantage. You should take into consideration your personal habits: What kind of sleeper are you; how well do you typically handle travel; will meals be manageable; and will there be access to work or family communication via text, phone, and email? For example, if you tend to be a "night owl," a red-eye flight can be an efficient way to travel; a window seat in an exit row is ideal. However, most "morning larks," or early risers, tend to struggle to sleep when traveling. If this is you, a red-eye can be a disruptive beginning, and if possible, you should instead opt for a daytime flight.

Daytime flights are ideal if you are hoping to be productive on the plane. Given that most flights have Wi-Fi service, you can fit in a lot of work while you're flying. Without interruptions, this time can be even more productive than your typical day in the office. You have to factor in time for commuting to the airport, walking through the terminal before and after your flight, collecting luggage, and getting transportation to the hotel after you reach your destination. However, if you want to be productive while you're in the air, that time can be a real advantage.

Make every effort to be well rested in the days prior to travel. If you can anticipate the stressors of travel at least one week out or more, you'll manage them better. Response to travel stress is highly individualized. If you are an older athlete, or you might have a slightly tougher time adjusting to the vicissitudes of travel, allow more time to rest before your trip. Athletes who seem to need slightly less sleep on a nightly basis tend to be more resilient to the rigors of travel and adapt more quickly. The bottom line is that you need to take into account your own quirks and preferences, and plan accordingly.

One of the keys to successful airline travel is to arrive at the airport as early as possible. The old question, "How late can I get to the airport and still make my plane?" is complete madness. This habit only compounds the hormonal stress when cortisol, a hormone released in response to stress, rises in your bloodstream. Can you get there later? Of course, but what is the point in doing so? You're much better off arriving at the airport ridiculously early, sitting down in a Wi-Fi-enabled lounge to answer a few emails and texts, and making sure you are relaxed, well nourished, and well hydrated so you can board your plane with reduced stress (you might even sleep!). Too many elements of the airport are out of your control: traffic, parking availability, oversized baggage check-in, security delays, crowded intra-airport transportation, and so forth. You often end up rushing to the gate and barely making your flight, which means you get on the plane sweating and uncomfortable. Save your adrenaline rush for the race.

When you're heading to the airport for a long flight, it's important to dress intelligently. Wear loose, comfortable clothing that won't catch on anything or complicate your ability to take off a layer or put on a layer during your flight. (If you're going for a meeting that begins hours after you arrive, you might need to wear business attire. However, even so, be as comfortable as possible. It's also a good idea to take off your shoes so you can flex your feet and wiggle your toes. Wear shoes that are easy to take off and don't smell! Compression gear, especially socks and tights, is helpful in reducing swelling when you travel. In fact, the original purpose of compression apparel was to help people avoid or reduce the effects of deep vein thrombosis (DVT). If you have a flight immediately after a race, use compression socks, sleeves, and/or tights to improve circulation, reduce swelling, and speed the recovery process. It's all about function over fashion; you want to have options to help regulate body temperature and prevent swelling.

Maintaining Nutrition and Hydration

Make it your mission to be appropriately fed, hydrated, rested, and as limber as possible. However, you don't want to consume too many calories. Going into a flight even a little bit hungry or semi-fasting is preferable to eating heavy foods like a burger and fries or fish and chips at the airport.

Interestingly, undereating prior to travel can help you acclimate to a new time zone more quickly, assuming you consume a meal at the appropriate local time you are adjusting to on arrival. If athletes have a long evening flight across several time zones, they could have a good-sized lunch and eat minimally before getting on the plane. Then, they can focus on staying hydrated and eating small, nutritious snacks without having to eat the meal served on the plane. When the athletes reach their destination, they will eat a full meal in the corresponding time zone. For example, if they arrive at their destination at 7 a.m., you would eat a proper, protein-rich breakfast. The brain's built-in starvation signal is synthetically reset or at least adjusted to the circadian rhythm, which helps diminish the time it takes to adjust to new time zones. The one caveat is that if they have to race within a day or two of reaching your destination, it's not great to approach travel in a semi-fasted state.

Many people eat because of boredom on flights or because various snacks, meals, and beverages are offered regularly. Avoid high-sodium foods (typically processed or packaged foods) and starchy carbohydrates because both can cause bloating, particularly uncomfortable while traveling. If possible, try to eat healthy snacks; instead of eating a package of chips or a sugary cookie, buy a small bag of nuts or baby carrots before you board. Whenever possible, carry on a sandwich and a piece of fruit rather than eat the sodium-laden meal provided.

Make sure some of the calories contain protein because it naturally helps to suppress the production of cortisol in response to low blood sugar.

As much as I emphasize that athletes should not live like monks while training, it's best to avoid drinking alcohol before or during a flight because of the increased stress to your body. Flying in the pressurized cabin of a plane is the equivalent of being at 9,000 feet. We know high altitude is a stressor both because it dehydrates the body and it can induce great fatigue. Alcohol exacerbates the effects of altitude. You want to arrive at your destination optimally hydrated, so you need to be cautious about alcohol consumption.

Also, limit your caffeine intake before and during a flight, though for daytime flights there's nothing wrong with having a couple of cups of coffee, or preferably some hot herbal tea, to keep your energy and productivity high. Coffee is less harmful as a diuretic than alcohol is, but it's not an effective hydration strategy. If you drink about 10 ounces of coffee, your body uses only about 6 ounces, or 60 percent, for hydration; the other 40 percent just passes through the urine. You certainly want to avoid caffeine entirely if it disrupts a normal night's sleep, particularly for red-eye flights. The quality and duration of your sleep will already be compromised when you are traveling, so it's best to minimize caffeine going into the flights.

If you are hydrating correctly, you should have to get up to pee a couple of times during a four- or five-hour flight. Even if it's annoying to your neighbor, it forces you to get up and move your body. While you're up, you can also do some light stretches and dynamic movements that will help maintain your energy and reduce any swelling.

Managing Your Environment

Sitting in cramped conditions for several hours does not allow you to replicate the normal routine or environment of your daily life. However, you can take action to help keep your stress low and stay rested.

First, set up your personal space as optimally as possible. When you sit for a prolonged period, it's helpful to support the small of your back. A lot of the pros and CEOs I coach travel with a firm, half-round, mini foam roller placed behind their lower backs. A rolled-up towel or sweatshirt can achieve the same purpose. You should also have a neck pillow to keep your posture in alignment if you plan to sleep. Falling asleep on an airplane is often difficult, but good neck support will ease that considerably and help you avoid awkward encounters with your neighbor.

Two more subtle but important factors to consider are the amounts of light and sound you absorb or deflect. Bright light, especially the fast-moving images on screens, will stimulate your brain and keep it engaged, therefore keeping you awake and in a heightened state of sensitivity. If you think you'll have a few hours before you'll sleep, then pack a paperback book or a magazine. If you want to sleep or even just relax, use eye masks to block the light. You can't control the light in the cabin or whether your neighbors use their reading lights or screens, but you can keep your own eyes covered. On the contrary, if you're planning to work or watch a movie on a laptop or a tablet, consider investing in an after-market screen cover to help reduce the blue light effect that signals daylight to your nervous system.

Perhaps the biggest challenge on a plane is that you're generally forced to absorb all of the sounds. Flying is a high-decibel experience thanks to the roar of jet engines. Studies have shown that the average interior noise level of an airplane is 95 to 105 decibels, roughly equivalent to that of a motorcycle or chainsaw. Add to this people talking and announcements on the sound system; food carts, utensils, and seatback trays clanking; and, of course, the teething, hungry, or otherwise cranky baby crying when you're trying to sleep. If you're sensitive to sounds, be sure to pack simple earplugs or noise-canceling headphones.

Executing Functional Movement and Specific Training

Breaking up long stretches of sitting benefits mental acuity, overall energy, and circulation. It improves your capacity to start training in the first day or so at your destination. The more you can move around on any flight, the better off you'll be when you arrive, regardless of whether you're headed to a race or traveling for business. If you take a red-eye flight, in the first hour, be sure to walk a bit and do some light stretching before you fall asleep, and do the same when you wake up or before you land. If it's a daytime flight, try to get up and move at least every hour. If you don't want to trouble the other passengers in your row, plan ahead and reserve an aisle seat.

I'm not suggesting that you try to do a sophisticated workout. Movement can be as simple as walking to the back of the plane to loosen your legs with some light squats, hip extensions, toe raises, and high-knee clutches. If you're on a plane with more room, you might also exercise with a foam roller. In the in-flight magazine in the seatback pocket, most airlines offer tips for doing yoga and easy stretches, another option for you to do a couple of times during your flight.

Your pretravel training is the final consideration as you prepare for your trip. It's good to work out on the day you travel, but I'd advise against doing anything too strenuous. Definitely avoid huge key sessions on the day of travel. I'm not in favor of athletes getting on a plane with muscular damage from a high-intensity workout, especially speed work at the track or hill running, which tend to cause muscular trauma. The significant dehydration and hormonal stress from which your body has to recover after one of these workouts is far too challenging when you are traveling. In other words, don't dig yourself a hole before you get on the plane. If a key session falls on the day you're supposed to travel, when you are planning your training for the week, make arrangements to do the workout a day earlier.

When you arrive at your destination, it is time to get moving. You want to get the blood flowing, and that can begin as soon as you get off the plane. Simply walking from the gate to the baggage claim area starts the blood moving, but you can speed up the recovery process by avoiding escalators and conveyor belts and walking instead. Given that there is often a wait to pick up your baggage, especially after international flights, take an extra 5 or 10 minutes to walk and do some light stretching and dynamic drills to help your mobility, flexibility, and agility.

When you get to your hotel or final destination, do some kind of light exercise as soon as you can. Keep this in mind when booking your travel. If you are traveling on business, try to build in time to go for a light run or do a gym workout before your first meeting starts. If you are traveling for a race, plan time for an easy run before you have to go to the check-in or other pre-race meetings.

Any exercise you do on the first day after traveling (no matter if it's swimming, biking, or running) should be easy but include neurological training with some fast building efforts, too. For example, if you go for an easy run, do a few 30-second buildups or striders in which you accelerate just to get your brain talking to your muscles. If you're swimming easy laps, throw in a couple of fast half-laps in which you accelerate from the center of the pool to the wall. If your flight arrives right before dinner (or late and you have to go straight to dinner) at least walk to dinner or after dinner. You need to keep your body moving; when you're not active, you feel worse the next morning. Anything you can do to get moving on the first day will be very helpful for the rest of your time at that destination.

Initially, you should expect to feel sluggish when you train, so don't judge yourself or get emotionally down. Just get through the first couple of days and focus on the bigger picture goals of the upcoming race or your business meetings. For example, if you live in New York and you're flying to Phoenix on Wednesday for Ironman Arizona on Sunday, don't expect to feel fit and energetic on Thursday. How you feel on that first day has no relevance to how you're going to race; it's just your body reacting to the fact that you were traveling all day on Wednesday. Dig into your toolbox for the habits that will speed recovery: set yourself up for good sleep, sound nutrition, sufficient fueling, and great hydration. Even though your body will feel off kilter, and you might have trouble with the time change, those building blocks will help offset the fatigue.

After that first easy exercise on your arrival day, the second day should include an endurance-focused workout. The actual session depends on your training schedule and whether you're traveling for work, a training camp, or a race. The best antidote to lingering sluggishness is to extend the warm-up and pre–main sets. As a rule, you should double your typical warm-up time. Let's say you have an interval running workout of 3 × 6 minutes in which you'll build up to race pace, and the warm-up would normally be 10 minutes of easy-to-moderate running. You might need 20–30 minutes of easy running to warm up to the point where you're running with good form and ready to do those intervals. The same goes for swimming and biking. Take a longer warm-up session at an easy pace before going into the pre–main set and the main set of the workout. However, don't expect to feel like a world-class triathlete on the second day, either. If you still feel sluggish even after the extended warm-up, you'll have to decide to adjust the progression of the harder effort and take solace in the fact that you got your body moving again.

On the third day, you can resume regular training with normal intensity. This might not apply to a business traveler who might be preparing to travel again, either back to the original point of departure or to a new destination. If you are traveling to attend a training camp or to have a weeklong lead-up to a race, this is useful to keep in mind. Travel demands pragmatism and willingness to shift training load as needed to retain energy and health. Don't try to play catch-up and squeeze in multiple key sessions back-to-back on your return home. Remain calm and realize that this week will likely carry fewer training hours, but you can retain some effectiveness from the workouts completed.

ACCLIMATING TO TRAVEL

Business travel often entails just a day or two at your destination. You might not want or need to acclimate to the new time zone, but you still want to be as effective as possible at your business and maintain your training. Sometimes travel means an extended period away, whether to race, to train, or to attend a business function. In these cases, you want to acclimate so that you can perform at your best. The mindset for how to deal with each of these scenarios is quite different.

Short Trips

For those times when you aren't trying to acclimate to your destination, you'll want to focus on simply mitigating the effects of travel. This kind of trip might involve traveling from your home near Los Angeles to a business meeting in New York or Tampa, Florida, and then returning 24–48 hours later. Because of the quick turnaround, you're not looking to adjust to Eastern Standard Time (EST). Instead, you want to maintain a performance-minded approach to life and training. Especially for these short trips, it's best to plan travel carefully so you can maintain your regular eating, sleeping, and training schedule if at all possible. If you normally get up early on a certain day of the week and exercise, stick to that timing.

On arrival you might feel sluggish, especially after a late-night or red-eye flight. Be disciplined about getting up to work out the next morning; your body will recognize the stimulus, and you will start to feel more like yourself. Your regular mealtimes might have to be adjusted slightly to accommodate meetings or scheduled business lunches or dinners, so be sure to pack small, healthy snacks (a bag of nuts or an apple) to keep hunger pangs at bay and maintain your energy between meals.

Do your best to manage the same lighting you're used to back home. If your home is brightly lit, turn on all of the lights in your hotel room. Also, if you typically do some work at night, then work on your computer or watch TV late for a few hours before going to bed at your corresponding time back home. If you've traveled to New York from Los Angeles, you might not feel tired until 11:30 p.m. or even later. Don't worry about it. As Dr. Chris Winter says, "It is easier to suppress a need instead of creating one." In other words, it's easier to deal with the awkwardness or inconvenience of keeping your schedule than it is to force yourself to eat or sleep at a different time. Maintaining your circadian rhythm, mealtimes, sleep times, and training times if possible will help you keep everything in balance before, during, and after your trip. You might have some lingering fatigue, but with some catch-up sleep, you should be able to jump right back into your training and work upon your return.

Extended Trips

When you're going somewhere to race or to train for an extended period, you want to be at your best (i.e., functioning as normally as possible) in the time zone of your destination. The focus shifts from stress mitigation to maintaining energy; alertness; critical thinking; and the ability to actually train and perform before, during, and after traveling. To accomplish that, you'll have to make slight adjustments before you leave home and continue acclimating the moment you arrive.

For a 9- or 10-hour shift in time zones, ahead-of-time acclimation is difficult to pull off; for example, if you're living in San Francisco, you can't change your window of sleep to 3–11 p.m. or eat your big meal of the day at 4 a.m. The change would be too drastic, and this attempt to bridge the gap would cause your system to go awry. That said, you might be able to shift your sleeping window and mealtimes by an hour or two over the course of a couple of weeks before you travel just to begin to get your circadian rhythms to adjust.

After you arrive, do what you can to adjust and be prepared for the worst. Nearly all travelers deal with jet lag in the first two days of their arrival, especially when flying from the West to the East. If your flight leaves the United States in the evening and arrives in Europe or South Africa in the morning or midday, it's best to avoid the urge to nap and get on with your meals at the appropriate time in that time zone. By that night, you'll be extremely tired. Prepare to go to bed at a decent hour, but know that you'll probably find yourself wide awake long before morning because your body's internal clock is confused. Acceptance is the best strategy; stressing over missed sleep only makes matters worse. Over the course of a few days, you will wind up sleeping through the night. Minimize simulated daylight from your electronic device screens before you go to bed at night, and maximize simulated daylight the moment you wake up in the morning to speed the transition.

TRAVELING TO RACES

If you travel to a race in a different time zone, you need to plan how many days in advance of the race you need to adjust your sleeping, eating, training, and recovery habits to acclimate to the new time zone. If you don't have the luxury of changing your schedule ahead of time or arriving at your destination with ample time for acclimation, you can make some subtle and not-so-subtle changes after you arrive.

Sleep is one of the most crucial factors and one of the most difficult to navigate given jet lag and general fatigue. Be prepared with activities that will put your body at ease, such as reading a paperback book or meditating. Avoid the bright light from your electronic devices if you are struggling to sleep. Sleep requires your mind and body to be "at rest," so focus on being still, calming your mind, and making your bedroom as dark as possible.

On the contrary, sometimes acclimating requires you to force yourself to stay awake longer. In these situations, you can use your devices, which signal your brain to be active and alert and keep grogginess at bay. You can also help your body adjust by controlling your environment. Make it light when you want to simulate daytime hours and dark when you want to simulate nighttime hours and get to sleep.

Start eating at the proper mealtimes in the destination's time zone as soon as possible. If you don't feel hungry, err on the side of eating lighter meals with high protein content and have healthy snacks to eat before the next mealtime. When you arrive at the new destination you will be considerably dehydrated, so you'll want to focus on rehydrating with water and electrolyte drinks.

It's extremely important to be on top of your schedule for the days leading up to the race, whether at home or at your destination. Review when you'll be training each day and what you'll be doing. Also, be aware of any additional obligations, especially the day before the race. Know when and where you need to check in, pick up your race bib, sign final waivers, attend safety meetings, and take your gear to the transition area. It's also a good idea to get familiar with the racecourse, including the start, the swim course, the bike course, and the run course. Consider these actionable items, as important as the adjustments you make for eating, hydrating, sleeping/recovery, and training.

Domestic Races

If you are doing a B race, not your goal race, only two or three time zones away from home (for example, within the continental United States), you don't need to arrive at the race destination more than four days in advance. It's perfectly fine to arrive on Thursday for a Sunday morning race. That enables you to do some easy exercise on the day you travel, have a low-stress endurance day on Friday, and do something short and easy on Saturday with some ramping efforts to remind your body of intensity. It might seem like more pre-race time is better, but I've found it often makes athletes nervous and tired.

Gradually start transitioning your life toward the new time zone the week before you travel. The key here is recognizing the things you can control and manage: what you eat, when you sleep, when you train, and the lighting optimal for your biorhythms. This can be challenging for busy triathletes, but if you know the time of the day at which you'll be racing in that time zone, you can benefit by starting to do some of your training in your native time zone during the corresponding hours in the destination time zone. You can also adjust your sleep time and some of your meals by a few hours. For example, if you live in San Francisco and are traveling to New York for Ironman Lake Placid, you can adjust by training at EST to help you out on race day. It would also be smart to go to bed a couple of hours earlier, get up a couple of hours earlier, and shift your meal times accordingly.

Because it's always more difficult to travel from West to East for a race than vice versa, starting to adjust to the destination time zone ahead of time makes a big difference. For example, if you're traveling from the West Coast to the East Coast, you'll be eating meals three hours earlier than your body is used to, and you won't be sleepy for three hours later than it is out East. Though East Coast athletes will be eating an evening meal around 6 p.m. or 7 p.m. and going to bed by 9 p.m. or 10 p.m., your internal body clock will initially be telling you that it's only 3 or 4 p.m., too early to eat, and that bedtime feels like only 6 p.m. or 7 p.m., again too early. If you start these adjustments before you leave home, you'll get a leg up on those changes.

On the contrary, it is much easier to travel from East to West for a race; for example, if New York athletes travel to California for a race, they can eat a smart, healthy snack while waiting the additional two or three hours for the 6–7 p.m. mealtime on Pacific Time (actually 9–10 p.m. according to their internal body clocks) and then go to sleep soon thereafter. Those athletes would still have to be smart about eating, sleeping, and training times, but the adjustments will be much easier to make.

International Races

At Purple Patch, we tell athletes that the best rule is to arrive at least one day in advance for every hour of time-zone shift when traveling to an international race. The longer the flight, the longer it will take you to physically and hormonally calibrate to the new time zone.

For example, if an athlete lives in New York, and he or she is planning to race in Berlin (a six-hour time-zone difference), then it would be ideal to get there six days prior to race day. If an athlete lives in San Francisco and is traveling to South Africa for the Ironman 70.3 World Championships, a 10-hour time-zone shift, then arriving 10 days before the race would be optimal. It's not always possible, especially financially, to arrive so early, but if you start thinking along these lines, you'll be better able to work through the challenges of adjusting, such as travel-related sluggishness and fatigue, sleep challenges that come with jet lag, or dietary and intestinal struggles.

Even with international travel, you can shift some of your training schedule in advance. For example, if you know the race time in South Africa corresponds to 5 p.m. in San Francisco, then you might start doing more of your training at that time a few weeks ahead. Although it might feel a bit awkward, it will definitely feel more normal when you arrive in South Africa. These scenarios reinforce the value of arriving a week to 10 days in advance of international races that require long flights.

CASE STUDY: **FAMILIARITY BREEDS CONFIDENCE**

Sam Appleton, a professional athlete I coach, is a young Australian who trains hard in Boulder, Colorado. He consistently arrives at his destinations three days before the race because that's what works for him. For the 2016 Ironman World Championships in Australia, he decided to arrive 10 days early. Rather than immediately going to the race site, where he risked getting caught in a media swirl that might contribute to nerves, wasting energy, and becoming fatigued, he stayed with his parents a few hours away to get over the jet lag and be optimally rested. After a few days he felt refreshed, and he was eager to get to the race site. I advised that he arrive on the Thursday before the Sunday event. "But it's the World Championships!" he protested. "So what?" I responded. "Just because the race has a grand title doesn't mean you have to change the approach that has consistently worked for you all year."

The key is that your best approach is not about what works for other athletes; it's about what works for you. Unless you have special commitments, such as visiting your family abroad or combining a business trip with a race, do what has proven effective for you over the course of the whole season in terms of timing your arrival. The only caveat is if your upcoming race is drastically different. What you've done to prepare for Ironman 70.3 Santa Cruz and Ironman 70.3 Santa Rosa might need to be reevaluated for Ironman South Africa. However, even for your key goal race, arrive when it feels best to you. If you have been thoughtful about your approach in your other races, and you've performed well, don't change your strategy just because it's your A race.

Sam flew to Australia 10 days early, got acclimated, and went to the race site three days before the event because that's part of his effective strategy. He had a great race, placing 5th in what turned out to be his breakout performance.

TRAVELING TO DIFFERENT CLIMATES

How do you prepare for a race in a drastically different climate than the one in which you live and train? Traveling to that race is just like any other travel, but your body will perform differently in that climate than it did during training back home. If you live in the relatively dry, high-altitude conditions of Boulder, Colorado, and you qualify to compete in the Ironman World Championships in Kona, Hawaii, you'll have to acclimate to that new environment to race at an optimal level.

Simulated heat training is an emerging science that offers great value, both physiologically and emotionally, in preparing for a race. At Purple Patch, the athletes I coach use two different kinds of heat training derived from environmental physiologists, including Dr. Stacy Sims's scientific research, and my own firsthand knowledge of how athletes respond to heat. I recommend incorporating heat training in a sauna or steam room in the final 10–14 days prior to traveling to your race.

The goal of heat training is to add the stressor incrementally, managing it in the context of your training and life. If it depletes your energy or performance to the point where you can't execute the intent of the prescribed training, there's no net gain. The discomfort of the heat is intended to give you exposure to that variable, but it's important that these sessions are executed according to protocol:

- When you are incorporating heat into your training sessions, avoid doing hard intervals and keep your efforts to an easy-to-moderate level. Alternatively, do a hard interval session and then go into the sauna/steam-room training.

- Heat sessions should be avoided on full recovery days because the hormonal stress is counterproductive to your recovery process.

- Finally, be sure to stop doing this heat training protocol two or three days before you travel so you don't begin your travel in a very dehydrated state.

You should evaluate simulated heat training on a cost/benefit basis. If you begin to feel excessively fatigued, if you aren't performing well in training, or if you are extremely uncomfortable, stop the session and hydrate so you can recover and return your body to equilibrium.

Postworkout Heat Simulation

To try simulated heat training after a workout, continue to follow your normal training plan, making sure to fuel and hydrate effectively beforehand and throughout the first part of the workout. Stop drinking fluids for the final 15 to 20 minutes of the session. After you are finished, spend 15–30 minutes in a sauna or steam room without attempting to rehydrate. Take in some calories via a recovery snack or energy bar if needed. Tolerate the heat and discomfort as long as you can, focusing on preparation for racing in a hot and humid destination. Follow your time in the sauna or steam room with a shower. Start hydrating with about 6–8 ounces of water with a pinch of salt and squirt of citrus juice, and then continue sipping fluids to restore full hydration status over the next four to five hours. Ensure you remember to promptly refuel with a postworkout meal in addition to commencing the rehydration process.

In-Training Heat Simulation

You can also simulate intense heat and humidity while on a bike trainer or a treadmill. Wear a good amount of clothing (a long-sleeved shirt over a baselayer T-shirt and maybe even long tights) and spin or run in a hot room with no fan or ventilation. It sounds primitive and uncomfortable (and it will be), but it will do the trick. Don't ride or run hard, but instead keep an easy-to-moderate intensity for 30–40 minutes (no more than 60 percent of your functional threshold power (FTP, or 60 percent of your best sustained effort over an hour), and hydrate as minimally as possible. You will become very thirsty in this session, perhaps uncomfortably so; take a few sips from a bottle if necessary. However, for the most part, ignore the urge to drink more and focus on how your body feels, reminding yourself that this is a race-preparation session, just not at race effort.

As with the postworkout simulated heat training in the sauna or steam room, take your time to shower, and then hydrate and eat a balanced meal. Once again, don't gulp excessive amounts of water immediately after getting off the bike or treadmill. Instead, drink a glass of water including that same pinch of salt and squirt of citrus juice, while eating your recovery meal. You can then continue sipping fluids to restore full hydration status over the next four to five hours.

It's undeniable that travel and environment are additional stress factors to be managed throughout training as well as in preparation for racing. Some extra planning and thought can go a long way to empowering you and limiting negative effects. Your best performance does not come from simply training hard and holding on to your routine. When you face disruptions and changes to your schedule, determine what factors you can control and continue to carefully manage your stress as part of your overall performance puzzle.

7

Executing Your Race Strategy

Races are the exciting part of your journey, an opportunity to put all of your training, focus, and intent into action. After months of dedicated, hard work amid the rest of your busy life, you have the chance to execute your goals. Although you might prioritize training around specific races (A versus B races), any race is a chance to prove your mettle on the racecourse.

With any race, no matter your goal, to achieve your best performance on that day you'll need to remain focused for many hours. Being present is the key to success. Racing is about planning, executing, then adapting to contingencies on the course. It's the reason for your race strategy, your fueling and hydrating strategy, your pacing in each discipline, your self-management throughout the race, your efficiency in transition areas, and your effectiveness at problem solving.

You can only accomplish all of those things to your fullest potential in a race if you're focused from start to finish. Given all that goes into an event, races are physically, mentally, and emotionally fatiguing. You can't show up on race day and expect to suddenly be uncompromisingly focused and effective at all of the tasks required. By continually practicing all of those aspects in your training, you can improve your proficiency and put yourself in a position to race to your trained potential.

Ultimately, even racing is about achieving the outcome you desire by focusing on the process. You might have a goal of finishing your first Ironman in less than 12 hours, but that's not your focus during the swim, bike, and run. Similarly, you might have a goal to improve your personal best Ironman 70.3 effort and break the 5-hour mark, but you can't have "5 hours" dancing through your head for hours on end. You have to be present at every point of the race, task-driven on the many smaller segments of the race. That means you will swim, ride, and run with good form, executing every portion as in your training.

You must have a race plan, but you can't expect everything to go according to that plan. Even in training, things go wrong or differently. Ultimately, you must execute a race with the cards you are dealt that day. A wide variety of situations can come up, and you need to be poised to respond. That's why we practice these scenarios in training.

PRIOR TO THE RACE

If you've been following a training plan, you are nearing the end of a race buildup, and you are preparing for a goal race, you should be able to sense the adaptations in your body. In the final weeks before race day your training load will decrease, which brings about different physical, mental, and emotional responses. As your overall stress level is temporarily reduced, your body should start to feel fresh and ready, especially as you try to get more quality sleep on a nightly basis. This in turn allows your mind to become more relaxed, too. However, with your excitement and anticipation mounting, it's also common for your stress level to increase. Be proactive in thinking about your race plan and envisioning your success, but avoid the natural propensity to become hyperanalytical about the training you have done.

In the lead-up to a race, I always encourage athletes to embrace their natural anxiety. Far from suppressing or hiding emotions, honesty is most important; simply accept the feelings as excitement to race instead of fear of results. Too many amateur athletes assume that pro athletes don't get nervous, but this isn't the case at all. In fact, anxiety is likely critical to having a great performance. Your body is readying itself for the race, and if not for nerves, lethargy would likely affect the performance. As soon as you realize that the race nerves are a part of the process, completely normal, and a symptom of race readiness, then you can shift them toward excitement.

As you approach a race, your training partners, friends, coworkers, family members, and significant other are bound to ask, "How do you feel?" or "Do you feel ready?" These questions come with good intent, but both the questions and your answers are irrelevant. During the final two weeks, you might feel antsy, flat, or a bit off. Resist the urge to become your own worst enemy and judge yourself, because this can be self-defeating. Five days out from a race, if you feel fantastic, that's great, but it doesn't matter. If you feel awful, don't worry, because that is also meaningless. Your body will go through different rhythms in those final two weeks, and it's important that you are not overly sensitive or reactionary toward them.

Avoid Validation Training

Be conscientious about how you approach training during the lead-up to race day. Some triathletes tend to avoid any amount of hard work in tapering, but that's not necessarily wise. This approach is common in sports such as competitive swimming and track and field, where so many events are shorter than four minutes. Triathlon, on the contrary, is an endurance sport, so approach the intent of race week with a similar physical, mental, and emotional rhythm in transition week training, with familiar workouts. Keeping some semblance of your regular training protocols will help your body maintain its normal rhythms amid the travel and excitement. As long as your training sessions are not depleting you, putting you into a hole before the trip, you'll be fine tackling a moderate training load.

Although you should maintain regular training and embrace some training load, don't keep pursuing fitness gains. You simply cannot improve your fitness with hard workouts in the final 10–14 days before a race. You should avoid extra hard workouts in which you seek even more positive adaptations. All it will lead to is fatigue. This is what I call validation training, and it is your enemy. You might feel like you have a lot of energy, given the decreased training load and additional rest, but you absolutely need to avoid using this energy to prove to yourself that you are truly primed for performance. Your proof is in your preparation over the preceding weeks and months, not the final two weeks.

I tell athletes I coach that it's all about "feel-good" training right before the race. If you're feeling fresh, do the work on your schedule, but stick to the prescribed intensity just as you have done throughout the season. If you're feeling even remotely fatigued, give yourself license to scale the workouts or even skip sessions if you feel you absolutely need to, but don't fight it or make it harder. Just go with the flow. If your workout metrics are not as high as you expect, don't worry about it. Do the work you can do, and rest up for the big day. As the final two weeks play out, you should start to put more of your time, focus, and energy into the logistics of race day, getting your gear and kit ready, and preparing to travel to the race site.

Mind Your Gear

In the days before you travel to the race (or in the week before local races), make sure your equipment is functional and clean. Take every precaution against avoidable mishaps. Tune up your bike and check your tires for slices and thorns. If your bike has an electronic shifting system, make sure it is charged. It sounds so simple, but it's another way to build confidence. After you get to the race site, you don't want to deal with equipment problems you could have resolved beforehand. Plenty of other logistical challenges will arise after you arrive and check in, so save yourself some stress and time.

Visualize Success

In the final two weeks, consider what success will look like for you on race day. Give yourself permission to confront your fears, either voicing them to a coach or training partner or writing them down. If you tend to overthink things, set aside 30 minutes every day to think through the race. Visualize the logistics of your day and your race plan (how you'll execute each discipline and the transitions). If a piece of the race is troubling you, close your eyes and think about it or even write it out. Creating a sense of familiarity with the discomfort will help you calm your nerves. Focus on the aspects within your control and how you can execute them.

After this 30 minutes has passed, you don't need to think or talk about the race for the rest of the day. Compartmentalize the stress and focus on the rest of your life. Of course, you'll think about it periodically, but you have nothing to gain by mentally chewing on it beyond that 30 minutes.

Know the Course

Start familiarizing yourself with the general logistics of the racecourse in the week leading up to the race. Look at the online course map and study the basics: swim start, swim course, T1, bike course, T2, run course, and finish line. Also think through the other details in your race plan:

- What's the course layout like overall?
- What's the terrain?
- What are the logistics of the transition area? (E.g., is the distance between the swim finish and the transition area short or long?)
- What is the typical temperature during the morning, midday, and afternoon?
- Will it be windy, and if so, on which part of the course?
- What's happened in your previous races?

Studying the course, going through some of the logistics, and understanding local environmental conditions in advance of arriving at the race site can help to prepare you and keep you focused on what you can control, without unnecessary concerns about the course. If you're prepared for anything (for example, if it is colder than you think when you arrive in the morning or if a thunderstorm comes out of nowhere when you're on bike), you will have a much less stressful time as you race. Whether you're a procrastinator or an easygoing individual who prefers not to think too much about a race, it is good to know what to expect.

After you arrive at the race site, familiarize yourself with the schedule (check-in times, safety meetings, course discussions, start times, etc.). Also become acquainted with the directional flow through the transition area, parking area, and portable toilets. You don't want to be wandering around wasting energy before a race or caught off guard after the race is under way.

SWIM COURSE

Not only do you need to know the swim course layout, you should also know the setup of the course. Seeing the course map or viewing it from a dock the day before the race can give you some idea of what to expect, but examine it a little further to understand some of the finer details. For example, what are the expected or current wind conditions, where does the sun typically rise, and is it normal to have fog on race mornings? These factors could influence your choice of goggles. Of course you'll want to know the direction you'll be swimming in, how the buoys are lined up, and where the relative halfway point will be. Pre-swimming some of the course is ideal because it doesn't take much of a wave to block your line of sight as you navigate the open water on race day.

BIKE AND RUN COURSES

Ride and run the main parts of those sections of the course and consider driving the entire route, if possible. You don't need to ride and run the whole course, and whatever you do before the race, it shouldn't deplete you. It's always less stressful when you see something for the second time and you know the way. If you become somewhat familiar with the course, your focus can be on terrain management and pacing instead of looking at the road ahead and asking how long before the next turn. Knowledge is power, allowing you to focus on what will return your best speed relative to your distribution of work and effort.

Sleeping, Fueling, and Hydrating

Even if you're preparing for a B race, stick with what's familiar and works for you. When it comes to arrival and logistics, if you have a pattern that has worked at other races (for example, if you typically arrive three days before the race), then follow that pattern and apply the same approach to eating and sleeping, too. Don't radically change your diet or adopt the sloth lifestyle and attempt to sleep 20 hours a day. Shift your emphasis to trying to get more quality sleep every night. Given your reduced training load, that should keep you energized. Try to maintain a similar eating schedule and diet to that of the previous weeks and months. Resist the urge to stuff yourself with big meals to top off your glycogen stores; you will end up bloated. Simply retain a healthy rhythm of eating: eat when you're hungry, eat healthy, and eat enough.

If you've been hydrating well on a daily basis, maintain your regular hydration habits. You don't have to walk around with three water bottles strapped to your body; your reduced training load will make sure that your cells are fully hydrated. Dumping liquids into your system in the days before a race is a stressor. Make sure you have a couple of glasses of water with breakfast, lunch, and dinner and have a glass of water whenever you're thirsty, but it's unnecessary to suddenly start pumping yourself full of fluids the day before the race.

The day before your race, eat simple, familiar foods. Avoid spicy foods or those you're not accustomed to eating. For lunch and dinner on the day before the race, focus on eating a mix of protein and carbohydrates, but avoid eating too much roughage and green leafy vegetables. Have a good breakfast, a solid lunch, and then an early dinner (closer to 5 p.m. as opposed to 7 p.m. or 8 p.m.). If you're hungry later in the evening, it's fine to eat a snack and drink some fluids before you go to bed.

Make an effort to get a full night's sleep on the eve of the race, but don't fret if you're too excited to fall asleep right away. When you wake up on race day, plan to eat a smallish breakfast about three hours before the race starts. Avoid anything that upsets your stomach, but do what works for you, whether that's coffee or a favorite breakfast food. There is no magic recipe, but it's smart to include some carbs and protein to set yourself up for the day until your fueling plan kicks in on the bike. Drink water with your meal. Have a bottle of water or an electrolyte drink with you en route to the race site, but be careful to avoid saturating yourself with fluid.

RACE DAY

Allow ample time to get to the race site on the morning of the race. There are plenty of opportunities for delay, not the least of which is parking your car. You'll have to finalize the gear you'll leave in the transition area, and it's always better to have more time for that. Make sure you know the temperature in the morning so you're not chilled before you start. If you checked in your bike the day before, it's worth double-checking your gear, especially the pressure in your tires. If it was a cold night, there's a good chance your tires lost pressure. After you have all of your gear, bottles, and accessories set, leave the transition area to focus on warming up and starting the race.

Warming Up

Many triathletes make a mistake on race day by not sufficiently warming up prior to the start. In the 30 minutes or so before the race starts, only a small percentage of the participants are running, swimming, or spinning on a bike trainer. It's interesting that most athletes don't make the same mistake in training. A warm-up session gets your system ready for the work ahead, and racing entails work. Executing a solid warm-up is crucial. The goals of a race warm-up session are to increase your core temperature to prime your body and to increase your heart rate so you'll be ready for the swim.

I am often asked what the best warm-up protocol is prior to the race. Ultimately, the answer is "the one you like; the one that makes you feel good." This requires you to practice, try different approaches, and learn what works for you, but athletes tend to be most prepared for a great performance when warming up in a familiar way they enjoy, which gives them self-confidence. Bearing this advice in mind, there are some general guidelines for priming yourself to perform. Depending on the logistics and the setup of the race site, you can start with an easy run just to get your blood moving. Some people like to do activation exercises, including mobility or core exercises to get their muscles moving and the brain engaged with the body, but an easy jog to bring up core temperature might be sufficient.

Then, put on your wetsuit, cap, and goggles and get in the water to warm up for the swim. Ideally, you'll want to do this as close as you can to the start of your race to avoid getting primed, then getting cold, between the warm-up and race start. Remember to double-check the position of the sun, the terrain, any waves or chop, and the buoy lines so you can be prepared to swim in a straight line, on course as much as possible. After you're in the water, prime your engine with a series of building efforts that alternate between easy and moderate/hard efforts.

An example of a warm-up might be something like this:

SWIM WARM-UP
40 sec. easy
30 sec. moderate/hard
20 sec. easy
10 sec. moderate/hard
20 sec. easy
30 sec. moderate/hard
40 sec. easy

The one caveat to a swim warm-up is that everyone has a personal threshold for cold, and it might be counterproductive to try to warm up in cold water. If the water temperature is below 58–59 degrees, you shouldn't get in the water. Even if you warm up a bit, the time you'll spend standing around before the start will just make you colder and more uncomfortable. In such a scenario, warm up on the run and consider using swim bands or a series of arm circles in place of your swimming warm-up. Also, in really cold water, consider wearing two swim caps. If you are prone to getting brain freeze from cold water, consider standing waist deep in the water and dipping your head under the water to avoid that sensation after the start. If you're not warmed up as well as you could be, opt for a more controlled start for the first quarter of the swim course.

Lining Up for the Swim

Before you line up, consider whether the race is a mass start or wave start, your relative swimming ability and overall confidence level, and relevant weather conditions. More races are adopting rolling swim starts, which limit the anarchy of a typical mass swim start and enable you to seed yourself with athletes racing at a similar speed. This makes the swim less congested, so you don't have to swim over people quite as much. Rolling starts also reduce the immediate pressure of the starting gun and can help eliminate the classic triathlete mistake of starting the swim too hard.

You always want to be in a place of power and control so you can get comfortable with your swimming as quickly as possible. Unless you are an elite swimmer, don't line up in the middle. Line up to the outside. If you're nervous at all or if you are a less accomplished swimmer, don't be in a rush to get going. Line up toward the back, and when the gun goes off wait there a few seconds and then gradually build into the swim to avoid putting yourself into distress. If you're a reasonable swimmer (45 minutes or less for 70.3 or 1:30 for an Ironman), you'll be eager to get going, so find your way to the outside.

EXECUTING THE SWIM

The biggest factor in whether you will swim to your trained potential is your ability to swim in a straight line. Although there has been much talk about drafting during the swim, most amateur triathletes are better off consistently swimming from buoy to buoy. If you do this and find you can swim with others, drafting is an added bonus. However, be advised that putting your race in the hands of another athlete or blindly following a person who passes you might put you in the wake of a bad navigator zig-zagging through the water.

I tell athletes that to navigate the swim course efficiently, they should plan to sight on every sixth stroke, which they can then adjust depending on conditions and their rhythm. This is just a baseline, but during an open-water swim it's easy to become distracted and forget to do it. When you first get going, you might need to sight more frequently, perhaps every fourth stroke, as you endure the splashing and flailing arms of hundreds of other swimmers. If conditions are calm and you are in a really good rhythm in the middle of the

How Important Is Bilateral Breathing?

Bilateral breathing can be a useful skill for triathletes in various situations on race day. If you are swimming on the outside of a group, the buoy line is to your left, and you can breathe only to the right, it will be much harder to keep track of the buoy line. Sometimes the conditions force you to breathe on your nondominant side; if the chop is coming from the right, it will be much easier to breathe on your left so you're not always breathing into the waves.

I don't recommend bilateral breathing as a regular breathing pattern because you are limiting the intake of oxygen, your body's biggest source of energy. A high stroke rate can negate this, but the majority of amateur triathletes have a lower stroke rate. Although many professionals have a stroke rate of 70 to 90 strokes per minute, most amateur triathletes have a stroke rate between 50 and 70 strokes per minute. If your stroke rate is approximately 60 strokes per minute, and you're breathing bilaterally every third stroke, you're taking only 20 breaths per minute. Replicate this when you're swimming and see for yourself whether it's a performance enhancement. With the same stroke rate, if you're breathing every two strokes, you will take 30 breaths per minute, which means you're getting 50 percent more oxygen every minute.

The bottom line is that swimming 1.2 or 2.4 miles in a triathlon is an endurance challenge, which means you need to maximize your oxygen and avoid putting your body into distress. It's great to have the skill of breathing from both sides, and it can come in handy, but you shouldn't feel forced to adopt the classic bilateral breathing pattern in the belief it will enhance your performance.

swim, you might be able to extend that to 10–16 strokes. Be aware that extending it can be detrimental to performance. I have watched swimmers take a more relaxed approach and sight every 20th to 25th stroke, and they meander all over the course, overswim, and get out of the water later.

To properly navigate a course, you need to understand the mechanics of sighting. Avoid looking into the sun as much as possible either by adapting your sighting strategy or perhaps by mixing in some bilateral breathing. If the sun is directly in line with a buoy line, you might need to look beyond the buoy line. Scan the exterior of the topography of the swim course to look for terrain features, buildings, telephone poles, or antennas that line up with the buoys. Are you swimming toward a land feature such as a peninsula, or are there some trees you can use to sight? You might look laterally at the shoreline or coast to gauge your forward movement in a straight line. In foggy or low-light conditions, you might need to look back at the buoy line to see the buoys you have already passed. Practice these scenarios as much as possible in your open-water swims. Use your observations to refine your strategy in the moments before your race begins.

Takeout Effort

No matter how strong a swimmer you are, be conscientious about the effort at which you start swimming. Whether it's the 1.2-mile swim of a 70.3 or the 2.4-mile swim of an Ironman, you're going to be out there for a long time, so you want to be careful about your takeout effort. You want to get off the line in good fashion, but you don't want to start out panicked with maximal effort, either. I call your takeout effort "easy speed," meaning it should be calm, fluid, and controlled, focused on swimming well in a straight line. You will still be traveling relatively fast (and possibly even keeping up with those panicked swimmers), but don't allow yourself to get to maximal effort.

Many people make the mistake of going out at a really hard effort because either they're so eager to start or they want to secure a good swim split. Unless they are elite swimmers, going hard doesn't usually correlate with going fast, or certainly not any faster than they would be if they remained calm. Think about being long and strong with length and strength; in other words, swimming with good form. If you do that, you'll actually swim as fast or faster than you would if you were going out as hard as possible and fighting the water and the other swimmers in your way. If you go out at an 80 percent effort, it will keep you calm and smooth. After swimming under control for a minute or two (about 100 strokes), you can reset your brain after the stress of the race start is behind you. This way you avoid the possibility of completely blowing up and having to recover and rebuild.

From a controlled, fluid start, you should ramp up to a steady and strong effort known as metronome swimming, a consistent rhythm dictated by your swimming fitness and abilities. Focus on swimming well and navigating the course in a straight line.

TRANSITION 1

When you're about 50 to 100 meters from the end of the swim, start thinking about the first transition area. Some athletes start to kick harder toward the end of the swim, claiming it improves blood circulation to their legs, but all it does is raise heart rate and put them in distress as they enter the point of the race when their heart rate is about to peak. Finish the swim the same way you started, calm and controlled heading into the transition.

The more habitual and automated your process is in transition, the better off you'll be. When you exit the swim, you go from a prone position in which your upper body is doing much of the work to an upright position in which your legs will be doing most of the work. Focus on remaining mentally and physically calm and do everything precisely the way you planned, without rushing. The pros are fast even through the transition area, but they're engaged in a different level of competition. As an amateur, you're engaged in an individual time trial. Being systematic in T1 is more important than being fast. If you get your heart rate down and avoid stress, you can ramp up into good riding more quickly when you get on the bike. T1 is all about making the best use of your time with as little energy expenditure as possible.

En route to the transition area, strip off the top of your wetsuit and remove your swim cap and goggles. Mentally review the process you're going to execute after you get to your bike. Take just enough time to put on your bike shoes, helmet, and sunglasses just as you practiced in training. The clock is running, but don't give in to panic; keep moving as calmly and efficiently as possible.

Many athletes feel as if they need to kick-start their fueling process in T1, but given the fact that your heart rate is likely at its highest point, your body's ability to absorb calories is at its lowest point. It's best to wait until you are out on the road and pedaling consistently, even though you haven't had any calories for a while. You might want to take in some water, especially if you consumed saltwater or lake water. Otherwise, your stomach is likely to have a high concentration of sodium and other electrolytes, so just drink water to quench your thirst and wait on the electrolyte drinks for the same reason you don't take in calories. Just be patient; there will be plenty of time to start your fueling and hydration process on the bike.

EXECUTING THE BIKE

When you first get on the bike as you are departing T1, you go from your highest heart rate to your highest likely level of stress. This is precisely why you want to use the first 10–30 minutes or so of riding to settle down, get comfortable on the bike, and focus on the task at hand. Ideally, this will be an extension of the habits you built in training: namely, riding your bike well.

For the initial period on the bike, focus on good cycling habits: establishing good pedal mechanics and maintaining a nice, supple posture from the tips of your fingers all the way to your toes. Keep your elbows, shoulders, and ankles loose so that you become one with your machine. If you practice this and it becomes habitual, it will be easier to implement during a race even though you've just completed the swim. Let your stomach settle for at least 20 minutes into the ride before you start your fueling strategy.

I train athletes to develop an internal pacing mechanism rather than targeting a specific power output or heart rate in an Ironman or 70.3. This allows you to be in tune with your body and maintain a good sense of strong effort, strong enough effort, and too strong of an effort throughout the race. Power output or heart rate might provide a baseline framework, especially for athletes prone to overpacing, but overemphasizing metrics can also diffuse your natural strength and paralyze your intuition. Furthermore, power output is easily influenced by the variables you face on race day (terrain, wind, temperature, altitude, humidity, etc.). Ultimately, the best athletes are riding the fastest, as opposed to producing the most power.

Bulldogs and Cricket Balls

I cannot possibly oversell getting set up on your bike. The key is getting fit for a sustainable, aerodynamic position. Take, for example, the Hawaii Ironman, where many athletes lose time over the final 35 miles of the bike, when they're coming back over rolling terrain and often riding into a headwind. Obviously, fatigue is creeping in, but the big reason their average power output goes down is they can't sustain the act of riding well over that terrain, retaining good body position on the bike. Many athletes sit on the bike differently as fatigue sets in. At Purple Patch we liken this change in bike position to a bulldog humping a cricket ball . . . it can get ugly fast.

As a result, when athletes get to the top of a roller, they don't accelerate over it. When they reach the bottom of a grade, they don't maintain or pick up speed. They wind up losing a few miles per hour simply because of poor posture leading to poor bike riding. That's why you need to get into a sustainable position that is as aerodynamic as possible.

Also, the bike fit is not a "set it and forget it" scenario. Your bike fit might change as you evolve through the season. Your mobility might increase, and you might wind up shedding some of the "junk in the trunk" throughout the season. Consequently, you might need to adjust your fit. However, you also have to train to retain your form, and ultimately your power output and efficiency, on the bike.

Pacing with Power

Many coaches tell you that on the bike portion of the race, you should simply plug into race power. The assumption is that if you hit your power target, you will maximize your race potential. By way of reference, the most common race efforts are promoted as:

- *Ironman bike racing:* 70 to 80 percent of functional threshold.

- *Ironman 70.3 bike racing:* 80 to 95 percent of functional threshold.

Note in both cases, the longer the ride takes, the lower the target will be. Although there is nothing wrong with shooting for a range of power that you can safely sustain, such a framework is not the whole story of triathlon bike riding.

For example, if a stretch of the road was consistently 5 percent uphill for 1 kilometer, then consistently 5 percent downhill for 1 kilometer, maintaining the same power uphill and downhill would not yield your fastest time. The grade on the uphill makes the production of power easier for most riders, and the speed return is great for little extra work. In contrast, forcing yourself to maintain the same power output downhill will cause metabolic stress with limited returns on the effort. The faster you go, the more work is needed to add incremental speed. The same law of diminishing returns goes for your cadence; it wouldn't be efficient to ride the same cadence over the 2 km distance. We haven't even begun to discuss the more valuable 6–10 pedal strokes athletes would deploy as they crest this hill to gain momentum and accelerate over the top. Although you might not experience a stretch of road just like this one, the example isolates the issue, giving us an opportunity to evaluate two different approaches to executing the ride.

CONSISTENT POWER	VARIABLE POWER
250W up the 1 km climb	280–300W up the 1 km climb
250W down the 1 km descent	165–185W down the 1 km descent
No focused acceleration over the crest of the hill	Conscious acceleration of 6–10 pedal strokes at the crest, perhaps with a form-based stand, at 320–370W

In this example, the variable power scenario is significantly faster, perhaps up to 30 seconds over the course of the 2 km. Of course, the terrain on a racecourse will not be so clear-cut, but imagine repeating shorter hills like this many times over rolling terrain. Over the duration of the entire race, your average power output might be lower, taking into account the relaxed output going downhill, but you will likely go a lot faster over the distance. To properly execute this strategy you must be specifically trained, adopt proper form and technique, and be focused enough to apply these skills to the actual terrain.

These concepts are tough to coach, especially remotely, so most coaches and writers simply return to overall output. Retaining power output up and down a grade is called flattening the course. If you were to apply this approach to the Ironman World Championships, you would either leave a lot of unused speed on the course or blow your energy with high effort going downhill.

Power Output on the Racecourse

To successfully use a power meter in a race, you need a solid understanding of how different terrain and conditions affect power output.

DIFFERENT GRADES

Athletes often have their own favorite grade, which allows them to generate an optimal power output for a given metabolic stress. If you ask any rider to perform a best effort time trial on flat terrain, then repeat the test on a smooth grade, the flat terrain will always produce less power. This means that holding the same power on the flats as you do on a grade isn't the fastest way to navigate the terrain.

HEADWINDS AND TAILWINDS

If you are sitting on a stretch of road with a strong tailwind, you will typically find it more challenging to maintain the designated power output than if you were riding in the opposite direction. Interestingly, retaining the high-power output with a tailwind typically nets minimal reward in terms of speed. Every 0.5 mph of speed you try to pick up will require disproportionately more power. If you hold your power output, you have a high risk of riding below your potential in headwinds and overworking in tailwinds with little speed to show for it. At the end of the day, efficiency will help you ride faster and run well off the bike.

ROLLING TERRAIN

Imagine a piece of rolling road with an uphill grade, a crest, a small descent, and finally a valley at the bottom leading into the next roller. Holding a tight power output range throughout this piece of road is not the fastest way to navigate this all-too-familiar stretch. If you instead push just above any power level heading up the grade, accelerate the bike over the crest of the hill with a small ramp up of power and/or cadence, then carry that speed down the back side of the roller and maintain it through the bottom of the valley, you will gain maximal speed over the stretch of road. Review your power graph when the ride is over, and you will see small surges of power that create acceleration.

Holding form is much more important than holding force and riding at a specific power number.

Ultimately, a cycling power meter is a great tool, but it is just that, a tool. It doesn't govern you or your riding, and using it successfully requires a real understanding of how different conditions and terrain will affect your power output. All of these scenarios require time in training to develop the skills to navigate terrain and conditions as efficiently as possible. So, you can use metrics as a framework early in the race and use them as a motivator later in the race, but you should never lose sight of the other intangibles.

Terrain Management

When it comes to the bike segment, one of the most important things you can do is to break the course down into sections. The ride constitutes the longest portion of the race and can be emotionally draining. Throughout the race, we prioritize process over outcome, and on the bike you can break it down to riding the bike well, listening to your intuition and managing feedback, and monitoring your fueling and hydration.

Remember to ride the bike well in the last quarter of the ride (that means sitting on the bike well, pedaling the bike well, managing the terrain well), and you'll be closer to your trained potential and less susceptible to muscular fatigue.

Most athletes see their power output dropping along with their speed and panic. They're chasing power levels, unaware that they're not sitting on the bike well, not pedaling well, and not managing the terrain well. Speed and efficiency are the result of riding the bike well. Double down on doing all of the little things right and stay in the moment as opposed to judging yourself, and you will maximize your speed potential.

Fueling and Hydration on the Bike

Your fueling protocol starts on the bike. To review, at 20, 40, and 60 minutes, take in 50 to 100 calories with water. At 10, 30, and 50 minutes of every hour, hydrate with a diluted electrolyte solution. An optimal solution has less than 4 percent carbohydrate with some electrolytes. From there it's about self-management; you have to be aware of your condition. If you are getting dizzy or weak or losing focus or motivation, you are calorie deficient. If you're 20 minutes into the bike segment, and you're feeling very weak, don't just hydrate; take in more calories because your body is asking for more. After your energy comes back, move to more hydration. On the contrary, if you start to burp and feel a little bloated or sick, don't keep piling in calories; drink your beverage so you can dilute the food in your stomach until it can be absorbed.

TRANSITION 2

Just as you did at the end of the swim, you should start to prepare yourself for T2 when you're near the end of the bike segment. For a 70.3 race, this begins with about 5 km to go; in a full Ironman, it's around 10 km to go. In both cases, you want to get your mind and body ready for transitioning to the run. The first

Be Good to Your Gut

Most athletes consume way too many calories during the race, especially relative to what they do in training and the demands of the day. This is why gastrointestinal (GI) distress is so common in Ironman racing. Your body experiences a high dose of physical stress, and even the emotional stress usually exceeds anything you have faced in training. It's better to be slightly underfueled than it is to consume too much; after all, catching up on calories is quicker and easier than dealing with the bloated feeling of underabsorption. Ironically, although most athletes overshoot their energy needs, they forget to hydrate, especially early on in the bike portion of the race. Find a sustainable approach to fueling that you can consistently execute. On race day, your fueling strategy is simple:

1. Consume and absorb enough calories to support the workload of your swimming, biking, and running.
2. Deliver yourself to T2 with minimal levels of dehydration.

Most research suggests that performance starts to decline after you're more than 4 percent below optimal hydration. When you're competing in an Ironman, particularly if it's hot, you will lose fluids, especially on the run. If you start out 3 percent below optimal hydration levels at T2, it is impossible to optimize your run performance. Even if you take in fluids at every aid station, you will quickly reach an overly dehydrated state.

This is why it's so important to hydrate on the bike. Ideally, you will get off the bike about 1 percent dehydrated. Then on the run you will continue consuming calories and hydration, but you'll still be shedding more than you take in.

step is to back off the intensity just a bit. That might mean letting your pace slow to 19 mph if you've been charging at 20 mph.

In addition, start to check in with yourself and think about where your body is tight and which muscles you need to loosen to be ready to run with good form. You can stand up out of the saddle a bit and cruise, stretching your hips, calves, lower back, shoulders, and neck. Otherwise, keep pedaling with good cadence and form on the way toward the bike finish. Also, do another check on your fueling and hydration needs: Do you need more calories? Are you feeling lightheaded or bloated? Do you need more hydration to clear your gut before you start to run?

As with the end of the swim, when you're moving into the transition you want a strong mindset going into T2. Think about precisely what you're going to do so you're as ready as you can be and not under duress. Focus on being calm and collected as you dismount your bike, carefully jog your bike to the rack, remove your helmet, and change into your running shoes, hat, and sunglasses. Feel free to execute some basic stretches or whatever works for you to help you feel good. The goal is to ramp up to your running potential as quickly as you can when you leave T2. Avoid taking in any calories, but drink some water and then head out on the course.

EXECUTING THE RUN

As with the swim and the bike, your first priority is to execute the run well. You only get one chance to set the tone of the run as far as posture is concerned. Don't fight the inevitable stress and awkwardness of coming off the bike. Good form starts with upright posture, shoulders slightly forward from your hips, a supple arm swing, and a quick cadence to generate the appropriate foot speed and propulsion. Remember that speed and efficiency will come out of good form, not harder effort.

Pacing on the Run

The biggest limit on the run in a 70.3 or Ironman race is typically mechanical fatigue. It's not usually the case that athletes run out of cardiovascular fitness or energy, but their legs no longer move as efficiently or effectively as possible because of muscular-skeletal fatigue. This forces athletes to make a decision: Walk or run?

At every Ironman event, including the Ironman World Championships in Kona, you'll see athletes walking during the run section. Many athletes scoff at that and do everything they can to keep jogging, even though it's barely faster than walking. Some people repeat the mantra "do not walk." Let it be understood: That's completely misguided. If you're spending the entire half-marathon or marathon running with poor form, you should consider taking a walking break. When you're running, you want to be running well, with the best form and speed possible. If that includes taking some strategic walking breaks to enable you to run the majority of the race well, it's in your best interest to do that. The run is an optimization challenge, not a toughness challenge. If you have to walk for 100 yards at a time or walk through aid stations to get yourself in position to run better, then do it. I've coached three-hour marathoners off the bike who have walked 10 to 15 times during the run

Donkey Dipped in Cement

For time-starved athletes looking to optimize their run on race day, it's all about being able to hold good running form despite fatigue. As soon as your form falls apart, you lose your efficiency and your speed. So much of the fatigue in Ironman (and Ironman 70.3) racing is mechanical or muscular fatigue, which happens when the big and small muscles in your feet, ankles, and lower legs get so tired that they don't allow you to hold good running form. So why do some age-group athletes wear super-light race shoes without any support if they're trying to avoid muscular fatigue? Yes, those shoes might feel great when you put them on, and for pros like Jessie Thomas or Sarah Piampiano or Kevin Collington, they might make sense. However, for amateur athletes who don't have the same depth of fitness or dynamic strength, it's much better to race in comfortable shoes that offer plenty of support and minimize mechanical fatigue. In other words, wear shoes that will be comfortable from start to finish, especially over the long haul of an Ironman or a 70.3 run section. That might be one of the models you have been training in or perhaps a marginally lighter model with similar characteristics.

portion of an Ironman. Remember, it's all about getting from Point A to Point B as fast as you can.

Although I support walking as necessary during a 70.3 or an Ironman, I am not a fan of a strict walking program. In other words, I wouldn't advocate running 4 minutes, then walking 1 minute, or whatever the case might be. This negates active energy management and doesn't take into account the terrain and opportunities it presents. If you're running along and your form is declining, it's better to take 15- to 20-second walk breaks to reset your form than it is to run with really bad form and have to take a 1- or 2-minute walk break because you pushed through 9 minutes of running. In addition, if you're running along and come to a steep hill, the speed penalty for walking up that hill rather than running up with a much higher heart rate and energy cost is minimal, so it makes sense to walk up that hill with purpose. On the contrary, the speed penalty for walking down a hill as opposed to running is huge. Decide when you need to walk relative to your energy level to retain good form given the terrain rather than when your watch tells you to do so.

During the run, you must relentlessly move forward with purpose no matter whether you're running or walking. Even if you're walking to relieve fatigue, you must be mentally present and execute proper form. A walk break is not a slow wander; it is purposeful, with good locomotion. The majority of the time you should be running with good form or walking with purpose, but you can also sprinkle in recovery walking just to bring your heart rate down before you move on to walking purposefully.

- *Running with good form:* Maintaining an upright posture and steady cadence

- *Walking for recovery:* 5- to 15-second walking sessions to lower stress, heart rate, anxiousness

- *Walking with purpose:* Vigorous speed-walking, swinging arms, driving off back foot, with good, consistent, forward locomotion (at 5-hour marathon pace) for 30 seconds to 2 minutes or until you can return to running with good form

Because the run is the last discipline in a triathlon, it can also be the most frustrating. Even if you've completed the swim and bike sections effectively, you might not be able to do much on the run because of mechanical fatigue or because you've reached the limits of your fitness. That's when you have to revert to the positive mindset you've held since the start of the season. When things go wrong, don't panic or give up. You have to do what's necessary to execute.

For some very fit, higher-level athletes, running in a triathlon is a pace-driven effort. Those athletes are able to execute consistent 6:45, 7:10, or 7:30 miles with good form for the entire run course. However, it's important to note that many athletes can't get their heart rate up as high as it needs to be to run that fast because of mechanical fatigue. Most athletes need to think about pacing the triathlon half-marathon or marathon differently than pacing a standard half-marathon or marathon. Rather than being focused on a consistent pace building to negative splits, think about running consistently and relentlessly driven by form, maximizing the time you are running with good mechanics.

Fueling and Hydration on the Run

In many ways, fueling and hydration is the last but not least aspect of the run. Much could be said on this topic, but the key is consistency. One of the biggest mistakes athletes can make on the run is following the fueling plan as it is written on a spreadsheet and not listening to their own bodies.

Responding to the body's signals is as important as any plan. There is no point in piling in more calories when your system is not absorbing what you've already consumed. GI stress is greatest on the run, so don't fuel to a point at which you throw up because that is dehydrating. Drink 6 to 10 ounces of water, give yourself time, and back off the intensity while you wait for your gut to clear.

CELEBRATE THE MOMENT

After you've crossed the finish line of a race, relish what you've accomplished. Whether your initial read on the race is good, bad, or indifferent, celebrate your finish and realize that every time you complete a race, it's an achievement. Take the time to remember why you compete and how fortunate you are. Remember all of the work you did to get to this point, and reflect on the sacrifices you made. Embrace the moment, and save your deep analysis for 24–48 hours later, after you've had a chance to let your feelings settle. You certainly don't want to make any big decisions in the 12 hours immediately following the race, unless, of course, you qualified for a spot in the Ironman World Championships in Hawaii.

CASE STUDY: EXECUTING A RACE PLAN WITH INTENT

By world-class standards, Purple Patch professional triathlete Sarah Piampiano is a mediocre swimmer, a strong cyclist, and an exceptional runner. Over the course of several years, she has become a consistent Ironman and 70.3 performer with several victories. Because of her swimming deficiencies, however, she's historically fallen into a mindset that she has a lot of ground to make up after the swim, which means chasing her competitors on the bike to get in better position for the run. She's done that many times with great success, but it's a strategy that can backfire with devastating effects. The simple truth is that spending so much energy on the bike can mean the demise of the run. For both amateurs and pros, it can lead to a loss of power and efficiency on the second half of the bike and all but eliminate the ability to run fast and efficiently.

For the 2015 Ironman World Championships in Hawaii, I set up a strategy for Sarah's race tailored more toward individual performance than the influence of competitors, which she could not control. Although it was against Sarah's natural, competitive instincts, I asked her not to chase to catch up as she came out of the swim. Before race day, we assumed that she'd be about 10 minutes behind the main group of female pros coming out of the water. The plan I detailed specifically had her execute her best ride, likely allowing a gradual move up on the bike, but delivered her to the run with great energy in her strongest discipline.

On race day, as it turned out, she got isolated in the ocean and hit shore with a much poorer performance and bigger deficit than either of us anticipated. She was more than 15 minutes behind the lead group. When your entire season of training is focused on one event, it would be natural for negative emotions to enter your mind at this time, and the allure of scrapping the plan on the bike might be too strong to avoid. Many athletes would have panicked and started furiously chasing to get back in the race; after all, this was Hawaii! Instead, Sarah smartly stuck to her plan, trusted her training, and realized that the poor swim was behind her and had little relevance to her ability to either bike or run. She rode with control and focus and ignored the influence of other competitors throughout the bike. Her ability to remain efficient on the bike paid huge dividends on the run, allowing her to run fast and efficiently with good form. She turned in one of the fastest run splits on a very hot day (3:07:04) and moved all the way up to 7th place overall, after coming out of the swim 2nd from last. It was a breakthrough performance that reflected her preparation and her ability to stay present on race day.

Despite Sarah's negative swim result, she had the courage and confidence to stick to her race plan and achieve a breakthrough effort. Had she tried to chase on the bike, I feel there was little chance she would have been able to run as strong as she did and certainly never would have broken into the top 10.

8

The Aftermath

After you've completed a big goal race, the next step is to reflect on how it all went and consider what you did well and not so well. This process will give you perspective and cues for improvement that you'll be able to apply as you continue on your journey. Remember, the promise of this book was twofold: to help address your long course triathlon challenges and to create a sustainable, life-affirming framework.

The ultimate goal is to achieve success in all areas of your life. In your post-race review, you should assess more than just your overall time as a standalone barometer of success or failure. Instead of examining various race-day metrics, you should take an honest look at all aspects of your life over the previous year. Of course, that should include a hard examination of both the raw numbers and mental and emotional nuances of your race as well as the path to get there.

This review is crucial because it represents your committed transition from the end of a goal race to the start of another training period or racing season that will build up to your next big event. It's especially important the first time you finish a race cycle because it will help you find numerous ways to improve as you go forward. As you continue to go through this introspection after subsequent race cycles, it will reaffirm the holistic approach outlined in earlier chapters and highlight subtle changes that will help you pursue your goals within a sustainable lifestyle. Only through persistent reinforcement of the framework and the application of lessons gained from each experience will you find continued progress. In other words, you can only continue to evolve if you understand what you did well and what you can improve in the future.

POST-RACE REVIEW

First, look at your race performance with a healthy dose of realism. Evaluate your results: what was good, what was bad. Although your final race time matters (especially if you recorded a new personal best for a given distance), the racecourse, the conditions, the relative performance of other competitors, and your overall journey are among the many other variables to consider. Your post-race reflection should be a comprehensive look into objective and subjective criteria as well as the many other nuances of your journey, your mindset, and how racing fits into your life.

Objective Review

How do you look at your race times and performance and determine whether it was a good or bad day? From a purely objective point of view, you can think about your swim, bike, and run splits and compare them with your expectations and possibly previous efforts on that same course. You should also compare your times with those of the top performers in your age group and to the average times in all categories. Look at the top age-group and average splits from previous years, and see how you would have stacked up against the field. You will gain a nuanced perspective about your results and determine if parts of the race were faster or slower than "normal."

For example, whether your swim split at Ironman 70.3 Oceanside or Ironman 70.3 Raleigh was 27:30 or 30:30, it would be much more telling to know if everyone in your age group swam relatively fast or slow that day compared with previous years on the same course. It allows you to understand whether your results were part of an overall trend or if you had an exceptional day. As those trends emerge, you might realize that the course was marked slightly short or long of the standard distance. (There can be small discrepancies from one year to the next.) Environmental conditions (temperature, wind, humidity, and so on) also play a role and can add up to big differences from the previous year's race.

In open-water swimming, the water level, current, or choppiness can have a significant impact on everybody's results. Even if you swam 30:30 one year and 27:30 the next year at the same 70.3 race, you can't interpret the result until you consider how those other variables affected all of the racers. If all conditions and course markings were relatively equal, you've certainly made a huge improvement over the previous year. However, if one or more of those variables signaled a trend of faster swimming or a shorter course, you likely improved but not by a three-minute margin.

Although comparative tactics work relatively well for the same event on the same course on a year-by-year basis, it's important to understand that comparing your most recent event with a previous event on another course is complete folly because there are so many differences between individual Ironman and 70.3 courses. First, no two courses have the same elevation profiles, climate conditions, road conditions, or location of aid stations and transition areas. This means even small discrepancies in the swim (water current, water temperature, wind, buoy placement, distance between the water and T1), bike (hills, wind, temperature, open versus closed roads), and run (elevation profile, wind, temperature, number of loops, crowd support, etc.) make comparing your splits from different events a futile effort.

The next step in your post-race self-analysis might be to look at the files generated from your power meter and review your pace data. If possible, compare those with your previous efforts on the same course. Just as with your raw swim, bike, and run splits, this is only a simple basis for comparison. Drilling down into other variables and course specifics, you might be able to determine a bit more about how well you actually swam, rode your bike, and ran, but the most effective measure is to break down the course into smaller segments. For example, if you compare your power output in 5-, 10-, 20-, and 30-minute segments and see how well distributed it was over 56 miles of a 70.3 course (or 112 miles of an Ironman course), you can determine how well you rode from the start, how well you rode hillier portions of the course, how well you kept efficient bike form, and even how well you were fueling. The same goes for your run splits, especially if you break them down in kilometers instead of miles. If your average pace increased or decreased at certain points of the run section, it could give clues as to your overall fitness, your fueling strategy, your ability to run off the bike, and the efficiency of your form and cadence.

Subjective Review

An equally important, or perhaps more important, part of your post-race analysis involves a subjective review of your performance, an honest reflection of how you managed your entire day. Examine where you had success, where you made mistakes, and where you just survived. One of the underlying principles of this book is the ability to be focused and present on a daily basis as you manage all parts of your life, especially in key training sessions, an essential (and trainable) skill you should absolutely carry into race day.

General, negative anxiety, not reframed as excitement, as well as a tendency to question your own preparation by doubting your training or dwelling on missed workouts are the two biggest factors that can sabotage your performance in the weeks and days leading up to race day. Remember when you arrived at the race site and think about how you managed your energy. What was your mindset the morning of the race? Were you confident in your abilities, and did you approach the race with exuberance? Alternatively, did you let nervousness and self-doubt cast a pall over your race that ultimately led to poor execution?

A couple of days after a race, I ask athletes this key question: If you were to go and do it again the following weekend, assuming your body was physically able to perform, what would you do exactly the same and what would you change? It's easy to discover the things you did well in a race. They bring you the most joy, especially in the days after your event when you're basking in your success. Even if you didn't achieve a personal best in a given race, you might have a new personal best swim split, faster and more effective transitions, optimal refueling and hydrating habits, better bike-handling skills on key parts of the course, or smarter pacing on the run.

The harder (but equally important) part of your race review entails identifying aspects that did not go well. Do a thorough review of your swim preparation, execution, and pacing; your bike fitness, execution, and position; and your run form and energy level. Consider specific aspects of the swim, bike, and run, including next-level details such as your ability to maneuver through the swim course, pacing consistency on the bike, bike-handling skills relative to the course, run cadence, and so forth.

Also, how well did you execute your fueling and hydration strategy? Did you take in enough calories? Did you continually hydrate, or were there big gaps when you forgot or just didn't feel like doing it? You might realize your fueling strategy needs to evolve. You might conclude that it was a really rough day in the water, or that you really need to work on your bike-handling skills. Work toward a realistic understanding of your race performance, and use it to improve in your next training cycle.

How well did you execute your overall race strategy? Were your fitness and functional strength enough to survive the final miles of the run, or did the cumulative fatigue from the swim and bike catch up with you on the run? Let's face it, no matter how your race day went, a lot of your perceived success or failure comes down to, for better or worse, how well you finished it on the run. Even in the case that you had a negative run result, broaden your perspective before making a new plan.

TROUBLESHOOTING THE RUN

It's not easy to finish an Ironman or 70.3 race with a strong run. In fact, the majority of age-group participants slog through it and underperform relative to their trained potential. As a result, one of the most common post-race perceptions for triathletes is that something went wrong in the run training before the race and that to improve, they need to "work on the run." It's a typical emotional, knee-jerk reaction based on an athlete's race-day run splits, but most athletes never discover what is really to blame for that poor run performance. Although your run might have been mediocre or relatively poor, it's usually not accurate to conclude that running is the discipline you need to work on the most. Regardless of how lousy you felt on the run, there is typically more to improving it.

When you have a disappointing run split, your running fitness or ability is potentially not the primary reason for your perceived demise. Run performance is dictated by fueling and hydration as well as various aspects of swim and bike preparation and execution. Running is also the most weight-bearing of the three disciplines, and because it is the last segment of a triathlon, fatigue comes into play. Your overall race performance in an Ironman or 70.3 race is conditional upon how many elements played out on race day and even in your training leading up to the race. It's likely that you haven't yet identified other areas of the race you need to improve in order to give yourself a better run. If you can fix those areas, several of which are outlined below, you're bound to have a run performance more in line with your expectations.

An especially strong swim and/or bike effort will often erode athletes' ability to run, even if running is normally their best discipline. Pacing relative to your overall strength, fitness, and race expectations can help moderate your effort in all three disciplines. By contrast, riding "scared," or chasing to catch up after executing what might be a poor swim result, can have a negative impact on your run because it can create too much intensity and take the focus off riding "well" (i.e., with good position), not to mention good fueling and hydration habits.

Riding in an inefficient bike position, or with poor posture, is one of the top causes for poor run performance, both because it forces you to expend too much energy on the bike and it leads to discomfort, cramping, and inefficient form on the run. Perhaps your bike isn't properly fit to your physique, or maybe your physique and fitness don't allow you to maintain good position for the duration of the bike section. Also, your bike position can change throughout the course of a training program as you lose weight, become stronger, and improve your bike fitness.

How well did you execute the bike course? Not riding the bike well on hilly terrain (for example, straining in a big gear or not holding an aero position when riding downhill) or chasing a specific power output will lessen the ability to run efficiently. Learning how to optimally ride in a triathlon relative to the course and that day's conditions, and therefore not being wedded to a specific power level, are two key ways to become more efficient on the bike.

The effects of poor fueling and hydration often don't present themselves until the run. Neglecting to refuel in the first 30 minutes of the bike ride, regardless of whether you feel good at the time, can lead to a quick downturn in energy early in the run. Ineffective hydration on the bike (especially on hot days) will lead to severe dehydration before the start of the run, and you cannot recover from this during the run.

REFLECTING ON THE JOURNEY

Although there are objective and subjective ways to review various aspects of race performance, results, and the overall outcome, based on the mindset we established early in this book, we know race results do not represent the total definition of success for a season. We also have to take a more holistic view of how we did along the way, and that requires a comprehensive look at the journey you were on for the previous year.

Looking back at your journey, recall what you did exceptionally well. Were you more consistent in executing your key workout sessions than in past seasons? Did you improve your bike-handling skills and your ability to ride in aero position? Did you run with better form than in previous race buildups? Were you able to effectively scale workouts when contingencies arose in your work or family life? It's easy to relish your success, but there should be a moment to look back and understand specifically what you did well and why you did it well. After you've identified those details, consider how you were able to translate those to race day.

It's equally important to review any disappointing days through an objective lens. In your review, look for lessons and insights that can shape your continued progression. Were there days during your journey in which you missed workouts, didn't sleep enough, or deviated from good nutrition habits? Did a last-minute, two-day business trip throw a wrench into your training for several days? Were you sick several times during the buildup to your race, or did you suffer pesky recurring or significant injuries? If so, what caused this to happen, and what did you learn?

Pre-Race Mindset

Because this approach is intended to be all about sustainability with bigger gains, it's important to look back at the final weeks before your race and evaluate your mindset. Were you able to hold on to the essence of this holistic approach, or did you start to break down physically, mentally, or emotionally? In the final 10–14 days before the race, did you feel healthy, excited, and vibrant? Did you feel strong, fit, and well rested? Or did you feel generally fatigued? It's natural for an athlete to feel flat in the final week or two before a race, given the reduced workload and additional free time while tapering workouts.

Plenty of athletes approach race day with a desperate "I have a race coming up, and I hope it goes well" kind of anxiety. We all express the pre-race nervousness in different ways, and nerves can be essential to getting yourself mentally prepared for an event. Ideally, though, you should feel confident, relaxed, energized, and even a bit loose as your race approaches. Any nerves should be labeled excitement and priming for your race instead of fear. That's exactly how pro triathlete Chris Lieto was just before he finished 2nd in the 2009 Ironman World Championships. Chris was fit, giddy with excitement, and ready to have a great day on the Kona course. He was also asking me whether he should plan on doing Ironman Arizona about six weeks later. This question, arriving in race week of the World Championships, was a clue that he was ready for a great performance in Hawaii. He was so invigorated that even before the biggest race of the season he was excited for what came next.

The reality is that not everyone feels so great in the weeks leading up to a race. A telltale sign might be a less-than-enthusiastic demeanor toward your race or even "I can't wait for this to be over so I can get this monkey off my back." Breaks are important after a big event, but if you have developed a love-hate relationship with triathlon, it's important to stop and take inventory of your situation.

If you struggled with fatigue or lack of enthusiasm in the weeks leading up to the race, it could be a sign that something was slightly out of line with one or more of the pillars of performance. Review your sleep habits to see how consistent you were in getting adequate rest. That's often the point where things begin to go out of whack. Even if you started your journey with good intentions of getting sufficient rest, it's usually the first casualty when you're deep into training, work projects, and family life.

Sustainability

Our task is to thrive in life. Results are important, but the other key indicator is whether this lifestyle is sustainable. Did you build consistency in your preparation? At some level, it's important to ignore your race outcome entirely and think through the methodology of your approach, your mindset, and how you set the lens on your available time. In which areas did you thrive and in which areas not so much? What stumbling blocks didn't you anticipate? How would you rate yourself in execution relative to your planning? Did you retain the intent, rhythm, and planning of the training? These are the building blocks of your training. How well did you complete your journey relative to your initial assessment of when you would be always available, sometimes available, and never available? How effective were you at training during those times?

Also, consider whether you managed to maintain balance in the rest of your life. What did your immersion into triathlon do to your family life and relationships? Did it improve your relationship with training? Did it boost your energy in life? After getting through the training program relative to your other experiences in life leading up to your race, did you feel more confident, more physically prepared, and more mentally prepared? Or did you feel undertrained because you were forced to miss too many training sessions? How did the impact of your training load affect you? Did you walk around like a zombie in your busy life? Did you not perform well at work? Did you not sleep as much? If you did not do well in any of these areas, what forced the situation, and what can change it?

Chances are that you've had concerns about some of these things in the past or you've gone through this journey before and certain things unhinged you. In your post-race analysis, it's important to identify where you became unhinged so that you can determine how to rectify those situations. For example, if you consistently missed swim workouts because 5:30 a.m. was just too early in the morning based on the variables of your life, then a simple scheduling change could help solve that problem. Or if you planned your run interval workouts on the same days as a morning strength session and found yourself skipping or scaling the workouts because of fatigue, you could reorganize your weekly training schedule going forward.

All of the information you gather from a review of your journey can help you begin to paint a picture of perfection versus reality. No one goes through a training cycle perfectly, not even the world's top pros. However, by creating that picture and understanding the contrast, you can get a sense of how things really went for you. Perhaps you'll look back and realize you did almost everything you could and had only a few minor challenges. Or maybe you realize you skipped or scaled the majority of your swim workouts, or you didn't do enough endurance sessions on the bike or long runs. You might realize you were trying to cram way too much training into your week, which was detrimental to your work performance, relationships, and your sleep. You might need to back off so you can be more consistent. If you were never sick, never overly fatigued, and never had injuries, you might have undertrained for your event and you might need to add more training to your regimen in the future. It's uncommon, but possible.

It's difficult to reflect on a journey, whether it is 10 or 20 or 52 weeks long, if you haven't tracked your workouts and reviewed the subjective and objective data. Use that information to understand how well you adhered to the training prescribed, how you pragmatically evolved your training (either by scaling, postponing, or skipping workouts), and what your mood and comments were both about specific workouts and at different times throughout your journey. Memories fade quickly, but tracking your training really helps. Being able to look back at your workouts with the perspective of your own feedback can empower you to understand what actually happened, especially as you're doing a post-race review.

You might need to consider other aspects of your life as well after a race. Although your race might have been a fun and positive experience, perhaps the path to get there was overwhelmingly challenging and dominated too much of your life. If that's the case, perhaps you need to go back to the start and reconsider how many hours during the week you have for training. It could be that you trained 15 or 16 hours per week, and, in reality, you really only had time for 12 or 13. If you wound up missing workouts, scaling workouts, or having challenges at work on a regular basis, those extra 3 to 4 hours of planned training every week might be the culprit. Reducing your training load by a few hours a week could pay huge dividends and keep your energy balanced across your entire life.

Another common element among many age-group triathletes is the desire to lose weight or improve your body composition. Maybe you approached a triathlon with the idea of getting fit. Did that happen? If you went through a training cycle and you followed everything correctly, you ate plenty, and you followed a good diet, but you still retained weight or had disappointing body composition, it could be that you have too much stress in your life. By fitting training into the scope of your life, getting sufficient sleep, and eating well, you'll be more successful in managing stress and likely have a better path toward the physical changes you seek.

Ultimately, when you look back at your journey, you'll want to look at all of these facets to get a global snapshot of your training cycle and race performance. Using that information, you can start to determine how you will make minor or major changes the next time around. If you went through this journey again, where would you place your focus? What would you improve next time?

CASE STUDY: **PASSION FOR THE JOURNEY**

I coached pro triathlete Meredith Kessler for 10 years. Over that time, she went from being a competitive age-group triathlete to a multiple Ironman champion. Her breakthrough professional race occurred in 2008 at Ironman St. George 70.3, where she raced brilliantly and became US national champion. She beat a stellar field, and her performance in St. George was the catalyst to enormous success in the second half of her career. Given the huge emotional lift, I assumed Meredith would take few days off to let it all sink in.

The next day I arrived to the early morning swim practice, and Meredith was already in the pool warming up, as usual the first athlete in the pool. I stopped her to ask what she was doing there, and she simply replied that she knew a swim would feel good, help recovery, and launch training for her next race. She wasn't wrong. Meredith loved the journey of the sport and always viewed training as a wonderful opportunity to improve, whether on tough days that provided lessons or easy recovery days such as this one that helped rejuvenation and adaptation. Her passion was her heartbeat of success, and failure or victory was simply a part of that journey.

WHERE TO GO FROM HERE

Ultimately, the path to success in long-distance triathlon begins with a proper mindset, grounded in pragmatism. This is especially true for a time-starved athlete with important business and family commitments that must be balanced on a daily and weekly basis. Although it can be tempting to squeeze in more workouts and make more sacrifices, the approach outlined in this book is decidedly the opposite. Although you might be limited to just 10 to 12 hours of training per week, if it helps accommodate the ebb and flow of life and the many demands and changes it brings, it will feel liberating, not limiting. Of course, this shouldn't leave you with the impression that the best way to train for an Ironman is a 10-hour weekly program. If that were the case, the professional triathletes I coach would spend more time in coffee shops and various other leisure activities.

The *Fast-Track Triathlete* program is all about finding the best training dose for you. It is a pragmatic approach that includes always being present to mindfully execute the intent and rhythm of workouts while also keeping the rest of your life in balance. The key to this, of course, is that it's entirely different for everybody. Sami Inkinen won the age-group title at the Ironman World Championships by training 12 hours per week, which was the optimized training prescription for him as a successful business entrepreneur and age-group Ironman phenomenon (see p. 19). He has amazing genetic gifts and a strong work ethic, but if I had given him a training workload of 16 hours per week, he surely would have failed. You have a similar optimization challenge, but your variables are based on your own reality. Ask yourself "How can I maximize the quality training I *can* do on a regular basis?"

By following a holistic approach that integrates the right amount of training into your life, you put yourself in a position to be optimally fit and ready to perform at your best on race day while also maintaining successful, positive relationships and outcomes in all other aspects of your life. In other words, the sustainable framework you foster in your journey goes way beyond just achieving success in your hobby; it goes well beyond triathlon performance. This is about developing and maintaining a better you through a performance lifestyle. Yes, you'll continue to progress in triathlon, but you'll also achieve better health, a better balance of energy and effectiveness in work, and greater presence and focus in your relationships.

I hope this book and the principles I've outlined can be a catalyst to a new approach to training that leads to your continued success in triathlon and in life. Although it will help facilitate a sustainable lifestyle, it doesn't make the journey easy. There are no shortcuts to success in triathlon or anything else in life. You still have to put in the hard work, continually manage and adapt to changes, and then execute with earnest intent in all aspects of your life. I truly believe that if you immerse yourself in pragmatism, and you can find the harmony of integrated performance, you will achieve success beyond your wildest dreams.

Characteristics of Excellence

In my coaching journey, I've been lucky to lead both elite professional athletes and a host of amateur athletes who are executive-level businesspeople from major companies; in other words, elite professionals in the business world. It's obvious that both of these types of people are elite performers, and it's clear that many correlated traits lead them to success in their fields. With that in mind, I have a saying: "Coach the pros like CEOs, and coach the CEOs like pros." So often the pros have all of the traits they need, but they need help with their executive management skills. On the contrary, the CEOs have great executive functionality, but they have trouble translating it to their own training and day-to-day functioning in triathlon. These two groups can learn an enormous amount from each other. I try to get the pros to think and act like executives and the C-level business executives to think and act like pro athletes because their processes are so aligned.

GOAL DRIVEN. Setting goals is not just about the classic results or outcomes as you might expect. Being driven is not about winning the Hawaii Ironman or a world championship, taking a company public or setting new highs for revenues or return on investments, although those goals are certainly important. These successful people thrive at whatever they're doing, and they tend to establish goals within a framework of what steps are necessary for their self-improvement or their company to be successful. In other words, even their goals involve a mindset of process. It's less about stating a goal of wanting to win the Hawaii Ironman and more about knowing they have to improve their bike performance based on specific criteria. Actionable goals aimed at self-improvement are effective because the goals set are the very actions that lead to the results. It comes down to identifying what you need to do to maximize your performance and creating goals that facilitate that progress.

PROCESS DRIVEN. Within the framework of goals, both CEOs and pro athletes tend to have an innate appreciation of the process and an ability to train a lens on the journey. Out of the process-driven approach comes the focus on controlling what they can, gaining proper perspective, and developing an ability to move past distractions. These two groups strive to understand what happened, take in that information, and move on without being bogged down in the negativity of a specific outcome. It's a learned skill that can be applied on race day, too.

APPRECIATE SUPPORT. Although individually successful, the best athletes and executives always have the capacity to value support. They are on a mission to surround themselves with resources that will help bring success. These individuals are very coachable because they have an ability to manage their egos and an innate understanding that they need to seek out answers from the appropriate sources. On the contrary, highly ego-driven people who give the impression of already having all the answers are typically not the most successful. The same goes for coaching, too. If a coach acts as if he or she always has all the right answers, it's usually a good sign to run the other way and find a new coach. Although most successful coaches are true to their training philosophies, most also consider additional resources, methodologies, and outside influences to help refine what is best for a particular athlete.

RESILIENCE AGAINST ADVERSITY. Despite the fact that both CEOs and pros are susceptible to nerves and fear, they seem to have an ability to remain task-focused and solutions based when adversity strikes. There are always many potholes on the journey, for both athletes and business executives. We always say there are a year's worth of business lessons in every Ironman race day. The pros are the best at maneuvering through those challenges, but most of the executives have the same quality lens and focus as the pros. If you have the ability to remain solutions-based, then you can navigate through anything triathlon throws at you.

FOCUS AND SPECIFICITY. The ability to filter out the noise of daily life and focus on what's important is invaluable. Pros and CEOs constantly ask and answer, "What is the most important thing I need to do?" Because they're so good at leaning into their coaching, they can easily go do the specific tasks. When the distractions increase, the very best pros and CEOs bear down with even more focus on the elements that will help them in their quest. With very high-functioning individuals, it's almost as if the chaos is the catalyst that enables their focus on being task-driven. This means a coach must be able to identify the focus to optimize their skills and traits despite any kind of static around them.

PASSION FOR THE JOURNEY. A single result, good or bad, seldom distracts a good CEO or pro from the passion of incremental improvement. The best certainly celebrate and embrace their success and enjoy the moment, but they also quickly move on to the next goal. If they have a disappointment, they assess what happened, do some self-analysis for perspective, and progress to an actionable focus instead of dwelling on a negative result that leads to a decline in confidence. The most dedicated athletes love the grind of the training and the battle of the races, and the gains just flow from that positive outlook. They understand that success comes from the process, and for that reason it's important to absolutely love the process.

EFFECTIVE WORK, NOT HARD WORK. We have all experienced the rigors of life and sport and the need for balance, rest, and recovery. The pro athletes often need the most help finding balance between their life components, whereas the CEOs need help in the health/sport department. However, their characteristics are similar in that both tend to embrace recovery in terms of its effectiveness. To the pros, it's all about doing what they need to do to be successful, and that's not more work or egregiously harder work just for the sake of racking up training hours and miles. They realize that balanced work is effective work that will pay off in the long run.

ASSESSMENT AND PLANNING. Chance and hope are not favorite words of most successful people. These concepts are too vague and therefore unreliable. The best will always do their homework, and in triathlon that's assessing course suitability and layout, planning a strategy for success, and using their ability to learn from what they've done well and what can be improved.

To successful athletes and executives, it's all about passion for the ongoing journey. People who aren't as successful often make the mistake of viewing challenges with a pass/fail mindset. However, it's about knowing these are opportunities to learn and improve. In any situation, whether it's an overwhelming success, an "epic fail," or somewhere in between, there's the chance to grow by constructively identifying those areas in which you can keep improving your race and your life simultaneously.

PART 2

THE PERFORMANCE PLAN

Functional Strength Training

Strength training is one of the pillars of performance, meaning it is critical to your evolution as a triathlete. Incorporating general strength training into your workload doesn't automatically make you a better swimmer, biker, or runner. A successful *functional* strength program uses resistance training to target the mobility, stability, and power required for the movements of swimming, biking, and running. This program will help you incrementally build functional strength and maximize your achievements at the three triathlon disciplines. Our bigger goal is to improve your functional health. Your commitment to strength training benefits your general health and equips you with more efficient, effective movements to meet the demands of daily life.

Correctly and purposefully integrating strength training into a training regimen, in a consistent manner, can be a challenge for most time-starved athletes. Many athletes do some type of strength training already with earnest intent, but it's important to know what each exercise does and how it functionally correlates to the movements of each discipline. We want to create a platform for improving strength, balance, synchronization, and kinesthetic awareness of the sport-specific movements of triathlon.

The best way to implement a strength-training program is to meet regularly with a good strength coach who can assess your current physique and athletic ability (taking into account your strengths, weaknesses, and discrepancies), develop a custom strength-training plan, and help you execute and adapt it on an ongoing basis. Just as you would benefit from having a coach's input before, during, and after every swim, bike, and run, you would also benefit from coaching on your functional strength program. As a time-starved athlete, though, it's not likely you have this luxury. Spending long hours at the gym doing strength training will cut into your swim, bike, and run training. What follows is a smart and effective alternative approach that I developed with our San Francisco–based strength expert, Brendon Rearick, to optimize the modest window of opportunity you have for strength training within the framework of your busy life. We maintain the optimization mindset in this program.

Naturally, the majority of your time should be spent training for swimming, biking, and running; heading to the gym for an hour is no replacement for the primary training required to facilitate endurance performance. However, it's crucial that you don't focus only on swim, bike, and run training and completely disregard strength training. That's not a sensible long-term approach because strength and conditioning leads to many benefits and provides a necessary foundational platform for success.

RATIONALE OF THE PROGRAM

This strength program will allow you to maximize the positive adaptations of your hard work, optimize your execution and movements across the three disciplines, and ultimately improve your race results. The program focuses on building foundational strength for total-body functional movement. Each exercise is set up as a progression, and you can start with the movement that you can complete with good form for the number of sets and reps specified.

For this to be an optimal strength-training program, you need to decide what you're hoping to get out of it and how consistently you can do the workouts. This program applies to 90 percent of the key areas of strength-and-conditioning development, in a way that meets the needs of 80 percent of the triathlete population. In other words, this program might be a little too advanced for some or not advanced enough for others. There are seven areas of focus and progression in a tiered structure that you should approach with patience and long-term diligence. If you are new to strength training and conditioning, it might take 18 to 24 months to reach the most advanced level in all seven areas. It is impossible to build a time-efficient program that accommodates every single need of every athlete, but this will give you a good start.

We've designed this program within the context of a typical, time-starved triathlete's daily life. You can do these exercises in a gym, at home, or even in a hotel room. If you have easy access to a gym, it will allow you to consistently execute the workouts. However, the program requires minimal equipment, potentially some replacement equipment, or even just body weight as resistance if you don't have any equipment available. If you wish to take these exercises and progressions to your own strength expert, he or she could add to or evolve them, with the understanding that these types of exercises are specifically designed to address the movement of a triathlete.

If you integrate this program into your busy life, you will experience some significant benefits. You will have a platform to support triathlon performance through the development of technical skills, strength, and mobility to maximize your physical resources, and musculoskeletal resilience and power potential. You will also have a reduced risk of injury as a result of building a stronger, more stable, and synchronized base. Ultimately, strength training will expand your performance potential and make you a more robust athlete.

EXECUTION OF THE PROGRAM

You will notice that most of the exercises in the program are performed on a single leg. Most life activities (including running and cycling) are based on single-leg movements. Single-leg exercises also reduce the need for training with heavy loads because you can use your body weight as the "load." Functional movements such as these will make you stronger for both life and sport.

- Consistency is key to this program. Do these functional strength workouts twice a week every week to see results.

- Choose one exercise (A, B, C) from each progression, and focus on mastering it before moving on to the next one. Learn to control your own body first before adding weights or difficulty. You'll be better in some categories than others based on your physique, experience, and skills, which means you'll progress in some categories faster than in others.

- The repetitions provided for each exercise are a benchmark. If you can't complete the full set of reps as indicated, get as many reps as you can with good form. Reps done with poor form don't count. If you get only five reps the first week, shoot for six the next week. Move on to the next progression after you've reached the benchmarked reps.

- There are seven exercises organized into a Tri Set and Quad Set. Do three rounds of each set as a circuit.

Equipment

- Wheel (for rollouts) ▪ Tennis ball ▪ Sliders ▪ Yoga block ▪ Resistance band
- Kettlebell or dumbbells—13 kg (25 lb.) for women, 16 kg (35 lb.) for men
- Bench (a chair will work for most exercises)
- Any exercise with sliders can be done with paper plates or towels on a wood floor or linoleum in place of sliders.

(These weight suggestions will apply to most triathletes. Adjust as needed.)

Single-Leg Squat Progression

Single-leg work is done to improve the strength, stability, force absorption, and resilience of the lower body. This is especially important in running, in which the ground impact is high, and you are at risk of injury if your body is not ready for the demands. This progression coordinates the mobility, balance, and strength of your ankles, knees, and hips.

PICK ONE: **A** , **B** , or **C**

A Single-Leg Hip Bridge

10 reps each side with 3-second hold per rep

The goal of the single-leg hip bridge is to use the glute, as opposed to the hamstring or lower back, to extend your hip. Clenching the tennis ball in the nonworking hip requires activation of the hip flexors and core, making it less likely that you will use your back to extend your hip.

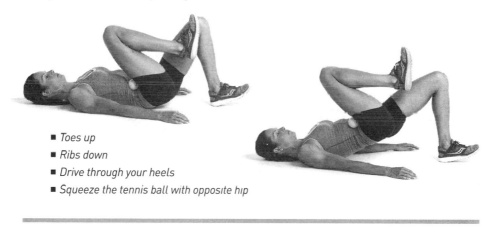

- *Toes up*
- *Ribs down*
- *Drive through your heels*
- *Squeeze the tennis ball with opposite hip*

DON'T *arch through your back or push through your toes.*

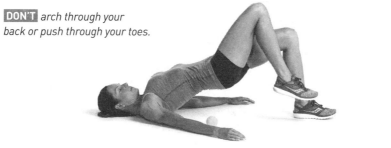

■ Kickstand Single-Leg Squat

8 reps each side

In this movement, the tennis ball allows you to learn the single-leg squat movement without the difficulty of balancing on one leg. You should rely on the tennis ball only during the "up" portion of the squat. The depth you are trying to achieve is 1 inch lower than parallel to the ground. If this is too difficult, use pads or a block to elevate the bench. Also be sure to progress the weight before beginning the next exercise.

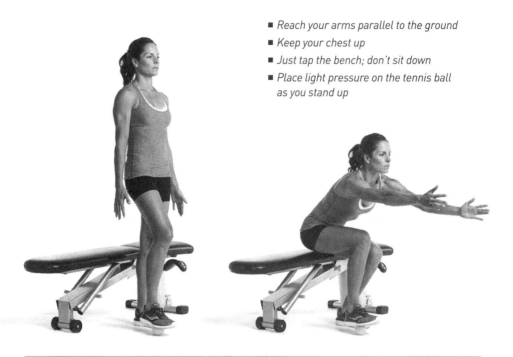

- *Reach your arms parallel to the ground*
- *Keep your chest up*
- *Just tap the bench; don't sit down*
- *Place light pressure on the tennis ball as you stand up*

DON'T *round your back or let your knee cave in.*

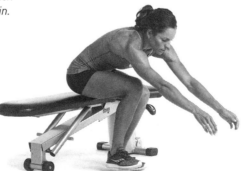

C Single-Leg Squat

8 reps each side

This is one of the most difficult exercises you'll perform in your strength program and one of the most important to master. It requires a great amount of both mobility and stability as opposed to bilateral exercises such as the squat and deadlift. As with the kickstand single-leg squat, the ideal depth of the squat is 1 inch lower than parallel to the ground. If this is too difficult, use pads or a block to elevate the bench. Avoid pistol squats (which entail the forward extension of your inactive leg) because they put additional stress on your knees, ligaments, core, and nervous system.

- *Keep the nonworking leg off the ground*
- *Reach your arms parallel to the ground*
- *Just tap the bench; don't sit down*
- *Keep your chest up*

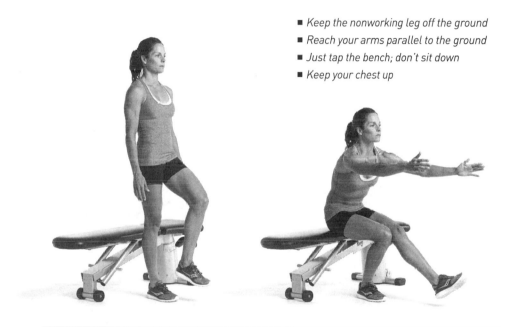

DON'T *round your back or do pistol-style squats.*

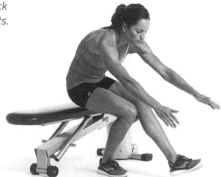

Anti-Extension Progression

Anti-extension exercises improve your core stability. Specifically, these help you to resist forces that create extension of your spine (e.g., sway back). They allow you to better transfer power from your arms and legs to propel you forward more efficiently and are key to creating postural endurance, both in the water and on the run.

PICK ONE: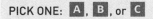

A Front Plank

1-minute max

The front plank builds core strength. Don't wear your planking ability as a badge of honor. This is an exercise where Herculean endurance efforts are wasted; instead move on to something more difficult.

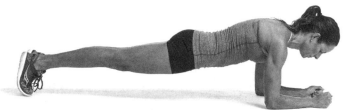

- *Your plank position should look like your standing posture*
- *Keep your toes flexed*
- *Lightly drive your elbows to your toes*

DON'T *let your hips rise or sag.*

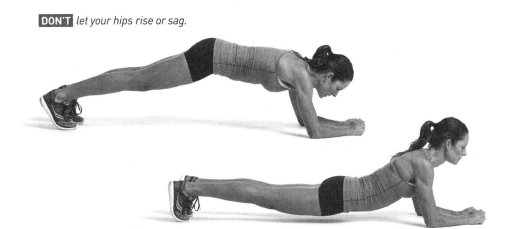

Body Saw

12 reps

The goal of a body saw is to slide your body back away from your arms in a good, front-plank position. This increases the lever arm and the demands from the anterior core. Use sliders under your feet to do this movement.

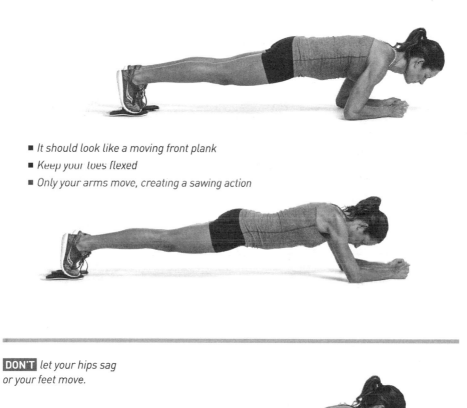

- *It should look like a moving front plank*
- *Keep your toes flexed*
- *Only your arms move, creating a sawing action*

DON'T *let your hips sag or your feet move.*

⊂ Wheel Rollouts

12 reps

This movement is the ultimate show of strength in the anterior core. A small amount of progress each month will pay big dividends. Place sliders or a pad under your knees if needed. Maintain neutral spinal position throughout the movement.

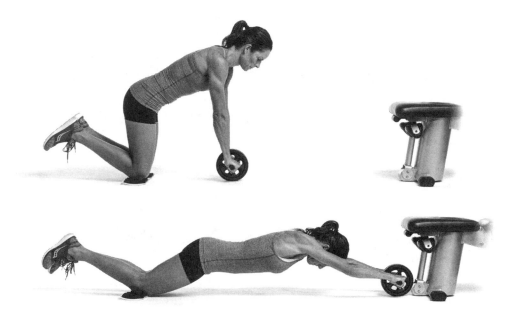

- Hold spinal position in neutral
- Use a wall to gauge your distance
- Hips go first, arms reach second

DON'T *use your lower back.*

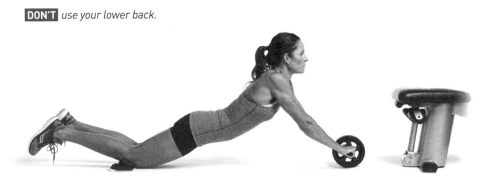

Push-Up Progression

These exercises strengthen your upper body and improve your postural strength. Specifically, they enhance your ability to transfer power from your arms to propel you forward as well as maintain your posture on the bike. Your ability to hold good form in a push-up directly correlates to your postural endurance in the water and on a run. Think of these exercises as moving plank exercises for your core, not chest exercises.

PICK ONE: **A** , **B** , or **C**

A Push-Up Taps

10 reps each side with a 2-second hold per rep

This movement engages your rotational core muscles and helps you become accustomed to being in the push-up position.

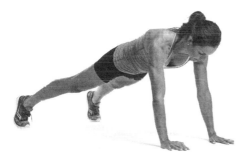 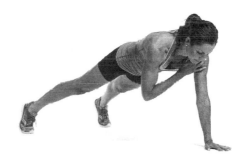

- *Keep hips in line with shoulders*
- *Shift your weight slowly to one side*
- *Place hand on opposite shoulder for 2 seconds*

- *Repeat the movement, alternating sides*

DON'T *let your hips shift from side to side.*

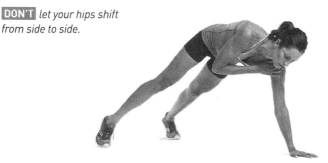

B Elevated Push-Ups

12 reps

For many athletes, maintaining a neutral core position during a push-up is more difficult than the actual pushing part. For that reason, it would be more appropriate to call them plank-ups. Elevating the hands during a push-up allows you to do this.

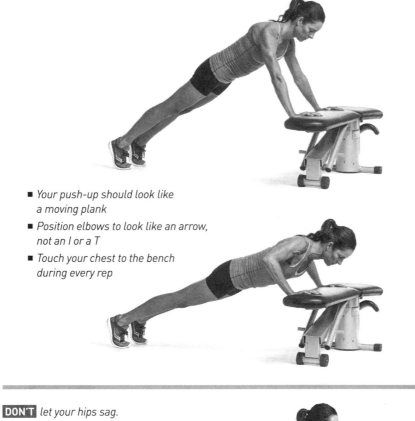

- *Your push-up should look like a moving plank*
- *Position elbows to look like an arrow, not an I or a T*
- *Touch your chest to the bench during every rep*

DON'T *let your hips sag.*

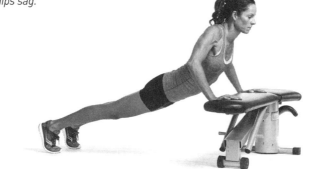

Push-Ups

12 reps

Use a foam block to ensure that you get the right depth every time.

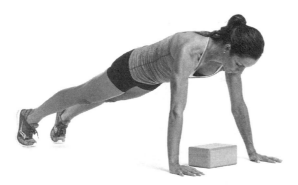

- *Your push-up should look like a moving plank*
- *Position elbows to look like an arrow, not an I or a T*
- *Touch the foam block every time, or it doesn't count*

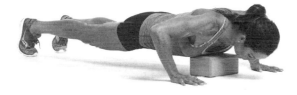

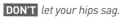

DON'T *let your hips sag.*

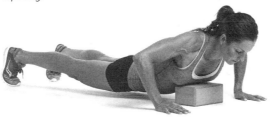

Quad Set   3 rounds

Split Squat Progression

This progression of exercises improves leg strength while allowing for a more upright torso than a traditional squat. It is less challenging in terms of technique and places less stress on the spine. Performing this movement properly also improves strength and mobility of the hips.

PICK ONE: **A**, **B**, or **C**

A Body Weight Split Squat

8 reps

Spare your lower back from heavy loads with this split squat, which allows you to tax your hips and legs using your own weight as an external load. Avoid spreading your feet too far apart so that you get a stretch; this is a strength exercise. Position a pad under your back leg if needed.

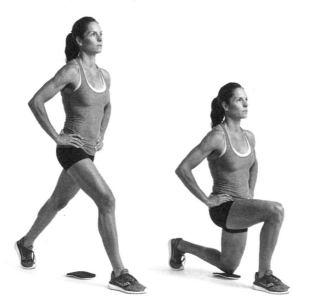

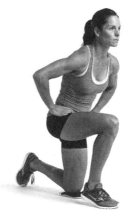

- *Set up in a split stance*
- *Stand tall, with the crown of your head to the ceiling*
- *Head, shoulder, hip, and knee should line up vertically*
- *Both legs at 90-degree angle*
- *Move up and down like a piston*

DON'T *move forward and back like a saw.*

B Goblet Split Squat

8 reps

Using a kettlebell or weight in the goblet position is ideal because it minimizes the stress on the lower back, reflexively engages the core, and increases the difficulty of the split squat. Again, avoid spreading your feet too far apart so that you get a stretch; this is a strength exercise. Position a pad under your back leg if needed.

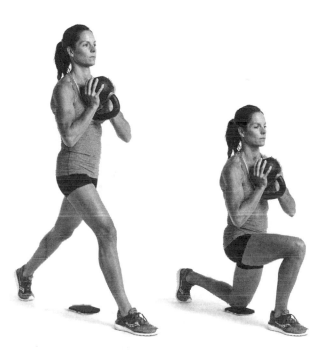

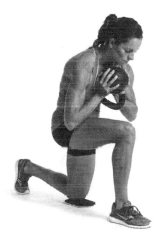

- *Set up as if you are on railroad tracks*
- *Stand tall, crown of head to the ceiling*
- *Hold the kettlebell like a goblet against your sternum*
- *Head, shoulder, hip, and knee should line up vertically*
- *Both legs at 90-degree angle, with knees under hips*
- *Move up and down like a piston*

DON'T *lean forward or back.*

c Rear-Foot Elevated Split Squat

8 reps

By elevating the rear foot in a split squat, you shift more weight to the front leg, creating more demand on the quad and glute of the down leg. Hold a kettlebell or weight in the hand opposite of the working (forward) leg. Position a pad or block under your back leg if needed. Again, avoid spreading your feet too far apart so that you get a stretch; it could cause knee pain on the back leg.

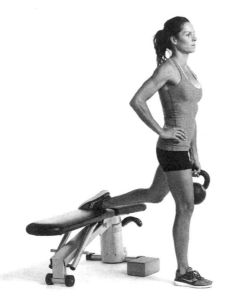

- *Body and shin angle should be the same*
- *Place your foot on the bench, laces down*
- *Move up and down like a piston*
- *Push through the front foot*

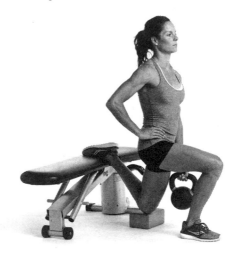

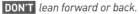

DON'T *lean forward or back.*

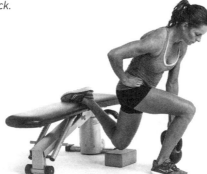

Hurdle Step Progression

This set of exercises combines hip mobility and core stability while layering strength training and ultimately dynamic work on top of these elements. Improvement in lower-body power production, while maintaining posture through the torso, allows for more powerful and efficient mechanics. This is where you transfer lower-body strength into movements that more closely mimic running.

PICK ONE: **A**, **B**, or **C**

A Lying Hip Flexion

3 reps each side with 10-second hold per rep

This movement should look like you're holding a running or sprinting position on your back. You can engage your inner-core musculature to maintain good spinal position. The band provides minimal resistance and emphasizes good form.

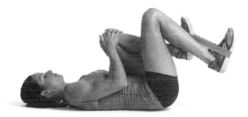

- Press your lower back into the ground
- Flex both toes toward your knees
- Place band around arches of your feet
- Pull in your knee as high as you can
- Keep the bottom leg straight

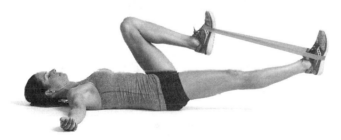

DON'T *let the knee drop below a 90-degree angle or flex your back.*

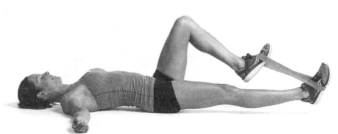

B Push-Up Position Slider Hip Flexion

12 reps alternating sides

This movement looks like you're a sprinter coming out of the blocks. The push-up position makes big demands on the core, and the moving leg mimics the hip flexion required during running.

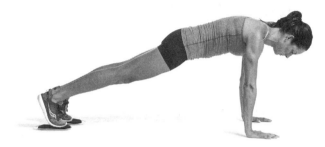

- *Start in plank position, with your feet on sliders*
- *Drive your big toe into the slider*
- *Bring your knee to your chest*
- *Keep hips in line with your shoulders*
- *Repeat movement, alternating sides*

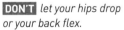

DON'T *let your hips drop or your back flex.*

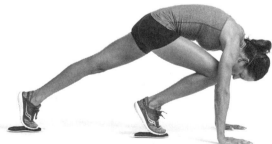

C Suitcase Walking Hip Flexion

10 steps in place each side with 3-second hold per rep

The pull of the kettlebell laterally on one side engages all of your small stabilizers. Holding the single-leg stance requires balance and focus, which are the first to go with age or injury.

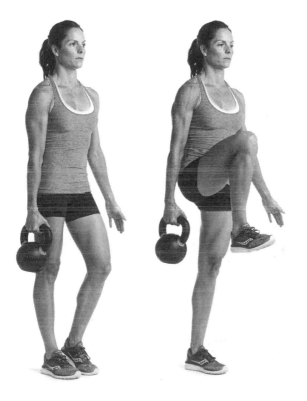

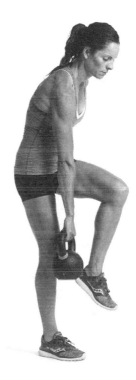

- *Hold the kettlebell 1 inch away from your leg*
- *Shift your weight onto one leg*
- *Bring your knee up to your chest*
- *Flex your toes toward your knee*
- *Hold each rep for 3 seconds*

DON'T *let the kettlebell lean against your body or pull you forward.*

Rotary Stability Progression

This progression improves core stability and the rhythm of opposite (reciprocal) arm and leg movements. These exercises work your full-body kinetic chains to better connect you through the core. Rotational and reciprocal movements are fundamental to improving stability and efficiency as an athlete, specifically in the swim stroke and running-form mechanics.

PICK ONE: **A** , **B** , or **C**

A Dead Bug

8 reaches each way

This exercise engages the core musculature, which creates a cross pattern or "sling" from one shoulder to the opposite hip. These are your swimming and running core muscles because these movements require action of the opposite hip and shoulder.

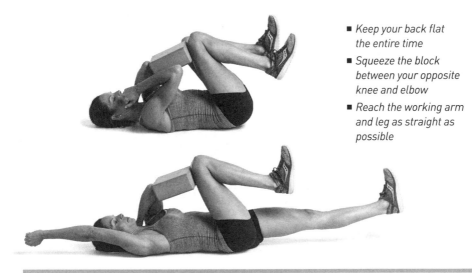

- *Keep your back flat the entire time*
- *Squeeze the block between your opposite knee and elbow*
- *Reach the working arm and leg as straight as possible*

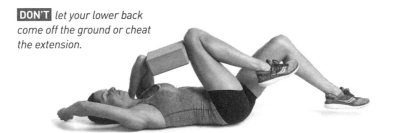

DON'T *let your lower back come off the ground or cheat the extension.*

B Bird Dog

8 reps each side with 3-second hold per rep

This movement creates high demand on the core musculature because the ground is no longer there to give your spine feedback, as in the dead bug. It is most important to prioritize your spine and core in this movement before you begin to move your arm or leg.

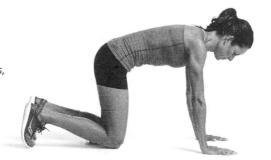

- Hands under shoulders, knees under hips
- Reach opposite arm and leg straight
- Keep your lower back flat and stomach tight

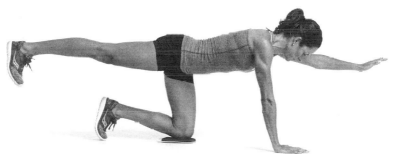

DON'T *use your lower back to extend your hip.*

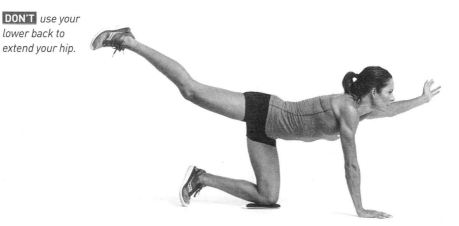

Bear Crawl

10 steps forward, then backward

This movement creates high demand on the core musculature, which creates a cross pattern or "sling" from one shoulder to the opposite hip. If your quad and core are sore after doing the bear crawl, you're doing it correctly.

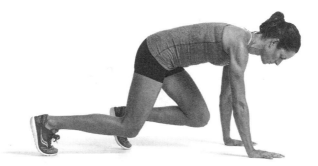

- *Place hands under shoulders, knees under hips*
- *Take steps with opposite hand and foot*
- *Keep your lower back flat and stomach tight*
- *You are a slow-moving tabletop*
- *Repeat movement backward to starting position*

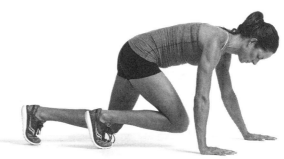

DON'T *use your lower back or hips to move forward. Also, don't go too fast; slow and steady wins the race here.*

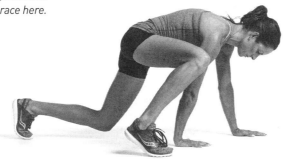

A Kettlebell Deadlift

12 reps

Engaging the posterior chain with deadlifts keeps your legs strong and back healthy. Learning how to safely pick up weight is important for everyone to master before moving on to the single-leg exercises that follow.

- *Line up the kettlebell with your heels*
- *Keep your back flat*
- *Squeeze the bell as if you're trying to break it; this gets your lats into position*
- *Stand up tall*
- *Squat back down with your legs and your back flat to set the weight down*

DON'T *collapse forward; use your back to lift the weight.*

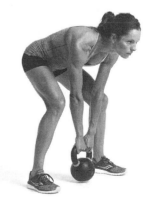

B Bench-Supported, Single-Leg Deadlift

8 reps each side

At some point the weights used in the deadlift start to become more dangerous than they are beneficial. Moving to exercises with one leg can still give you all the benefit of deadlift without all the load and stress on the lower back. First practice this movement without weight.

- *Put a slider on top of the bench*
- *Hold the weight in the opposite hand from the working leg*
- *Keep a soft bend in your working knee*
- *Straighten out your back leg on the slider, using the bench for support*
- *Keep your back flat*
- *Bring the kettlebell down to the floor*

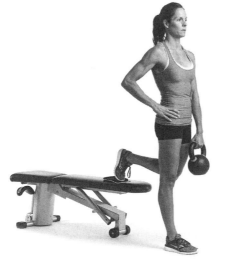
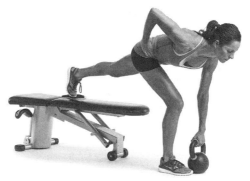

DON'T *round your lower back.*

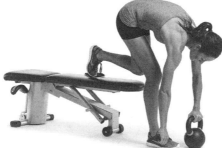

C Single-Leg Deadlift

8 reps each side

This is one of the best leg exercises you can do consistently. It puts high demand on the most important posterior chain and challenges your core and your balance. Be sure you can do this movement with good form before adding the weight.

- *Hold the weight in the opposite hand from the working leg*
- *Bring the kettlebell down to the floor*
- *Keep your extended leg straight, high enough to be parallel to the ground*
- *Flex your foot, toes point down*
- *Keep your back flat*
- *Have a soft bend in your working knee*

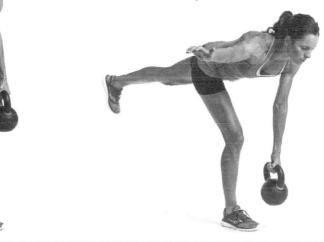

 DON'T *round your lower back or let your hips rotate.*

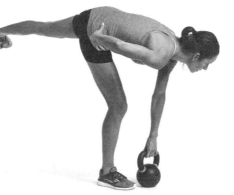

The Fast-Track Training Progression

The following is an overview of a season of training, encompassing the postseason, preseason, and race-specific phases in a progressive approach to:

1. Prepare you for race day. The specific training that leads to race readiness, focused specifically on the designated A races.
2. Develop you as an athlete. The overall goal here is to achieve ongoing improvement from one season to the next.

Take into consideration your background, hours available, goals, and races, then plan a progressive season of training that facilitates your race readiness and development. As you make your own plan, keep in mind the goals and purpose of each phase of training and the intent of the different blocks of training prescribed.

POSTSEASON PHASE: THE OFF SEASON

The true "start" of your season comes on the heels of a break at the end of the prior season. The postseason phase can be 4 to 12 weeks, depending on your experience level, when your previous season finished, and your race plans for the upcoming season. You should not be at full training capacity during the postseason. Even if compressed in time, your training load should be nowhere near your max. In addition, you can enjoy a degree of flexibility in this phase. Although hitting every intensity during every week and phase of the year is important, it is all about how much intensity. In these weeks, you will do very little threshold work and will not have event-specific focus.

Here are the key points to remember when you approach postseason work:

Preparatory: This block of work is all about preparing for strong upcoming training. So the aim is to gently build fitness and muscular resilience as well as to strengthen the tendons and ligaments. When your training does ramp up, you should be prepared to accept the load as the best opportunity to adapt to the hard work, avoiding injury.

Technical: This is a great time to focus on refinements of habits, technique, and form. Physical stress should be lower, which opens the door for more technical focus.

Equipment fit: Choose new equipment, change your bike fit, or upgrade your shoes or wetsuit. The postseason provides plenty of time to adapt to such changes within the context of a ramping training load.

Low physical stress: As mentioned, global stress is low. Even if you are time starved, you should operate at a lower training load (in weekly training hours as well as intensity of key sessions).

Flexibility: Put the time-trial bike aside for now. You'll have plenty of leeway to integrate some fun and associated activities, such as mountain biking, cross-country skiing, hiking, trail running, and so forth. Enjoy it. In the meantime, spend some time on your road bike. It is a more intuitive machine that facilitates work on handling skills and terrain management.

Embrace intensity: It sounds like a paradox, but do some high-intensity work. It is all in the pursuit of neurological conditioning and technical development, so think about form over force especially during the postseason.

Begin the strength habit: You must learn and refine the key movements with which you will load heavy and explosive strength training. To effectively embrace the benefits of season-long strength and conditioning, you need to adopt these habits now.

Add key sessions: You will have a heavy load after emerging from this preparatory phase, so you must get ready for the upcoming sessions. Include neuromuscular power work on steep grades in some key runs, touch on low-rpm strength work on the bike, and hit some fast, paddle-based swimming sessions. This readies you for the tough work coming.

Goals for Postseason Success

- Emerge with good baseline, but not prime, fitness levels.
- Build a resilient musculoskeletal system.
- Establish positive habits to carry through the season.
- Be emotionally fresh and eager to add hours and training load.
- Commit to integrated strength training.

KEY WORKOUTS

	KEY SWIM #1	KEY SWIM #2	KEY BIKE #1
WEEK 1	**TECHNICAL Prep** 4 rounds of: 2 × 100 with snorkel, with 10 sec. rest 2 × 200 with good form, retaining tempo	**ENDURANCE Short Intervals** 20 × 50 at 80%, good tempo with 5 sec. rest	**END-OF-RANGE Strength-Endurance** On trainer: 4 × 3 min. Z3 at <65 rpm 4 × 2 min. Z3 at <65 rpm 4 × 1 min. Z3 at <65 rpm 1 min. Z1 spin with good form between intervals
WEEK 2	**TECHNICAL Form** 1–2 rounds of: 200 with snorkel, with 30 sec. rest 3 × 100 form-focused, progress 1 to 3 with 15 sec. rest 100 with snorkel, with 30 sec. rest 3 × 50 form-focused, progress 1 to 3 with 15 sec. rest	**ENDURANCE Short Intervals** 30 × 50 at 80%, good tempo with 5 sec. rest	**END-OF-RANGE Strength-Endurance** On trainer: 10–14 × 2 min. Z3 at <60 rpm 1 min. Z1 spin at faster rpm between intervals
WEEK 3	**TECHNICAL Speed and Power** 3–5 × 400: 75 smooth, 25 strong, 75 smooth, 25 very strong, 75 smooth, 25 MAX, 100 smooth 30 sec. rest between intervals	**ENDURANCE Short Intervals** 40 × 25 at 90%, good tempo with 2–3 sec. rest	**END-OF-RANGE Strength-Endurance** On trainer: 3 × 4 min. Z3 at <65 rpm 3 × 3 min. Z3 at <65 rpm 3 × 2 min. Z3 at <65 rpm 3 × 1 min. Z3 at <65 rpm 1 min. Z1 spin with good form between intervals
WEEK 4	**TECHNICAL Prep** 4 rounds of: 3 × 100 with snorkel, with 10 sec. rest 2 × 200 with good form, retaining tempo	**ENDURANCE Short Intervals** 30 × 50 at 80%, good tempo with 5 sec. rest	**END-OF-RANGE Strength-Endurance** On trainer: 14–16 × 2 min. Z3 at <60 rpm 1 min. Z1 spin at faster rpm between intervals
WEEK 5	**TECHNICAL Form** 1–2 rounds of: 300 with snorkel, with 30 sec. rest 3 × 100 form-focused, progress 1 to 3 with 15 sec. rest 150 with snorkel, with 30 sec. rest 3 × 50 form-focused, progress 1 to 3 with 15 sec. rest	**ENDURANCE Short Intervals** 40 × 50 at 80%, good tempo with 5 sec. rest	**END-OF-RANGE Strength-Endurance** On trainer: 4 × 7 min. all at strong effort: 1 min. at 70 rpm, 1 min. at 60 rpm, 1 min. at 50 rpm, 1 min. at 40 rpm, 1 min. at 50 rpm, 1 min. at 60 rpm, 1 min. at 70 rpm 1 min. Z1 spin with good form between intervals
WEEK 6	**TECHNICAL Speed and Power** 3–5 × 400: 75 smooth, 25 strong, 75 smooth, 25 very strong, 75 smooth, 25 MAX, 100 smooth 30 sec. rest between intervals	**ENDURANCE Short Intervals** 60 × 25 at 90%, good tempo with 2–3 sec. rest	**END-OF-RANGE Building** On trainer: 4 × 7 min. all at 40–55 rpm: 1 min. Z2/Z3, moderate effort, 1 min. Z3, moderately strong, 1 min. Z3/Z4, strong, 1 min. Z4, very strong, 1 min. Z3/Z4, strong, 1 min. Z3, moderately strong, 1 min. Z2/Z3, moderate effort 1 min. Z1 spin with good form between intervals

KEY BIKE #2*	KEY RUN #1	KEY RUN #2
ENDURANCE General Endurance On trainer: 4 × 10 min. with every 3rd min. at <65 rpm 2 min. Z1 spin at high rpm between intervals	**TECHNICAL Prep Run** 40–70 min. Add 6 × 20 sec. blast fast, form-based 1 min. easy between efforts	**ENDURANCE General Endurance** On trail: Up to 75 min., form-based Softer surface is ideal, hike steep sections with good form
ENDURANCE General Endurance On trainer: 5 × 10 min. with every 3rd min. at <65 rpm 2 min. Z1 spin at high rpm between intervals	**TECHNICAL Prep Run** 40–70 min. Add 6 × 20 sec. blast fast, form-based 1 min. easy between efforts	**ENDURANCE General Endurance** On trail: Up to 75 min., form-based Softer surface is ideal, hike steep sections with good form
END-OF-RANGE High Cadence On trainer: 2 rounds of: 8 × 20–30 sec. high effort at high rpm 1 min. easy between efforts 10 min. Z2 smooth between rounds	**INTERVALS Strength** 45–60 min. 2 rounds of: 4 × 20–30 sec. blast with bounding power on hill Walk downhill and recover completely between each effort 5–10 min. endurance between rounds	**ENDURANCE General Endurance** On trail: Up to 85 min., form based Softer surface is ideal, hike steep sections with good form
ENDURANCE General Endurance On trainer: 6 × 10 min. with every 3rd min. at <65 rpm 2 min. Z1 spin at high rpm between intervals	**TECHNICAL Prep Run** 40–70 min. Add 9 × 20 sec. blast fast, form-based 1 min. easy between efforts	**ENDURANCE General Endurance** On trail: Up to 85 min., form-based Softer surface is ideal, hike steep sections with good form
END-OF-RANGE High Cadence On trainer: 2 rounds of: 8 × 20–30 sec. high effort at high rpm 1 min. easy between efforts 10 min. Z2 smooth between rounds	**INTERVALS Strength** 45–60 min. 2 rounds of: 4 × 20–30 sec. blast with bounding power on hill Walk downhill and recover completely between each effort 5–10 min. endurance between rounds	**ENDURANCE General Endurance** On trail: Up to 75 min., form-based Softer surface is ideal, hike steep sections with good form
ENDURANCE General Endurance On trainer: 6 × 10 min. with every 3rd min. at <65 rpm 2 min. Z1 spin at high rpm between intervals	**TECHNICAL Prep Run** 40–70 min. Add 9 × 20 sec. blast fast, form-based 1 min. easy between efforts	**ENDURANCE General Endurance** On trail: Up to 95 min., form-based Softer surface is ideal, hike steep sections with good form

*Note: You can always replace KEY BIKE #2 with an outside ride. Add intensity as you are able.

KEY WORKOUTS

	KEY SWIM #1	KEY SWIM #2	KEY BIKE #1
WEEK 7	**TECHNICAL Prep** 4 rounds of: 4 × 100 with snorkel, with 10 sec. rest 3 × 200 with good form, retaining tempo	**ENDURANCE Short Intervals** 40 × 50 at 80%, good tempo with 5 sec. rest	**END-OF-RANGE Strength-Endurance** On trainer: 6 × 7 min. all at strong effort: 1 min. at 70 rpm, 1 min. at 60 rpm, 1 min. at 50 rpm, 1 min. at 40 rpm, 1 min. at 50 rpm, 1 min. at 60 rpm, 1 min. at 70 rpm 1 min. Z1 spin with good form between intervals
WEEK 8	**TECHNICAL Form** 1–2 rounds of: 400 with snorkel, with 30 sec. rest 3 × 100 form-focused, progress 1 to 3 with 15 sec. rest 200 with snorkel, with 30 sec. rest 3 × 100 form-focused, progress 1 to 3 with 15 sec. rest	**ENDURANCE Short Intervals** 50 × 50 at 80%, good tempo with 5 sec. rest	**END-OF-RANGE Building** On trainer: 6 × 7 min. all at 40–55 rpm: 1 min. Z2/Z3, moderate effort, 1 min. Z3, moderately strong, 1 min. Z3/Z4, strong, 1 min. Z4, very strong, 1 min. Z3/Z4, strong, 1 min. Z3, moderately strong, 1 min. Z2/Z3, moderate effort 1 min. Z1 spin with good form between intervals
WEEK 9	**TECHNICAL Speed and Power** 3–5 × 400: 75 smooth, 25 strong, 75 smooth, 25 very strong, 75 smooth, 25 MAX, 100 smooth 30 sec. rest between intervals	**ENDURANCE Short Intervals** 60–80 × 25 at 90%, good tempo with 2–3 sec. rest	**END-OF-RANGE Strength-Endurance** On trainer: 4 × 11 min. all at strong effort: 1 min. at 70 rpm, 2 min. at 60 rpm, 2 min. at 50 rpm, 1 min. at 40 rpm, 2 min. at 50 rpm, 2 min. at 60 rpm, 1 min. at 70 rpm 1 min. Z1 spin with good form between intervals
WEEK 10	**TECHNICAL Speed and Power** 3–5 rounds of: 250 at 70%, 150 at 80%, 50 at 90% All with 10–15 sec. rest	**ENDURANCE Short Intervals** 50 × 50 at 80%, good tempo with 5 sec. rest	**END-OF-RANGE Building** On trainer: 4 × 11 min. all at 40–55 rpm: 1 min. Z2/Z3, moderate effort, 2 min. Z3, moderately strong, 2 min. Z3/Z4, strong, 1 min. Z4, very strong, 2 min. Z3/Z4, strong, 2 min. Z3, moderately strong, 1 min. Z2/Z3, moderate effort 1 min. Z1 spin with good form between intervals

KEY BIKE #2*	KEY RUN #1	KEY RUN #2
END-OF-RANGE High Cadence On trainer: 10 sec. at MAX, 50 sec. easy spin, 20 sec. at MAX, 50 sec. easy spin, 30 sec. at MAX, 50 sec. easy spin, 40 sec. at MAX, 50 sec. easy spin, 50 sec. at MAX, 50 sec. easy spin, 60 sec. at MAX, 10 sec. off, 50 sec. at MAX, 20 sec. off, 40 sec. at MAX, 30 sec. off, 30 sec. at MAX, 40 sec. off, 20 sec. at MAX, 50 sec. off, 10 sec. at MAX	**INTERVALS Strength** 45–60 min. 2 rounds of: 6 × 20–30 sec. blast with bounding power on hill Walk down and recover completely between each effort 5–10 min. endurance between rounds	**ENDURANCE General Endurance** On trail: Up to 95 min., form-based Softer surface is ideal, hike steep sections with good form
ENDURANCE General Endurance On trainer: 3 × 16 min.: 1: Every 4th min. at fast rpm 2: Every 4th min. at slow rpm 3: Build rpm every 4 min., on last 4 min. >100 rpm 4 min. Z1 spin at high rpm between intervals	**TECHNICAL Prep Run** 40–70 min. Add 9 × 20 sec. blast fast, form-based 1 min. easy between efforts	**ENDURANCE General Endurance** On trail: Up to 75 min., form-based Softer surface is ideal, hike steep sections with good form
END-OF-RANGE High Cadence On trainer: 10 sec. at MAX, 50 sec. easy spin, 20 sec. at MAX, 50 sec. easy spin, 30 sec. at MAX, 50 sec. easy spin, 40 sec. at MAX, 50 sec. easy spin, 50 sec. at MAX, 50 sec. easy spin, 60 sec. at MAX, 10 sec. off, 50 sec. at MAX, 20 sec. off, 40 sec. at MAX, 30 sec. off, 30 sec. at MAX, 40 sec. off, 20 sec. at MAX, 50 sec. off, 10 sec. at MAX	**INTERVALS Strength** 45–60 min. 2 rounds of: 6 × 20–30 sec. blast with bounding power on hill Walk down and recover completely between each effort 5–10 min. endurance between rounds	**ENDURANCE General Endurance** On trail: Up to 95 min., form-based Softer surface is ideal, hike steep sections with good form
ENDURANCE General Endurance On trainer: 3 × 16 min.: 1: Every 4th min. at fast rpm 2: Every 4th min. at slow rpm 3: Build rpm every 4 min., on last 4 min. build to >100 rpm 4 min. Z1 spin at high rpm between intervals	**TECHNICAL Prep Run** 40–70 min. Add 9 × 20 sec. blast fast, form-based 1 min. easy between efforts	**ENDURANCE General Endurance** On trail: Up to 95 min., form-based Softer surface is ideal, hike steep sections with good form

*Note: You can always replace KEY BIKE #2 with an outside ride. Add intensity as you are able.

POSTSEASON

PRESEASON PHASE: CONDITIONING

Following the preparatory postseason work you begin to truly work hard for the first time, although the key races of the year are likely still relatively far away. This is called the *building block* phase because many of the sessions here are the foundation for effective event-specific training. The mission is to continue your focus on technique and carry through the good habits you have established in recent weeks. Now you begin a drive to improve fitness, muscular endurance, and resilience. Because you have plenty of time before your key races, you are able to integrate less event-specific training, including higher power output, speed, and sprint training to help build the muscles' capacity.

In the preseason, you also develop overall cardiovascular fitness; continue your focus on technical skill, form, and technique; and include elements of the focused work for race preparation (including end-of-range training and very low and very high rpm work on the bike). In general, the season is a series of progressive, but moveable parts to fit your life, schedule, fatigue level, and so on. You could easily extend it to 16, 18, or 20 weeks as needed, depending on how your race season is planned.

Here are the key points to remember when you approach preseason work:

Maintain technical focus: While you ramp up your workload, your goal should always be *form over force,* so embrace the focus on technical development from prior training and keep it a priority here.

Carry the habits: You must not forget those promises with which you likely began the season: Fueling? Sleeping? Whatever positive habit you chose for the season, it is now time to double down so that it can become a habit!

Pursue resilience and endurance: Much of your strength and resilience will be established in this block of work. Preseason will bring the first concerted, strength-based training in the bike and run. This means low rpm on the bike and some hill work in your running. It is important to understand *how* to execute this training well and balance it with some other end-of-range training, such as fast-rpm cycling and fast downhill running.

Get unspecific: You are training for endurance events, but the preseason opens the door to improve your muscles' capacity to do the work, with some higher-intensity power output and speed work. Plenty of higher-intensity training will improve the effectiveness of your more endurance-driven miles, which come closer to the key races.

Be strong like a bull: Assuming you have already hit some movement-based strength training in previous weeks, the preseason will bring some overload strength work. Some high-load work, even explosive exercises, will enable you to develop real strength.

Swim fit: Our sport is swim/bike/run, so bring a swim focus to the forefront at this part of the year. Great swim fitness has solid cross-over properties for overall conditioning, provides low musculoskeletal stress, and builds a base of swim fitness to rely on when later months call for extended bike and run hours of training.

Goals for Preseason Success

- Emerge with great fitness and musculoskeletal fitness, but not quite in "race ready" form.
- Retain the good habits you established.
- Layer several weeks of consistent training without injury.
- Maintain a routine of strength and mobility training.
- Set a baseline of sustainable power output and speed that is ready to be extended to event-specific work.

KEY WORKOUTS

	KEY SWIM #1	KEY SWIM #2	KEY BIKE #1
WEEK 1	**ENDURANCE Short Intervals** 50 × 50 at 80%, good tempo with 5 sec. rest	**TECHNICAL Speed and Power** 2–3 rounds of: 6 × 25 MAX, with 20 sec. rest, 6 × 100 smooth, with 15 sec. rest 1 min. rest between rounds	**END-OF-RANGE Strength-Endurance** On trainer: 4 rounds of: 5 min. strong at <60 rpm, 1 min. low stress at >90 rpm, 5 min. strong at <60 rpm, 1 min. low stress at >90 rpm 5 min. Z1 spin between rounds
WEEK 2	**ENDURANCE Short Intervals** 80–100 × 25 at 90%, good tempo and rhythm with 2–3 sec. rest	**ENDURANCE Building** 8 × 150, with 30 sec. rest Progress effort and speed every 2 intervals, with last 2 intervals at 95%	**ENDURANCE General Endurance** On trainer: 6 × 10 min. with every 3rd min. at <65 rpm 2 min. Z1 spin at high rpm between intervals
WEEK 3	**ENDURANCE Short Intervals** 2 rounds of: 20 × 50 at 80%, good tempo with 5 sec. rest, 300 straight, holding same tempo with 1 min. rest	**ENDURANCE Over-Distance** 200 at 80%, 100 with toys 400 at 80%, 300 with toys 600 at 80%, 100 with toys Toys here are paddle, buoy, ankle strap All with 1 min. rest	**END-OF-RANGE High Cadence** On trainer: 6 rounds of: 2 min. easy low at >95 rpm, 1 min. strong at <60 rpm, 2 min. easy low at >95 rpm, 1 min. strong at <60 rpm 3 min. Z1 easy spin between rounds
WEEK 4	**ENDURANCE Short Intervals** 3 rounds of: 16 × 50 at 80%, good tempo with 5 sec. rest, 300 straight, holding same tempo with 1 min. rest	**TECHNICAL Speed and Power** 2–3 rounds of: 4 × 50 MAX, with 30 sec. rest, 6 × 100 smooth, with 15 sec. rest 1 min. rest between rounds	**ENDURANCE General Endurance** On trainer: 1–2 rounds of: 12 min. with every 3rd min. at <65 rpm, 9 min. with every 3rd min. at <65 rpm, 6 min. with every 3rd min. at <65 rpm 2 min. Z1 spin at high rpm between intervals and rounds
WEEK 5	**ENDURANCE Short Intervals** 60–100 × 25 at 90%, good tempo and rhythm with 2–3 sec. rest	**ENDURANCE Building** 8 × 200, with 30 sec. rest Progress effort and speed every 2 intervals, with last 2 intervals at 95%	**END-OF-RANGE Building** On trainer: 4 × 4 min. at <60 rpm Build from moderately strong to the last 10 sec. at MAX effort 5 min. Z1 spin between intervals 1 × 15 min. Z2 steady endurance
WEEK 6	**ENDURANCE Short Intervals** 3 rounds of: 16 × 50 at 80%, good tempo with 5 sec. rest 300 straight, holding same tempo with 1 min. rest	**ENDURANCE Over-Distance** 200 at 80%, 100 with toys 400 at 80%, 200 with toys 600 at 80%, 200 with toys 800 at 80%, 100 with toys Toys here are fins and snorkel All with 1 min. rest	**END-OF-RANGE High Cadence** On trainer: 6 rounds of: 2 min. easy low at >95 rpm, 1 min. strong at <60 rpm, 2 min. easy low at >95 rpm, 1 min. strong at <60 rpm 3 min. Z1 easy spin between rounds

KEY BIKE #2	KEY RUN #1 (OR SUPPORTING)	KEY RUN #2
ENDURANCE General Endurance Outside: 90 min. smooth and steady ride On trainer if needed, 75–90 min.	**ENDURANCE** General Endurance 45–75 min. supporting run, form-based	**ENDURANCE** General Endurance Hilly trail run 60–90 min.
END-OF-RANGE Building On trainer: 3 × 4 min. at <60 rpm Build from moderately strong to the last 10 sec. at MAX effort 5 min. Z1 spin between intervals 1 × 15 min. steady endurance	**INTERVALS** Strength 3 rounds of: 3 × 30–40 sec. power uphill with easy run down, 2 min. rest between intervals 6 min. hilly endurance loop, form-based running between rounds	**ENDURANCE** General Endurance Trail run 60–90 min.
ENDURANCE General Endurance Outside: 90 min. smooth and steady ride On trainer if needed, 75–90 min.	**ENDURANCE** General Endurance 50–80 min. supporting run, form-based	**ENDURANCE** General Endurance Hilly trail run 60–90 min.
END-OF-RANGE Strength-Endurance On trainer: 5 rounds of: 5 min. strong <60 rpm, 1 min. low stress >90 rpm, 5 min. strong <60 rpm, 1 min. low stress >90 rpm 5 min. Z1 spin between rounds	**INTERVALS** Strength 3 rounds of: 3 × 30–40 sec. power uphill with easy run down, 2 min. rest between intervals 6 min. hilly endurance loop, form-based running between rounds	**ENDURANCE** General Endurance Trail run 60–100 min.
ENDURANCE General Endurance Outside: 90 min. smooth and steady ride On trainer if needed, 75–90 min.	**ENDURANCE** General Endurance 50–80 min. supporting run, form-based	**ENDURANCE** General Endurance Hilly trail run 70–110 min.
ENDURANCE General Endurance Outside: 90 min. smooth and steady ride On trainer if needed, 75–90 min.	**INTERVALS** Strength 3 rounds of: 2 × 30 sec. blast uphill with 1 min. easy run down, 3 × 3 min. at 4% grade 5 min. form-based flat running between rounds	**ENDURANCE** General Endurance Hilly trail run 60–90 min.

KEY WORKOUTS

	KEY SWIM #1	KEY SWIM #2	KEY BIKE #1
WEEK 7	**ENDURANCE Short Intervals** 3 rounds of: 20 × 50 at 80%, good tempo with 5 sec. rest, 400 straight, holding same tempo with 1 min. rest	**TECHNICAL Speed and Power** 2–3 rounds of: 8 × 25 MAX, with 15 sec. rest, 6 × 100 smooth, with 15 sec. rest 1–2 min. rest between rounds	**ENDURANCE General Endurance** On trainer: 6 × 10 min. with every 3rd min. at <65 rpm 2 min. Z1 spin at high rpm between intervals
WEEK 8	**ENDURANCE Short Intervals** 80-100 × 25 at 90%, good tempo and rhythm with 2-3 sec. rest	**ENDURANCE Building** 8 × 250, with 30 sec. rest Progress effort and speed every 2 intervals, with last 2 intervals at 95%	**END-OF-RANGE Building** On trainer: 5 × 4 min. at <60 rpm Build from moderately strong to the last 10 sec. at MAX effort 5 min. Z1 spin between intervals 3 × 6 min. Z3 at <60 rpm 3 min. Z1 spin between intervals
WEEK 9	**ENDURANCE Short Intervals** 12 × 50 at 80-85%, with 5 sec. rest 12 × 25 at 90%, with 2-3 sec. rest 12 × 50 at 80-85%, with 5 sec. rest 12 × 25 at 90%, with 2-3 sec. rest 30 sec. rest between sets	**ENDURANCE Over-Distance** 200 at 80%, 100 with toys 400 at 80%, 200 with toys 600 at 80%, 200 with toys 800 at 80%, 100 with toys Toys here are paddle, buoy, ankle strap All with 1 min. rest	**END-OF-RANGE High Cadence** On trainer: 8 rounds of: 3.5 min. easy low at >95 rpm, 1 min. strong at <60 rpm 3 min. Z1 easy spin between rounds
WEEK 10	**ENDURANCE Short Intervals** 16 × 50 at 80-85%, with 5 sec. rest 16 × 25 at 90%, with 2-3 sec. rest 16 × 50 at 80-85%, with 5 sec. rest 16 × 25 at 90%, with 2-3 sec. rest 30 sec. rest between sets	**TECHNICAL Speed and Power** 2–3 rounds of: 8 × 50 MAX, with 30 sec. rest, 6 × 100 smooth, with 15 sec. rest 1–2 min. rest between rounds	**ENDURANCE General Endurance** On trainer: 1–2 rounds of: 12 min. with every 3rd min. at <65 rpm, 9 min. with every 3rd min. at <65 rpm, 6 min. with every 3rd min. at <65 rpm 2 min. Z1 spin at high rpm between intervals and rounds
WEEK 11	**ENDURANCE Short Intervals** 3 rounds of: 20-30 × 25 at 90%, with 2-3 sec. rest, 500 straight, holding same rhythm and tempo with 2 min. rest	**ENDURANCE Building** 8 × 250, with 30 sec. rest Progress effort and speed every 2 intervals, with last 2 intervals at 95%	**END-OF-RANGE Strength-Endurance** On trainer: 4 rounds of: 4 min. strong at <60 rpm, 1 min. strong at >90 rpm, 4 min. strong at <60 rpm, 1 min. strong at >90 rpm 5 min. Z1 spin between rounds
WEEK 12	**ENDURANCE Short Intervals** 16 × 50 at 80-85%, with 5 sec. rest 16 × 25 at 90%, with 2-3 sec. rest 16 × 50 at 80-85%, with 5 sec. rest 16 × 25 at 90%, with 2-3 sec. rest	**ENDURANCE Over-Distance** 200 at 80%, 100 with toys 400 at 80%, 200 with toys 600 at 80%, 200 with toys 800 at 80%, 100 with toys 1000 at 80%, 100 with toys Toys here are fins All with 1 min. rest	**END-OF-RANGE Strength-Endurance** On trainer: 8 rounds of: 3.5 min. easy low at >95 rpm, 1 min. strong at <60 rpm 3 min. Z1 easy spin between rounds

KEY BIKE #2	KEY RUN #1 (OR SUPPORTING)	KEY RUN #2
END-OF-RANGE Strength-Endurance On trainer: 4 rounds of: 5 min. strong <60 rpm, 1 min. low stress >90 rpm, 5 min. strong <60 rpm, 1 min. low stress >90 rpm 5 min. Z1 spin between rounds	**ENDURANCE General Endurance** 50–80 min. supporting run, form-based	**ENDURANCE General Endurance** Hilly trail run 70–110 min.
ENDURANCE General Endurance Outside: 90 min. smooth and steady ride On trainer if needed, 75–90 min.	**INTERVALS Strength** 2 rounds of: 4 × 3 min. at 4% grade, form-based, 3 min. at 1% grade or flat road 5–7 min. smooth, form-based running between rounds	**ENDURANCE General Endurance** Hilly trail run 70–120 min.
ENDURANCE General Endurance Outside: 90 min. smooth and steady ride On trainer if needed, 75–90 min.	**ENDURANCE General Endurance** 50–80 min. supporting run, form-based	**INTERVALS Strength** 3 rounds of: 2 × 30 sec. blast uphill with 1 min. easy run down, 3 × 3 min. at 4% grade 5 min. form-based flat running between rounds
END-OF-RANGE Building On trainer: 5 × 4 min. at <60 rpm Build from moderately strong to the last 10 sec. at MAX effort 5 min. Z1 spin between intervals 3 × 6 min. Z3 at <60 rpm 3 min. Z1 spin between intervals	**INTERVALS Strength** 2 rounds of: 4 × 3 min. at 4% grade, form-based, 3 min. at 1% grade or flat road 5–7 min. smooth, form-based running between rounds	**ENDURANCE General Endurance** Trail run 70–110 min.
ENDURANCE General Endurance Outside: 90 min. smooth and steady ride On trainer if needed, 75–90 min.	**ENDURANCE General Endurance** 50–80 min. supporting run, form-based	**ENDURANCE General Endurance** Hilly trail run 80–120 min.
ENDURANCE General Endurance Outside: 90 min. smooth and steady ride On trainer if needed, 75–90 min.	**INTERVALS Strength** 3 rounds of: 3 × 3 min. at 4% grade, form-based, 3 min. at 1% grade or flat road 5–7 min. smooth, form-based running between rounds	**ENDURANCE General Endurance** Trail run 80–120 min.

KEY WORKOUTS

	KEY SWIM #1	KEY SWIM #2	KEY BIKE #1
WEEK 13	**ENDURANCE Short Intervals** 4 rounds of: 16 × 50 at 80%, good tempo with 5 sec. rest, 300 straight, holding same tempo with 1 min. rest	**TECHNICAL Speed and Power** 2–3 rounds of: 4 × 100 MAX, with 45 sec. rest, 3 × 200 smooth, with 30 sec. rest 1 min. rest between rounds	**END-OF-RANGE High Cadence** On trainer: 10, 9, 8, 7, 6, 5, 4, 3, 2, 1 min. as: Even intervals: steady state Z3 endurance Odd intervals: smooth and ramp rpm to fast 1 min. Z1 spin at high rpm between intervals
WEEK 14	**ENDURANCE Short Intervals** 3 rounds of: 20–30 × 25 at 90%, with 2–3 sec. rest, 500 straight, holding same rhythm and tempo with 2 min. rest	**ENDURANCE Building** 8 × 250, with 30 sec. rest Progress effort and speed every 2 intervals, with last 2 intervals at 95%	**END-OF-RANGE Building** On trainer: 5 × 4 min. at <60 rpm Build from moderately strong to the last 10 sec. at MAX effort 5 min. Z1 spin between intervals 3 × 6 min. Z3 at <60 rpm 3 min. Z1 spin between intervals

Race-Specific Phase: Race Preparation

Many, if not most, athletes have more than one Ironman-distance or Ironman 70.3 race in the season, so our job is to develop a progression that allows solid racing throughout the lead-up to the A race as well as get you optimally prepared for B races along the way. As you transition to race-specific training, you can expect not only to retain some of the elements of previous developmental training but also to build the overall focus with race readiness.

Expect to go through one, two, or even three cycles of race-specific training within a calendar year. Each cycle might last between 8 and 14 weeks depending on the layout and progression of your racing schedule. Following this training, take a break of 1 to 2 weeks, then ramp back up with some progressively building work before restarting the process of race-specific training for the next goal race. Of course, in round two, you will have learned from the great, good, and indifferent weeks. What worked? What didn't? Through your experience and analysis, your evolution and progression occurs. As you become more familiar with each aspect of preparation, you can better focus on execution, make adjustments that work for you, and enjoy greater predictability of your performance. Consider some key points when you approach race-specific work:

KEY BIKE #2	KEY RUN #1 (OR SUPPORTING)	KEY RUN #2
END-OF-RANGE Strength-Endurance On trainer: 4 rounds of: 4 min. <60 rpm, 1 min. >90 rpm, 4 min. <60 rpm, 1 min. >90 rpm 5 min. Z1 spin between rounds	ENDURANCE General Endurance 50–80 min. supporting run, form-based	ENDURANCE General Endurance Hilly trail run 70–90 min.
ENDURANCE General Endurance Outside: 90 min. smooth and steady ride On trainer if needed, 75–90 min.	INTERVALS Strength 3 rounds of: 3 × 3 min. at 4% grade, form-based, 3 min. at 1% grade or flat road 7–10 min. smooth, form-based running between rounds	ENDURANCE General Endurance Trail run 80–120 min.

Translate to race readiness: Your focus here is on translating all the building-block training you already completed in the postseason and preseason into being truly prepared for your best racing performance. This means you have plenty of event-specific intensity and focus.

Continue strength-endurance focus: An important element of training to retain your gains is the strength-based endurance training. You can expect to see plenty throughout the early stages of a race-specific phase and even some in race-prep sessions closer to the race.

Turn strength therapeutic: You won't get stronger now, so your focus shifts to retaining the strength gains and keeping your joints healthy. You'll retain two to three weekly core and stability sessions, but "real" strength training can only be completed once weekly.

Get fueled: It is time to dial in race pace, race fueling, and hydration plans and other elements that can facilitate a positive expression of your hard work and readiness.

Stay healthy: Load is higher, with an emphasis on leaning into the bike and run sessions each week, so ensure that you have superb supporting habits (sleep, fueling, hydration, and recovery) to retain health and maximize adaptations and readiness.

Think through the sessions: There is no more important time to understand the intention of the prescribed sessions, executing them as intended and remaining present and focused. You are creating great economy, with the mission of being able to retain *form under fatigue*, central to racing success.

Simulate: Be ready to simulate the intensity, experiences, and sensations you will encounter on race day. This will include specific, open-water, racing-focused swim sessions; bike intervals at and above race effort; and runs designed to help you find posture, form, and pace immediately following the bike effort. You must merge this with practice in fueling and hydration aligned with intentions for race day.

Goals for Race-Specific Success

- Arrive on race day as fit as your life and training allows, healthy, and with energy to maximize your effort.
- Be confident of your preparation and start races with little that leaves you guessing.
- Approach racing as an opportunity to let all your hard work and commitment express itself when it counts.

Training Modules

Whether getting ready for an Ironman or 70.3, you can follow a progression we have devised at purplepatch and adds the "special sauce" that allows readiness for these events. The mission is to have you arrive to your race very fit, ready for the demands of the race, *and* emotionally and physically fresh so you can perform to your trained potential. You can get very fit over 14 weeks, but you don't want that fitness at the expense of becoming physiologically or emotionally stale. That's a high risk for the busy and committed athlete, but you now understand the intent behind each week in ensuring the training is variable enough to retain your interest by shifting training loads to help keep you fresh.

To ensure that gains from those other intensities remain intact, we have created a modular final 14-week road map leading into the race, with an array of training blocks with different themes. Although there is a clear week-by-week focus, this approach is meant to be a flexible framework that allows a coach or athlete to change the weekly focus to integrate it with lead-in races, work responsibilities, business travel, and other extenuating circumstances of life, as you will see in the case studies that follow.

Here is an overview of each of the weekly themes and how they fit into the overall context of the pre-race buildup.

BUILDING

In these training programs, I have provided a two-week, introductory, building phase to bring in the range of cadence, effort, and strength-based endurance that becomes a feature across the program. These weeks allow a steady ramp up into training and include highly accessible strength-based sessions to improve your awareness of the tools available in riding and running.

Key point: If I were individually coaching an athlete, we would likely integrate these building weeks into training earlier. However, it is important to ramp up to the final race buildup if that type of training is newer to you or if you are relying heavily on the 14-week approach as the lion's share of your training after a less-intensive preseason phase.

STRENGTH-ENDURANCE (SE 1 AND SE 2)

These strength-endurance-based blocks of training are the special sauce of what we do at purplepatch. I have found that it is effective to target both strength-based riding and running in the same weeks, with each week of SE work having a slightly different theme.

Key point: We can typically hit only about two weeks in a row of SE-focused work before we need to shift the load to less strength-based training. Of course, we can then revisit the work as needed after the system and legs are refreshed.

TRANSITION

This week should follow a familiar pattern of training to freshen up and sharpen your skills. Although a typical transition week will carry more overall training load than race week, the *rhythm and intent* will be similar. As you go through the process of training, I encourage you to track and learn what works for you. What helps you feel good while leaning into the important weekend training? Carry those lessons into race week, which should look *similar.* This helps predictability of performance readiness. You will see these transition weeks throughout the road map, added to break up the load, sharpen your form, or even lead into a B race or race simulation to ready yourself for the bigger A race.

Key point: Don't call it a recovery week. Although I discuss removing some of the overall load in these weeks, it is better not to view them as recovery weeks. A transition week is still moving you forward and providing training stimulus but not digging a deeper hole by repeating the heavy load of strength-based or event-specific training. It holds high value in the training progression.

EVENT-SPECIFIC (ES 1 AND ES 2)

These event-specific weeks are as you would expect, with the key sessions focused on event-specific training and simulations. This is a wonderful chance to practice race fueling and hydration, with much of the load similar to a race-day experience. Notice that we still integrate some of the lower-cadence and higher-cadence (rpm) end-of-range riding even in race simulations. I have found this highly effective, if challenging. Be prepared for very specific running off the bike in these weeks.

Key point: We aim to hit two weeks of event-specific training load before freshening up and sharpening form with a shift in focus to speed and power. The range of intensity and overall load are helpful in maintaining progression but remove *some* of the intensity from this training week.

ENDURANCE

I place this endurance and resilience in the middle of the program for padding. There are many ways to skin a cat, but the biggest fear for athletes, especially those on a time-sensitive approach, is whether they have a suitable number of "miles in the legs." To develop resilience and confidence in a safe manner, I will often add a two-week block of endurance-focused load. We begin with a transition-type few days of lower stress, but then ramp up into multiple days of run-focused endurance training. Consistent accumulation of running hours on variable terrain and softer surfaces, if possible, provides a less-specific boost to muscular resilience than that required by running off the bike. Following five to six days of running-focused endurance, the mission is to be able to transfer and hit two to three days of riding miles. This is one of those weeks that requires planning and allotment of additional training hours.

Key point: The actual training hours in an endurance week can be less specific, mostly free of intervals and designed to develop pure resilience. We often refer to the small riding blocks as riding "tours," a chance to explore, have fun, and enjoy riding without obsessing over the metrics.

A 14-Week Roadmap to Success

With these modules of training, we can showcase a few different ways of outlining a road map into a race. First is the master progression, with some notes added to help you navigate the main plan. How the actual flow of an race-specific phase looks is completely dependent on your race planning and schedule, but a typical approach is outlined in the chart that follows.

WEEKS OUT	FOCUS	NOTES
14	Building	Introduction to the range of training focus, with an endurance running focus on the weekend
13	Building	Progression of ramping effort and range of training, with an endurance riding focus on the weekend
12	SE 1	Strength-endurance (SE) and end-of-range training
11	SE 2	Strength-endurance (SE) and end-of-range training
10	Transition	Freshen up and remove some of the SE work
9	Endurance	Final prep for a 70.3 B race or race simulation
8	Transition	Recuperation and sharpening
7	ES 1	Event-specific sessions with SE work integrated
6	ES 2	Event-specific sessions with SE work integrated
5	Transition	Freshen up and remove some of the work
4	ES 1	Event-specific week
3	ES 2	Event-specific week
2	Transition	Freshen up and remove some of the work
1	Race week	Final prep for an Ironman or 70.3 A or B race

Of course, your life might not mesh directly with the progression of this road map either because of travel, work, and family commitments or because of other races you might have entered. If you grasp the meaning and intent of each of the training we eks, it is not overly difficult to manage the progression differently. Let's look at a couple of examples where I manipulated the training progression to fit the nuances of the specific life challenges of these two individuals.

Case Study: Ashley, an Amateur Age-Group Athlete

This plan shows how an athlete can smartly fit in a 70.3 B race in the nine-week lead-up nine weeks to a 70.3 A race. The key here is to plan transition weeks on each side of the B race before getting back into event-specific work.

WEEKS OUT	FOCUS	NOTES
14	Building	Introductory building week with an endurance-focused run on weekend
13	Endurance	Build resilience with a run-focused endurance week into a riding tour
12	SE 1	A few lighter days' recuperation from the endurance week, then heavy SE work
11	SE 2	Heavy SE work
10	Transition	No SE the week prior to race week to avoid too much fatigue
9	Race week	Final prep for an Ironman 70.3 B race
8	Transition	A few days recuperation, then ramp up into weekend training
7	ES 1	Event-specific week
6	ES 2	Event-specific week
5	Transition	Freshen up
4	ES 1	Event-specific week
3	ES 2	Event-specific week
2	Transition	Freshen up and remove some of the work but still maintain the rhythm and intensity
1	Race week	Final prep for an Ironman 70.3 A race

Case Study: Pat, a Corporate Executive Who Travels Frequently

Just because you have a 14-week road map to your A race in front of you doesn't mean it will be easy to follow that plan entirely, especially if you're a time-starved athlete with a big life. This example of a real-life, imperfect road map shows how a logistically challenged athlete can remain on a path to success. Remember, juggling travel on a regular basis brings additional stress, so the goal is to keep moving forward while also maintaining good health, which means the casualty is some of the heavy work. It is better to adjust, evolve, and retain productivity than to cram in workouts and force fatigue and staleness. This is known as performance within the context of life and, specifically, the context of *your* life.

For this type of athlete, the road map might also require resetting the lens to match the reality of frequent business trips. The athlete highlighted in this real example was traveling from the United States to Europe and Asia on a regular basis, raising capital for a new company. Despite that regular travel, we adapted his schedule to optimize his training to maintain his fitness and race readiness. As a result, he didn't have the huge breakthroughs that he had in previous years when he wasn't traveling, but his performance didn't decline drastically, either. In many ways, his success was managing not to regress (or to stop training entirely) amid the added stress and complications of constantly being in different time zones with limited ability to train consistently.

WEEKS OUT	FOCUS	NOTES
14	Building	Introduction to the range of training focus
13	Transition (travel)	Pat's first big trip requires removal of some of the load and intensity
12	SE 1	Strength-endurance (SE) and end-of-range training using the two weeks at home to hit some backbone training
11	SE 2	More SE work and end-of-range training
10	Transition (travel)	Freshen up and remove some of the SE work, but the travel might not allow real recuperation; red flags for fatigue here
9	Transition	Despite being home, Pat stays *feeling* fresh by holding back on very heavy SE work
8	Endurance	Pat is worried about race readiness, so an endurance-run and riding tour week for resilience and confidence; only weekend he clears his schedule for both days
7	Transition (travel)	Another week of international travel, but he leaves feeling good about himself with the "miles in his legs"
6	Transition	Despite being home, Pat stays *feeling* fresh by holding back on very heavy ES work
5	ES 1	Pat gets two weeks at home, with a chance to make up some lost ground with ES work
4	ES 2	Another week to bank event-specific focus, which adds to Pat's confidence
3	Transition (race)	Loading more event-specific training this close to the race can be challenging, but the aim is to keep Pat's body resilient and his mind confident; added a local Olympic-distance race so he can execute with a high effort, but it won't negatively affect his key race in two weeks
2	Transition	Recover from the Olympic-distance race and begin to freshen up for the A race
1	Race week	Race-prep week

The Master Plan

What follows is a blueprint of the key sessions in each week of training leading up to your Ironman (pp. 232–233) and 70.3 Ironman (pp. 290–291). It is important to remember we're only highlighting the main session of each day, not the additional supporting sessions on most days. Typically, we keep Mondays as lighter days of recuperation and Fridays as prep days, or bridges, for the bigger training workload on the coming weekend. Supporting sessions on these days do not appear on the matrix. The remaining days have the central focus session but might include additional supporting sessions where it illustrates important aspects of your preparation. Of course, not many time-starved athletes will be able to get in 13 sessions detailed in the full training plan (see Ironman-Distance Race-Prep Program, pp. 234–288, and Ironman 70.3-Distance Race-Prep Program, pp. 292–346), but it gives you an example of how such a week might look. Make this plan work for your life: If that means Mondays are harder days and Tuesdays are lighter days, so be it.

Ironman-Distance
Race-Prep Program

IRONMAN Overview of Key Workouts in the Race-Prep Phase

	WEEK TYPE	M	T	W	TH
WEEK 1	BUILD		KEY SWIM #1 Endurance, Building	KEY BIKE #1 End-of-Range, Strength-Endurance (low rpm)	KEY RUN #1 Event-Specific, Intervals
WEEK 2	BUILD		KEY SWIM #1 Endurance, Short Intervals	KEY BIKE #1 + RUN End-of-Range, Strength-Endurance (low rpm)	Supporting Swim Endurance, Short Intervals
WEEK 3	STRENGTH- ENDURANCE		KEY SWIM #1 Event-Specific, Threshold	KEY BIKE #1 + RUN End-of-Range, Strength-Endurance (low rpm)	KEY RUN #1 Intervals, Strength
WEEK 4	STRENGTH- ENDURANCE		KEY SWIM #1 Endurance, Building	KEY BIKE #1 + RUN End-of-Range, Strength-Endurance (low rpm)	KEY SWIM #2 Event-Specific, Threshold
WEEK 5	TRANSITION to Endurance		Supporting Swim Technical, Form	KEY BIKE #1 + RUN End-of-Range, High Cadence (max sprints)	KEY SWIM #1 Event-Specific, Pyramid
WEEK 6	ENDURANCE		KEY SWIM #1 Endurance, Over- Distance	KEY RUN #3 *Continues weekend work* General Endurance (1-2 hr.) + Optional Evening Run	Supporting Swim Endurance, Short Intervals
WEEK 7	TRANSITION		Supporting Swim Endurance, Short Intervals	KEY BIKE #1 + RUN End-of-Range, High Cadence (max sprints)	KEY SWIM #1 Intervals, Building
WEEK 8	EVENT-SPECIFIC		KEY SWIM #1 Endurance, Over-Distance	KEY BIKE #1 + RUN End-of-Range, High Cadence (high/low rpm)	Supporting Swim Endurance, Short Intervals
WEEK 9	EVENT-SPECIFIC		KEY SWIM #1 Intervals, Building	Supporting Bike Technical, Prep	KEY RUN #1 Intervals, Strength
WEEK 10	TRANSITION		Supporting Swim Endurance, Short Intervals	KEY BIKE #1 + RUN End-of-Range, High Cadence (max sprints)	KEY SWIM #1 Intervals, Building
WEEK 11	EVENT-SPECIFIC		KEY SWIM #1 Endurance, Building	KEY RUN #1 Intervals, Speed	Easier Supporting Sessions (Swim, Bike)
WEEK 12	EVENT-SPECIFIC		KEY SWIM #1 Endurance, Over-Distance	KEY BIKE #1 + RUN Event-Specific, Intervals	KEY RUN #1 General Endurance (building effort)
WEEK 13	TRANSITION		KEY BIKE #1 + RUN End-of-Range, High Cadence (max sprints)	Supporting Swim Endurance, Short Intervals	KEY SWIM #1 Endurance, Over-Distance (Ironman form)
WEEK 14	RACE		KEY BIKE #1 + RUN Technical, Prep	KEY SWIM #1 Intervals, Building (feel-good) Supporting Run Technical, Activation	Supporting Bike Technical, Recovery

F	SA	SU	TOTAL TIME (HR.)
	KEY BIKE #2 + RUN Event-Specific, Intervals	KEY SWIM #2 Event-Specific, Threshold	6–8.5
	KEY RUN #1 Intervals, Tempo	KEY BIKE #2 + RUN Endurance, Over-Distance	7.6–11.3
	KEY BIKE #2 + RUN Event-Specific, Intervals	KEY SWIM #2 Endurance, Over-Distance	7.3–8.6
	KEY RUN #1 Intervals, Strength	KEY BIKE #2 General Endurance (2–5 hr.)	6.4–10.4
	KEY RUN #1 General Endurance (1.5–2 hr.)	KEY RUN #2 General Endurance (75–100 min.)	5.7–7.3
KEY BIKE #1 End-of-Range, Strength-Endurance *Double trainer ride*	KEY BIKE #2 + RUN Endurance, Over-Distance Riding Tour (3–6 hr.)	KEY BIKE #3 General Endurance (2–4 hr.) KEY SWIM #2 Event-Specific, Simulation	10.8–17.75
	KEY BIKE #2 + RUN End-of-Range, Building	KEY SWIM #2 Event-Specific, Pyramid	5.4–7.8
	KEY RUN #1 Intervals, Tempo	KEY BIKE #2 General Endurance (2–4 hr.) KEY SWIM #2 Endurance, Over-Distance	8.2–12.75
	KEY BIKE #1 + RUN End-of-Range, Strength- Endurance (high/low rpm)	KEY SWIM #2 Endurance, Over-Distance	7–9.5
	KEY BIKE #2 + RUN End-of-Range, Building	KEY SWIM #2 Event-Specific, Pyramid	6.25–8.5
	KEY SWIM #2 Endurance, Building	KEY BIKE #1 + RUN Event-Specific, Simulation (rpm mix)	8.75–12.2
	KEY SWIM #2 Endurance, Over-Distance KEY RUN #2 Intervals, Tempo	KEY SWIM #3 Event-Specific, Simulation	9.25–10.4
	KEY BIKE #2 + RUN End-of-Range, Building	KEY SWIM #2 Event-Specific, Pyramid KEY RUN #1 Event-Specific, Intervals	7.4–8.7
Supporting Bike + Run Technical, Prep	KEY SWIM #2 Technical, Prep KEY BIKE #2 Technical, Activation	**IRONMAN RACE**	3.6–4.6

233

FOCUS This is a building week to prepare you for the challenging strength-endurance work ahead. The key sessions are similar to preseason training—building blocks with a touch of speed and intensity.

WEEKLY OVERVIEW

	M	T	W	TH	F	SA	SU	TOTAL
S1	50 min.	45–60 min.	95–105 min.	45–75 min.	45–60 min.	2–2.5 hr.	1–1.5 hr.	11.25–
S2	—	40–60 min.	30 min.	45–70 min.	30 min.	—	70–110 min.	14.8 hr.

MONDAY

SESSION ONE

SUPPORTING BIKE
TECHNICAL Activation, 50 min.

Warm-Up 10 min. easy spin

Pre-Main
10 min. ramp effort from Z1 to Z3

Main 3 rounds of:
2 min. Z1 ramp rpm to fast, 30 sec. easy,
90 sec. Z2 ramp rpm to fast, 1 min. easy,
1 min. Z3 ramp rpm to fast, 90 sec. easy,
30 sec. Z4 ramp rpm to fast, 2 min. easy

Scale for Time Trim as needed or skip if unable to complete.

Scale for Fatigue You should not have heavy fatigue today.

SESSION TWO

PM OFF

TUESDAY

SESSION ONE

KEY SWIM
ENDURANCE Building, 1800–3350

Warm-Up 5–10 min. easy with mix of strokes

Pre-Main 3–6 rounds with paddles and fins:
50 at 75%,
50 at 85%,
50 at 95%
Always 10 sec. rest

Main
9 × 150–250
Increase effort/pace every 2 intervals:
1 and 2 at 65%, 3 and 4 at 75%, 5 and 6 at 85%,
7 and 8 at 95%, 9 at MAX
Always 30 sec. rest

Add-On 200 cool-down

Scale for Time Drop Main set to 6 intervals: 1 at 65%, 1 at 75%, 1 at 85%, 1 at 95%, 2 at best effort.

Scale for Fatigue Drop Main set to 6 intervals and only build to 85%.

SESSION TWO

SUPPORTING RUN
ENDURANCE General Endurance, 40–60 min.

Warm-Up 10 min. easy
Add dynamic warm-up if possible.

Main
30–50 min.
Every 4th min. or so, check on form, posture, etc.
Aim for best MFP (minimal form pace). Do not exceed Z2 effort.

Scale for Time Scale duration as needed.

Scale for Fatigue Trim duration or skip if needed.

WEDNESDAY

KEY **BIKE**
END-OF-RANGE Strength-Endurance, 95–105 min.

Warm-Up 10 min. easy spin

Pre-Main 2 rounds of:
4 min. Z2 build rpm to fast,
3 min. build effort Z1 to Z3/Z4,
2 min. Z2 build rpm to fast,
1 min. build effort Z1 to Z3/Z4

Main 3 rounds Z3/Z4 at low rpm, progress as:
3 min. at 65 rpm,
2 min. at 55 rpm,
1 min. at 45 rpm,
2 min. at 55 rpm,
3 min. at 65 rpm
5 min. Z1 between rounds

10–15 min. at IM effort
2 min. easy
5–10 min. at IM effort

Scale for Time Cut the 4 min. interval from the Pre-Main set and trim the number of intervals in the Main set.

Scale for Fatigue Maintain the Pre-Main set but convert the Main set to 4 rounds Z2 build rpm to fast on each.

STRENGTH & CONDITIONING
30 min.

Scale for Time Be sure you hit at least 5–10 min. of mobility.

Scale for Fatigue This is a floating session that can occur any day.

THURSDAY

KEY **RUN**
EVENT-SPECIFIC Intervals, 45–75 min.

Warm-Up 15 min. of smooth build to MFP with 2 min. recovery

Main
5 min. at IM effort, smooth
4 min. at half-IM effort, strong
3 min. at 10K effort, very strong
4 min. at half-IM effort, strong
5 min. at IM effort, smooth

6 min. smooth form to finish

Add-On 30 min. MFP run

Scale for Time Trim Warm-Up and drop the MFP run at the end of the workout.

Scale for Fatigue Begin very easy and do a gradual ramp in effort, but can convert to a feel-good endurance run.

SUPPORTING **SWIM**
ENDURANCE Short Intervals, 2450–3300

This is a recommended session.

Warm-Up 300–600 with non-free on every 4th lap

Pre-Main Pull set with paddles, snorkel, and buoy:
200, 175, 150, 125, 100, 75, 50, 25
All with 10 sec. rest
Progress effort as you go to feel good.

Main
25–30 × 50 at 85% effort with 5–7 sec. rest
Choose a send-off interval and aim to leave on the same time each 50.

Add-On 12 × 25 with paddles, do as 3 rounds of:
1 easy form, 2 building effort to fast, 3 and 4 fast
Always 15 sec. rest

Scale for Time Reduce the number of 50s you complete with good form and rhythm.

Scale for Fatigue Reduce Main set to 20 × 50 at 80% and complete with good form and rhythm.

FRIDAY

SUPPORTING **BIKE**
TECHNICAL Prep, 45–60 min.

This is a recommended session.

Main
45–60 min.
First and last 10 min. at >95 rpm with minimum power to maintain chain tension.
Include 4–6 × 30 sec. build to Z5 effort (10 sec. at Z3, Z4, and Z5)
3-4 min. spin between each 30 sec. build

TRAINER OPTION

Warm-Up 10-20 min. Z1 spin

Pre-Main
5 × 90 sec. Z1 at very fast rpm
30 sec. spin between intervals

Main 3–7 rounds of:
30 sec. build as 10 sec. at Z3, Z4, then Z5,
2 min. Z3 steady and smooth riding (aiming to settle post Z5 effort)
2 min. Z1 spin between rounds

Scale for Time This is an optional ride.

Scale for Fatigue Remove the Z5 work, but moving the body will help. Do something that feels good.

STRENGTH & CONDITIONING
30 min.

Scale for Time Be sure you hit at least 5–10 min. of mobility.

Scale for Fatigue This is a floating session that can occur any day.

SATURDAY

KEY **BIKE + RUN**
EVENT-SPECIFIC Intervals, 2–2.5 hr.

Warm-Up 30–45 min. smooth

Pre-Main
6 min. as 4 × 90 sec. in Z1, Z2, Z3, Z4 to open the engine

Main 3 rounds of:
8 min. Z2 smooth,
6 min. Z3 strong,
2 min. Z4 very strong
5 min. spin between rounds

5 min. at IM effort (no data)

Add-On 15 min. smooth home with good form

RUN OFF THE BIKE

3 min. ramp to Z3, 1 min. MFP
2 min. Z4, 1 min. MFP
1 min. Z5, 2 min. MFP
1 min. Z4, 1 min. MFP
3 min. Z3

Scale for Time Trim Warm-Up to 15-20 min. and do just 2 rounds of Main set.

Scale for Fatigue Transition to a feel-good endurance ride.

PM OFF

SUNDAY

KEY **SWIM**
EVENT-SPECIFIC Threshold, 2400–2700

Warm-Up 10 min. easy with mix of strokes

Pre-Main
100 smooth
2 × 75 build to fast
3 × 50 build to fast
4 × 25 fast
All with 15 sec. rest

Main With paddles and buoy:
100 at 70% with 20 sec. rest
100 at 80% with 10 sec. rest
1 × 100 at 90–95% with 5 sec. rest

100 at 70% with 20 sec. rest
100 at 80% with 10 sec. rest
2 × 100 at 90–95% with 5 sec. rest

100 at 70% with 20 sec. rest
100 at 80% with 10 sec. rest
3 × 100 at 90–95% with 5 sec. rest

100 at 70% with 20 sec. rest
100 at 80% with 10 sec. rest
4 × 100 at 90–95% with 5 sec. rest

100 easy to finish

Add-On 12 × 25 with paddles and fins, swim as
4 rounds of: easy, MAX, MAX
Always 10 sec. rest

Scale for Time Finish the Main set at 3 × 100 and
skip the Add-On 25s.

Scale for Fatigue Maintain the rhythm and intent,
but scale intensity for hard 100s to 80–85% effort.

SUPPORTING **RUN**
ENDURANCE General Endurance, 70–110 min.

This is a recommended session.

Warm-Up 10 min. easy

Main
60–100 min.
MFP run on variable terrain. If you are injury-prone,
a softer surface is ideal.
Take short 20–40 sec. walk breaks as needed to
retain form and manage heart rate.

For capable runners, control overall pace with
inclusion of downhill leg speed and form-based
activation: bench strides, bounding, challenging
terrain, etc.

Scale for Time Reduce duration as needed, but it is
important to get this run in.

Scale for Fatigue Include more walk breaks and
keep the effort conversational. Make total run no
more than 60 min.

IRONMAN

RACE SPECIFIC

FOCUS This week develops the initial strength-based running that will feature heavily in the program. The midweek bike focuses on maintaining a low rpm at progressively harder efforts, which builds strength-endurance.

WEEKLY OVERVIEW

	M	T	W	TH	F	SA	SU	TOTAL
S1	50 min.	1–1.5 hr.	2.25 hr.	45–70 min.	45–60 min.	1–1.5 hr.	2.5–5 hr.	12–
S2	—	40–70 min.	30 min.	—	30 min.	70–85 min.	—	16.5 hr.

MONDAY

SESSION ONE

SUPPORTING BIKE
TECHNICAL Recovery, 50 min.

Warm-Up 10 min. easy spin

Pre-Main
10 min. ramp effort from Z1 to Z3

Main 3 rounds of:
2 min. Z1 ramp rpm to fast, 30 sec. easy,
90 sec. Z2 ramp rpm to fast, 1 min. easy,
1 min. Z3 ramp rpm to fast, 90 sec. easy,
30 sec. Z4 ramp rpm to fast, 2 min. easy

Scale for Time Trim as needed or skip if unable to complete.

Scale for Fatigue If you are very sore you can maintain all the rpm builds in the Main set as Z1 to Z2 and keep it low power/effort.

SESSION TWO

PM OFF

TUESDAY

SESSION ONE

KEY SWIM
ENDURANCE Short Intervals, 3500–4100

Warm-Up 5–10 min. easy with mix of strokes

Pre-Main 2 rounds with buoy and snorkel:
200 at 70%,
2 × 100 at 75%,
2 × 50 at 80%,
2 × 25 at 90%
All with 10 sec. rest

Main
12 × 25 at 90% with great tempo and rhythm with 2–3 sec. rest right into:
6 × 50 with 10 sec. rest

12 × 25 at 90% with great tempo and rhythm with 2–3 sec. rest right into:
3 × 100 with 20 sec. rest

12 × 25 at 90% with great tempo and rhythm with 2–3 sec. rest right into:
2 × 150 with 30 sec. rest

12 × 25 at 90% with great tempo and rhythm with 2–3 sec. rest right into:
300 straight swimming

Maintain rhythm and form of the 25s on longer distances.

Add-On Up to 3 rounds with paddles (parachute or ankle strap OK):
2 × 25 MAX with 20 sec. rest, 50 easy float, 50 MAX with 30 sec. rest, 2 × 25 easy

Scale for Time Trim Pre-Main to a single round. Do Main set as 12 × 25, then skip the next 2 sets and go straight to 3 × 100. Then trim the 25s if needed.

Scale for Fatigue Trim Pre-Main to one round, then complete Main set through the end of the 100s.

CONTINUES…

TUESDAY

SESSION TWO

SUPPORTING RUN
ENDURANCE General Endurance, 40–70 min.

This is a recommended session.

Warm-Up 10 min. easy
Add dynamic warm-up if possible.

Main
30–60 min.
Aim for best MFP. Every 4th min. or so check in on form, posture, etc. Do not exceed Z2 effort.

Keep the effort down by adding leg speed, striding/bounding, and activation; also practice the run/walk protocol.

Scale for Time Simple scale of duration as needed.

Scale for Fatigue Trim duration or skip if needed.

WEDNESDAY

SESSION ONE

KEY BIKE + RUN
END-OF-RANGE Strength-Endurance, 2.25 hr.

Warm-Up 10 min. at >90 rpm

Pre-Main
1 min. Z2 smooth at 65 rpm,
3 min. Z2 smooth at 65 rpm,
5 min. Z2 smooth at 65 rpm
All with 3 min. Z1 at >95 rpm

Main
5 × 6 min. at <65 rpm, progress as:
1 smooth, 2 strong, 3 very strong,
4 strong, 5 smooth
5 min. Z1 at >95 rpm between intervals

15 min. IM (no data) and smooth home

RUN OFF THE BIKE

5 min. ramp to IM effort, 2 min. easy
3 min. at above IM effort, 2 min. easy
3 min. well above IM effort, 2 min. easy
3 min. at above IM effort, 2 min. easy
5–10 min. IM effort, form-focused

Scale for Time Trim the Main set to 3 intervals: 2 strong, 1 very strong. Convert the run to 15 min. Build to above IM effort by feel.

Scale for Fatigue Maintain the Pre-Main but convert the Main set to 4 × 10 min. Z2; build rpm to fast on each. Remove all work from the brick run and convert to smooth 15 min. with good form. Shift run to 10 min. form-based off the bike.

SESSION TWO

STRENGTH & CONDITIONING
30 min.

Scale for Time Be sure you hit at least 5–10 min. of mobility.

Scale for Fatigue This is a floating session that can occur any day.

THURSDAY

SESSION ONE

SUPPORTING **SWIM**
ENDURANCE Short Intervals, 2700–3800

This is a recommended session.

Warm-Up 300–600, swim every 4th lap as non-free

Pre-Main Pull set with paddles, snorkel, and buoy: 200, 175, 150, 125, 100, 75, 50, 25
All with 10 sec. rest
Progress effort as you go to feel good.

Main
30–40 × 50 with 5-7 sec. rest
Choose a send-off interval and aim to leave on the same time each 50. Always swim at 85% effort with heightened focus on rhythm and intent of the session.

Add-On 12 × 25 with paddles, swim as 3 rounds of: 1 easy form, 2 building effort to fast, 3 and 4 fast
All with 15 sec. rest

Scale for Time Reduce the number of 50s you complete with good form and rhythm.

Scale for Fatigue Skip the Add-On session and reduce the Pre-Main set to begin at the 150. You can still complete the Main set, but with a focus on form rather than hitting 85% (reduce to 70–75% effort).

SESSION TWO

PM OFF

FRIDAY

SESSION ONE

SUPPORTING **BIKE**
TECHNICAL Activation, 45–60 min.

Main
45–60 min.
First and last 10 min. at >95 rpm with minimum power while retaining chain tension. Focus on posture and good pedaling.
Include 4–6 × 30 sec. build to Z5 effort (10 sec. at Z3, Z4, and Z5)
3–4 min. spin between each 30 sec. build

Finish with smooth endurance ride home

TRAINER OPTION

Warm-Up 10–20 min. Z1 easy

Pre-Main
5 × 90 sec. Z1 at very fast rpm
30 sec. spin between intervals

Main 4–6 rounds of:
15 sec. build to Z5 effort (5 sec. at Z3, Z4, and Z5)
3 min. Z1 spin between intervals

Scale for Time Scale duration as needed.

Scale for Fatigue Remove the Z5 effort work. Do something that feels good.

SESSION TWO

STRENGTH & CONDITIONING
30 min.

Scale for Time Be sure you hit at least 5–10 min. of mobility.

Scale for Fatigue This is a floating session that can occur any day.

SATURDAY

SUPPORTING **SWIM**
ENDURANCE Over-Distance, 3300–3600

This is a recommended session.

Warm-Up 10 min. easy with mix of strokes

Pre-Main
100 smooth
2 × 75 build to fast
3 × 50 build to fast
4 × 25 fast
All with 15 sec. rest

Main
100 with toys, 200 swim at 80%,
200 with toys, 400 swim at 80%,
300 with toys, 600 swim at 80%,
200 with toys, 800 swim at 80%
All with 1 min. rest
Toys are snorkel and buoy to help retain form.
In the solid swims, sight 3 times per lap.

Add-On 12 × 25 with paddles and fins, do as
4 rounds of: easy, MAX, MAX
All with 10 sec. rest

Scale for Time Remove the speed Add-On, as well
as trim the Main set to finish at the 600 as needed.

Scale for Fatigue Remove the additional speed at
the end, and trim the Main set to the 600.

KEY **RUN**
INTERVALS Tempo, 70–85 min.

Warm-Up 10 min. at MFP

Pre-Main
3 × 2 min., build by 30 sec. to strong
30 sec. rest between intervals

Main
2 × 15 min. sustained Z3+, strong but sustainable
10 min. at MFP between intervals

Add-On 10–15 min. easy endurance running at
the end

Scale for Time Remove any additional endurance
running and scale Warm-Up as needed.

Scale for Fatigue Transfer into a variable trail run
up to 75 min. with walk breaks on the steep grades.

SUNDAY

KEY **BIKE + RUN**
ENDURANCE Over-Distance, 2.5–5 hr.

Main
2–4.5 hr.
After at least 30 min. build in with variation as
terrain allows:
5 × 6 min. at <65 rpm strong in aero position
5 min. Z2 at >80 rpm between intervals

Carry on from the last effort into 15 min. IM effort
(no data) at choice of cadence.

TRAINER OPTION

Warm-Up 30 min., build from Z1 to Z3

Pre-Main 2 rounds:
2 min. Z2/Z3, 30 sec. easy,
90 sec. Z3, 30 sec. easy,
1 min. Z3/Z4, 30 sec. easy

Main
5 × 6 min. Z3 at <65 rpm
4 min. Z1 spin at fast rpm between intervals

Add-On 15 min. build by 5 min. (5 min. at Z2,
Z2/Z3, and Z3)

RUN OFF THE BIKE

20–30 min. with good form at smooth to moderate
(steady) effort

Scale for Time Trim Warm-Up and do 1 round of
Pre-Main set. Change Main set to 3 × 6 min. at low
rpm, then 15 min. form-based run.

Scale for Fatigue Transition to a feel-good
endurance ride.

PM OFF

FOCUS These are building block sessions that mix low- and high-rpm work as you evolve your fitness and progress toward the main race. A challenging low-rpm bike ride is the main feature of this strength-endurance week.

WEEKLY OVERVIEW

	M	T	W	TH	F	SA	SU	TOTAL
S1	40–60 min.	1–1.5 hr.	2 hr.	45–70 min.	45–60 min.	2.5–2.75 hr.	1–1.5 hr.	12.5–16 hr.
S2	—	40–80 min.	30 min.	50 min.	30 min.	—	80–110 min.	

MONDAY

SESSION ONE

SUPPORTING RUN
ENDURANCE General Endurance, 40–60 min.

Warm-Up 10 min. easy
Add dynamic warm-up if possible.

Main
30–50 min. smooth
Focus on form and posture. No more than Z2 effort.

MFP running with walk breaks as needed to retain the ability to run with form and maintain a conversational and endurance-focused performance.

Scale for Time Trim as needed or skip if unable to complete.

Scale for Fatigue If your muscles are sore from last week, convert to a 30–45 min. flush/spin on the bike or a very easy 1–2 km swim.

SESSION TWO

PM OFF

TUESDAY

SESSION ONE

KEY SWIM
EVENT-SPECIFIC Threshold, 2400–4850

Warm-Up 10 min. easy

Pre-Main 2–3 rounds with snorkel:
300 at 70% with 30 sec. rest,
3 × 50 form-based swimming, building tempo, effort, and stroke rate throughout
All with 10 sec. rest

Main With paddles (and ankle-strap for advanced swimmers):
15–30 × 100 at 80%, keep stroke rate up, swim every 5th 100 very strong (Z4)
All with 10 sec. rest

Add-On 2 rounds of power:
4 × 25 MAX with paddles,
150 form-based swimming

Scale for Time Trim Pre-Main to one round and reduce the number of 100s if needed.

Scale for Fatigue Trim Pre-Main to one round. Use fins for Main set and trim to 10–20 × 100.

SESSION TWO

SUPPORTING RUN
ENDURANCE General Endurance, 40–80 min.

This is a recommended session.

Warm-Up 10 min. easy
Add dynamic warm-up if possible.

Main
30–70 min. Z2
Every 4th min. or so check in on form, posture, etc.
Do not exceed Z2 effort.

Scale for Time Simple scale of duration as needed.

Scale for Fatigue Trim duration or skip if needed.

WEDNESDAY

KEY **BIKE + RUN**
END-OF-RANGE Strength-Endurance, 2 hr.

Warm-Up 10 min. at >90 rpm

Pre-Main
1 min. Z2 at 65 rpm,
3 min. Z2 at 65 rpm,
5 min. Z2 at 65 rpm
All with 3 min. Z1 at >95 rpm

Main
5 × 6 min. at <65 rpm, progress as:
1 smooth, 2 strong, 3 very strong,
4 strong, 5 smooth
5 min. Z1 at >95 rpm between intervals

5 min. at IM effort (no data) and smooth home

RUN OFF THE BIKE

3 min. ramp to Z3, 1 min. MFP
2 min. Z4, 1 min. MFP
1 min. Z5, 2 min. MFP
1 min. Z4, 1 min. MFP
3 min. Z3

Scale for Time Trim Pre-Main set to one round and reduce the Main set intervals and rests (e.g., 3 on, 2 off). Convert the run to 15 min., build to above IM effort by feel.

Scale for Fatigue Evolve the Main set to 4 × 10 min. Z2, build rpm to fast on each interval. Remove all work from the run and convert to a 15 min. smooth, form-based run.

STRENGTH & CONDITIONING
30 min.

Scale for Time Be sure you get at least 5–10 min. of mobility.

Scale for Fatigue This is a floating session that can occur any day.

THURSDAY

SUPPORTING **SWIM**
ENDURANCE Short Intervals, 2150–3200

Warm-Up 10 min. easy

Pre-Main 5–7 rounds with fins:
50 at 70% with 10 sec. rest,
50 at 80% with 5–7 sec. rest,
50 at 90% with 3–5 sec. rest

Then, 2 rounds of:
2 × 25 fast, 50 easy,
50 fast, 2 × 25 easy
All with 15 sec. rest

Main With paddles:
40–70 × 25 at 85–90% with only 2–5 sec. rest between intervals

Scale for Time Scale Pre-Main and Main as needed.

Scale for Fatigue Cut Main set to 20–40 × 25 at 80%, without paddles.

KEY **RUN**
INTERVALS Strength, 50 min.

Warm-Up 5–10 min. easy

Pre-Main Prep with feel-good builds, up to 2 rounds of:
40 sec. moderate, 30 sec. easy,
30 sec. strong, 30 sec. easy,
20 sec. strong, 30 sec. easy,
10 sec. very strong, 30 sec. easy

Main 2 loops of hill running:
3 min. flat and smooth, MFP
90 sec. at 4% grade, very strong and sustained powerful running
30 sec. MAX at 6–10%, driving off the toes, arms pumping behind, eyes up
2 min. downhill on shallow grade (2–4%), pick up leg speed but not hard
Note: If you cannot find a loop, run on the treadmill. Use 1% for flat and 0% for downhill.

Finish with 20 min. steady form-based running above IM Z3 to Z3+ feeling good.

Scale for Time Trim Warm-Up and skip the final 20 min. of the Main set.

Scale for Fatigue Begin easy and gradually ramp effort. Convert to a feel-good endurance run on rolling hills if needed.

FRIDAY

SUPPORTING **BIKE**
TECHNICAL Prep, 45–60 min.

Main
45–60 min.
First and last 10 min. at >95 rpm with minimum power to maintain chain tension. Focus on posture and good pedaling.
Include 4–6 × 30 sec. build as 10 sec. at Z3, Z4, and Z5
3–4 min. between each 30 sec. build

Steady endurance, smooth home

TRAINER OPTION

Warm-Up 10-20 min. Z1 spin

Pre-Main
5 × 90 sec. Z1 at very fast rpm
30 sec. spin between intervals

Main 4–6 rounds of:
15 sec. build as 5 sec. at Z3, Z4, and Z5
3 min. Z1 spin between intervals

Scale for Time Scale duration as needed.

Scale for Fatigue Remove the Z5 effort work. Do something that feels good.

STRENGTH & CONDITIONING
30 min.

Scale for Time Be sure you get at least 5–10 min. of mobility.

Scale for Fatigue This is a floating session that can occur any day.

SATURDAY

KEY **BIKE + RUN**
EVENT-SPECIFIC Intervals, 2.5–2.75 hr.

Warm-Up 30–45 min. smooth

Pre-Main
6 min. build to open the engine as 90 sec. at Z1, Z2, Z3, Z4

Main 3 rounds of:
25 min. Z2/Z3 to Z3, IM effort,
5 min. stronger (Z3+), above IM effort

RUN OFF THE BIKE

2 rounds of:
4 min. form-based running,
3 min. at IM effort,
3 min. above IM effort,
3 min. at IM effort

Scale for Time Trim Warm-Up and shift the Main set to: 1 under, 2 at, 1 above race effort, on both the bike and the run.

Scale for Fatigue Transition to a feel-good endurance ride.

PM OFF

SUNDAY

KEY **SWIM**
ENDURANCE Over-Distance, 3300–4700

Warm-Up 10 min. easy with mix of strokes

Pre-Main
100 smooth
2 × 75 build to fast
3 × 50 build to fast
4 × 25 fast
All with 15 sec. rest

Main With paddles (add ankle strap for advanced swimmers):
100 with toys, 200 at 80%,
200 with toys, 400 at 80%,
300 with toys, 600 at 80%,
200 with toys, 800 at 80%
100 with toys, 1000 at 80% (for advanced swimmers)
All with 1 min. rest between intervals
In the solid swims, sight 3 times per lap.

Add-On 12 × 25 with paddles and fins, do as
4 rounds of: easy, MAX, MAX
Always 10 sec. rest

Scale for Time Remove the speed Add-On, and trim the Main set to finish at the 600 or 800 as needed.

Scale for Fatigue Finish the Main set at the 600.

SUPPORTING **RUN**
ENDURANCE General Endurance, 80–110 min.

This is a recommended session.

Warm-Up 10 min. easy

Main
70–100 min.
Low-stress endurance run on variable terrain. If you are injury prone, a softer surface is ideal.
Take short 20–40 sec. walk breaks as needed to retain form.

Scale for Time Scale duration as needed.

Scale for Fatigue Include more walk breaks and keep the effort purely conversational. Run no more than 60 min.

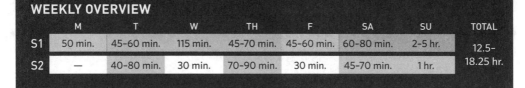

WEEK

4

FOCUS Strength-endurance work is very challenging, especially Saturday's Key Run where you are asked to maintain great form and posture while running very hard uphill. Midweek highlights include the strong, end-of-range ride with a run-off-the-bike and the beginning of event-specific swimming.

WEEKLY OVERVIEW

	M	T	W	TH	F	SA	SU	TOTAL
S1	50 min.	45–60 min.	115 min.	45–70 min.	45–60 min.	60–80 min.	2–5 hr.	12.5–
S2	—	40–80 min.	30 min.	70–90 min.	30 min.	45–70 min.	1 hr.	18.25 hr.

MONDAY

SESSION ONE

SUPPORTING BIKE
TECHNICAL Prep, 50 min.

Warm-Up 10 min. easy spin

Pre-Main
10 min. ramp effort from Z1 to Z3

Main 3 rounds of:
2 min. Z1 ramp rpm to fast, 30 sec. easy,
90 sec. Z2 ramp rpm to fast, 1 min. easy,
1 min. Z3 ramp rpm to fast, 90 sec. easy,
30 sec. Z4 ramp rpm to fast, 2 min. easy

Scale for Time Trim as needed or skip if unable to complete.

Scale for Fatigue If you are very sore maintain the rpm builds in the Main set, but keep it low power/effort, Z1/Z2.

SESSION TWO

PM OFF

TUESDAY

SESSION ONE

KEY SWIM
ENDURANCE Building, 1800–3350

Warm-Up 5–10 min. easy with mix of strokes

Pre-Main 3–6 rounds with paddles and fins:
50 at 75%,
50 at 85%,
50 at 95%
All with 10 sec. rest

Main
9 × 150–250, progress every 2 intervals as:
2 at 65%, 2 at 75%, 2 at 85%, 2 at 95%, and last one at MAX
As effort increases, the pace should, too.
Always 30 sec. rest

Option to add paddles for this strength-focused set. Advanced swimmers can add an ankle strap.

Add-On 200 cool-down

Scale for Time Drop Main set to 5 intervals: 1 at 65%, 1 at 75%, 1 at 85%, 1 at 95%, 1 at MAX.

Scale for Fatigue Drop to 6 intervals in Main set, only building to 85%.

SESSION TWO

SUPPORTING RUN
ENDURANCE General Endurance, 40–80 min.

This is a recommended session.
Warm-Up 10 min. easy
Add dynamic warm-up if possible.

Main
30–70 min. low stress
Every 4th min. or so, check in on form, posture, etc.
Aim for best MFP. Do not exceed Z2 effort.

Scale for Time Simple scale of duration as needed.

Scale for Fatigue Trim duration or skip if needed.

WEDNESDAY

SESSION ONE

KEY BIKE + RUN
END-OF-RANGE Strength-Endurance, 115 min.

Warm-Up 10 min. at >90 rpm

Pre-Main
1 min. Z2 at 60 rpm,
3 min. Z2 at 60 rpm,
5 min. Z2 at 60 rpm
All with 3 min. Z1 at >95 rpm

Main
5 × 8 min. at <60 rpm, progress as:
1 smooth, 2 strong, 3 very strong,
4 strong, 5 smooth
3 min. Z2 at >95 rpm between intervals

10 min. IM effort (no data) and smooth home

RUN OFF THE BIKE

3 min. ramp to Z3, 1 min. MFP
2 min. Z4, 1 min. MFP
1 min. Z5, 2 min. MFP
1 min. Z4, 1 min. MFP
3 min. Z3

Scale for Time Cut the first two intervals of the Pre-Main set (1 min., 3 min.) and trim the number of intervals in the Main set.

Scale for Fatigue Evolve the Main set to 4 × 10 min., Z2 build rpm to fast on each interval. Remove all work from the run and convert to 15 min. smooth, form-based run.

SESSION TWO

STRENGTH & CONDITIONING
30 min.

Scale for Time Ensure you hit at least 5–10 min. of mobility.

Scale for Fatigue This is a floating session that can occur any day.

THURSDAY

SESSION ONE

KEY SWIM
EVENT-SPECIFIC Threshold, 3100–3400

Warm-Up 10 min. easy with mix of strokes

Pre-Main
100 smooth
2 × 75 build to fast
3 × 50 build to fast
4 × 25 fast
All with 15 sec. rest

Main With paddles and buoy:
100 at 70% with 20 sec. rest
100 at 80% with 10 sec. rest
1 × 100 at 90–95% with 5 sec. rest

100 at 70% with 20 sec. rest
100 at 80% with 10 sec. rest
2 × 100 at 90–95% with 5 sec. rest

100 at 70% with 20 sec. rest
100 at 80% with 10 sec. rest
3 × 100 at 90–95% with 5 sec. rest

100 at 70% with 20 sec. rest
100 at 80% with 10 sec. rest
4 × 100 at 90–95% with 5 sec. rest

100 at 70% with 20 sec. rest
100 at 80% with 10 sec. rest
5 × 100 at 90–95% with 5 sec. rest

100 easy to finish

Add-On 12 × 25 with paddles and fins, do as
4 rounds of: easy, MAX, MAX
Always 10 sec. rest

Scale for Time End Main set at 4 × 100.

Scale for Fatigue End Main set at the 4 × 100. Build efforts to 70%, 75%, and 80% only. Keep the fast 25s at the end.

SESSION TWO

SUPPORTING RUN
TECHNICAL Activation, 70–90 min.

Warm-Up 10 min. easy

Main
60–80 low stress
Endurance run on variable terrain. If you are injury prone, a softer surface is ideal.
Include 6 × 20 sec. blasts with 90 sec. form-based running between intervals.
Take short 20–40 sec. walk breaks as needed.

Scale for Time Reduce Main set to 30–50 min.

Scale for Fatigue Reduce Main set to 30–50 min.

FRIDAY

SESSION ONE

SUPPORTING BIKE
TECHNICAL Prep, 45–60 min.

Main
45–60 min.
First and last 10 min. at >95 rpm with minimum power while retaining chain tension. Focus on posture and good pedaling.
Include 4–6 × 30 sec. build to Z5 effort (10 sec. at Z3, Z4, and Z5)
3–4 min. spin between each 30 sec. build

TRAINER OPTION

Warm-Up 10–20 min. Z1 spin

Pre-Main
5 × 90 sec. Z1 at very fast rpm
30 sec. spin between intervals

Main 4–6 rounds of:
15 sec. build as 5 sec. at Z3, Z4, Z5
3 min. Z1 spin between intervals

Steady and smooth home

Scale for Time Trim duration as needed.

Scale for Fatigue Remove the Z5 effort from Main set, building as Z2, Z3, Z4. Moving the body will help. Do something that feels good.

SESSION TWO

STRENGTH & CONDITIONING
30 min.

Scale for Time Ensure you hit at least 5–10 min. of mobility.

Scale for Fatigue This is a floating session that can occur any day.

SATURDAY

SESSION ONE

KEY RUN
INTERVALS Strength, 60–80 min.

Warm-Up 10–15 min. easy and smooth

Pre-Main Up to 3 rounds, until you feel ready for work:
90 sec. smooth, 30 sec. easy,
1 min. steady, 30 sec. easy,
30 sec. strong, 30 sec. easy

Main 3 loops of hill running:
3–4 min. flat with great form at smooth endurance (Z2/Z3)
3 min. sustained hill at very strong sustained effort with great form (bounding)
30 sec. MAX effort on steeper grade (5–8%) to finish hill
3 min. downhill running on shallow grade (3–5%), pick up feet and float down with fast foot speed
No breaks. This will be very tough. If you cannot find a loop, run on the treadmill. Use 1% for flat and 0% for downhill.

Finish with 20–30 min. smooth tempo at IM effort, running with great form

Scale for Time Trim Warm-Up and skip the final 20 min. of the Main set. The hills are the meat and potatoes today.

Scale for Fatigue Do a 50–75 min. feel-good endurance run over rolling terrain.

CONTINUES...

SATURDAY CONTINUED

SESSION TWO

SUPPORTING **SWIM**
ENDURANCE Short Intervals, 2950–4050

Warm-Up 300–600, swim every 4th lap as non-free

Pre-Main Pull set with paddles, snorkel, and buoy:
200, 175, 150, 125, 100, 75, 50, 25
All with 10 sec. rest
Progress effort as you go to feel good.

Main
35–45 × 50 at 85% with 5–7 sec. rest
Choose a send-off interval and aim to leave on the same tight time each 50. Strong push-off and streamlines on every wall.
Paddles are OK if you can retain stroke rate.

Add-On 12 × 25 with paddles, do as 3 rounds of:
1 easy form, 2 build effort to fast, 3 and 4 fast
Always 15 sec. rest

Scale for Time Reduce the number of 50s you complete with good form and rhythm.

Scale for Fatigue Reduce the Warm-Up and begin Pre-Main set at 150. Complete the Main set without paddles, and focus on form over hitting 85% (reduce to 70-75% effort).

SUNDAY

SESSION ONE

KEY **BIKE**
ENDURANCE General Endurance, 2–5 hr.

Main
2–5 hr.
Endurance ride on variable terrain

TRAINER OPTION

Warm-Up 30 min. stepper, building very easy to steady

Main Up to 4 rounds of:
15 min. Z2 smooth,
5 min. Z3 strong,
2 min. Z3+ stronger,
3 min. Z1 easy

Scale for Time Reduce Warm-Up to 15 min. stepper. Reduce rounds in the Main set as needed.

Scale for Fatigue Reduce the Warm-Up to a 15 min. stepper. Main can be 2 rounds.

SESSION TWO

SUPPORTING **SWIM**
EVENT-SPECIFIC Pyramid, 2600–3700

This is a recommended session.

Warm-Up 10 min. easy with mix of strokes

Main
100 with toys, 100 at race pace
200 with toys, 200 at race pace
400 with toys, 400 at race pace
200 with toys, 800 at race pace
100 with toys, 1000 smooth endurance (for advanced swimmers)
200 race pace
Always 30 sec. rest

The idea is to use the swim toys in the sequence that promotes best connection with the water for free swims (e.g., start with snorkel, paddles, and fins). Strip off a toy per set then add buoy and band.

Scale for Time Stop Main set after the 800.

Scale for Fatigue In the Main set, do the race pace intervals as smooth endurance swim.

FOCUS We remove some of the muscular-loading strength and endurance work early in the week and freshen up. At the end of the week we begin 8 days focused on endurance with an endurance run weekend. The goal is 3 longer endurance runs over 5 days to build resilience before the upcoming block of work.

WEEKLY OVERVIEW

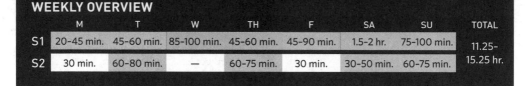

	M	T	W	TH	F	SA	SU	TOTAL
S1	20–45 min.	45–60 min.	85–100 min.	45–60 min.	45–90 min.	1.5–2 hr.	75–100 min.	11.25–15.25 hr.
S2	30 min.	60–80 min.	—	60–75 min.	30 min.	30–50 min.	60–75 min.	

MONDAY

SESSION ONE

SUPPORTING **BIKE**
TECHNICAL Recovery, 20–45 min.

Main
20–45 min.
Very low stress with first and last 10 min. at fast rpm, in a small gear.
If you ride outside, practice cornering and handling skills to refine control and comfort on the bike.

Scale for Time Trim as needed or take a rest day.

Scale for Fatigue It may still be worth fitting in the ride not for fitness, but to enhance recovery and adaptations.

SESSION TWO

STRENGTH & CONDITIONING
30 min.

Scale for Time Be sure you get in at least 5–10 min. of mobility work.

Scale for Fatigue This is a floating session that can occur any day.

TUESDAY

SESSION ONE

SUPPORTING **SWIM**
TECHNICAL Form, 3150–3550

This is a recommended session.

Warm-Up 10 min. easy

Pre-Main 15 × 50 with fins and snorkel, do as 5 rounds of:
25 kick on back, 25 free at 70% effort,
25 kick on back, 25 free at 80% effort,
25 kick on back, 25 free at 90% effort
Always 10 sec. rest

Main With buoy (no paddles, as we want to retain stroke rate):
100, 150, 200, 250, 300,
250, 200, 150, 100
All with 45 sec. rest
The first 25 of every swim is fast sighting 3 times per lap. The rest of the swim is smooth, endurance-focused swimming at 70%.

Add-On 400 with fins, alternate kick-swim by 25

Scale for Time Drop intervals in the Main set to 100, 150, 200, 200, 150, 100.

Scale for Fatigue Drop intervals in the Main set to 100, 150, 200, 200, 150, 100.

SESSION TWO

SUPPORTING **RUN**
ENDURANCE General Endurance, 60–80 min.

Warm-Up 10 min. easy
Add dynamic warm-up if possible.

Main
50–70 min. low stress
Every 4th min. or so check on form, posture, etc.
Aim for best MFP. Do not exceed Z2 effort.

Scale for Time Adjust duration as needed.

Scale for Fatigue Adjust duration or skip if needed.

WEDNESDAY

KEY **BIKE + RUN**
END-OF-RANGE High Cadence, 85–100 min.

Warm-Up As needed, include a few ramps to higher output so you can select work gear for Main set.

Main Up to 2 rounds of MAX sprints:
10 sec. MAX, 50 sec. easy,
20 sec. MAX, 40 sec. easy,
30 sec. MAX, 30 sec. easy,
40 sec. MAX, 20 sec. easy,
50 sec. MAX, 10 sec. easy,
60 sec. MAX,
10 sec. easy, 50 sec. MAX,
20 sec. easy, 40 sec. MAX,
30 sec. easy, 30 sec. MAX,
40 sec. easy, 20 sec. MAX,
50 sec. easy, 10 sec. MAX
7 min. easy spinning between rounds
Do MAX efforts as best effort at >90 rpm
Use the same gear for each work effort. Cadence decreases as set progresses. Shift from recovery gear 3 sec. before work starts.

Cool-down 5–15 min. spin

RUN OFF THE BIKE

5 min. ramp to IM effort
5 min. form-based running
5 min. above IM effort
5 min. form-based running
5 min. at IM effort
5 min. smooth and floating

Scale for Time Reduce Warm-Up and trim run-off to 15 min. build to above IM effort.

Scale for Fatigue Remove the MAX sprint efforts and replace with an easy ride.

PM OFF

THURSDAY

KEY **SWIM**
EVENT-SPECIFIC Pyramid, 2650

Warm-Up Smooth 10 min. light, then 400 pull smooth with choice of equipment at 70%

Main
Progressive building effort with medium-duration swims: 1850 swim with variable pace. Always 20 sec. rest, followed by a form-based swim interval.

200 steady at 85%, 150 form-based Z2 at 70%
150 strong at 90%, 150 form-based Z2 at 70%
100 very strong at 95%, 150 form-based Z2 at 70%
50 MAX with good, tidy hold on the water
(no panic)
150 form-based Z2 at 70%, 100 very strong at 95%,
150 form-based Z2 at 70%, 150 strong at 90%,
150 form-based Z2 at 70%, 200 steady at 85%

400 pull smooth to finish

Scale for Time Reduce form-based swim interval to 100. Reduce performance pyramid to be: 100, 75, 50, 25, 50, 75, 100 (each interval is half the original distance).

Scale for Fatigue Evolve to an endurance interval session with all intervals at 70–80%.

SUPPORTING **BIKE**
TECHNICAL Activation, 60–75 min.

Warm-Up 30 min. smooth

Main 2–3 rounds of:
5 min. smooth,
2 min. spin higher rpm in a small gear,
3 min. steady,
2 min. spin higher rpm in a small gear,
1 min. strong,
2 min. spin higher rpm in a small gear

TRAINER OPTION

Warm-Up 10 min. spin

Pre-Main
5 × 3 min. smooth, ramp rpm by 1 min. to fast rpm

Then complete Main set detailed above.

Scale for Time Simple scale of duration as needed.

Scale for Fatigue Trim duration or skip if needed. Remove the neurological high-cadence work if needed.

FRIDAY	SATURDAY

FRIDAY

SESSION ONE

SUPPORTING **BIKE**
TECHNICAL Prep, 45–90 min.

This is a recommended session.

Do a feel-good ride, whatever that is for you: more, less, building intervals, spinning, etc. Be aware and look for patterns to better manage readiness. Here is a possible option, but do what works for you.

Main
45–90 min. smooth
Include 4 × 3 min., ramp by 1 min. to strong but not deep effort.
3–4 min. spin between intervals

Scale for Time Adjust duration as needed.

Scale for Fatigue Remove the ramping effort, but moving the body will still help.

SESSION TWO

STRENGTH & CONDITIONING
30 min.

Scale for Time Be sure you get in at least 5–10 min. of mobility work.

Scale for Fatigue This is a floating session that can occur any day.

SATURDAY

SESSION ONE

KEY **RUN**
ENDURANCE General Endurance, 1.5–2 hr.

Main
1.5–2 hr.
This is the first of 3 endurance runs in 5 days, focused on building muscular endurance, so harder is not better.

Retain form under fatigue. Hills are good. Very steep grades are also fine, but just hike these sections with great form. Finish pleasantly fatigued, but without soreness.

Scale for Time Trim to 1 hr. and do PM run.

Scale for Fatigue This is all feel-good work today, so you are under no pressure to run hard.

SESSION TWO

SUPPORTING **RUN**
ENDURANCE, General Endurance, 30–50 min.

This is an optional run to be added only if you ran short in the morning session.

Main
30–50 min. low stress and focused on resilience
All easy endurance; walk breaks are OK.

Aim for best MFP; keep the effort down by consciously subtracting leg speed or push off, and practice the run/walk protocol.

Scale for Time Skip entirely if you ran 2 hr. in morning workout.

Scale for Fatigue Optional workout; trim duration or skip if needed.

SUNDAY

SESSION ONE

KEY RUN
ENDURANCE General Endurance, 75–100 min.

Main
75–100 min.
Hills are great. Variable terrain and a soft surface is optimal. Walk breaks are OK as needed to retain form under fatigue. Finish pleasantly fatigued, but without soreness.

Very steep grades are fine in this run; just hike these sections with great form.

Scale for Time Simple scale of duration.

Scale for Fatigue This is all feel-good work today, so you are under no pressure to run hard.

SESSION TWO

SUPPORTING SWIM
TECHNICAL Form, 3050–3750

This is a recommended session.

Warm-Up 300–600, swim every 4th lap as non-free

Pre-Main 15 × 50 with fins and snorkel (to help flush the legs), do as 5 rounds of:
50 at 70% effort,
50 at 80% effort,
50 at 90% effort
Always 10 sec. rest

Main With buoy (no paddles, as we want to retain stroke rate):
100, 150, 200, 250, 300,
300, 250, 200, 150, 100
All with 45 sec. rest
The first 25 of every swim is fast sighting 3 times per lap. The rest of the swim is smooth, endurance-focused swimming at 70%.

Add-On 400 with fins, alternate kick-swim by 25

Scale for Time Reduce the Main set pyramid to a distance that allows completion within time available.

Scale for Fatigue Convert to a Warm-Up of 500 easy, then Main is 1000 with buoy and snorkel.

FOCUS We retain the endurance focus, while integrating some strength-endurance work into the load. We have one endurance run remaining, then we transition to a weekend focused on riding to bank some miles and resilience. For the time-starved athlete, the trainer option can be used to sneak in some miles.

WEEKLY OVERVIEW

	M	T	W	TH	F	SA	SU	TOTAL
S1	20–45 min.	1–1.5 hr.	1–2 hr.	45–70 min.	95 min.	3–6.5 hr.	2–4 hr.	14–22.3 hr.
S2	—	50–80 min.	30 min.	1 hr.	1 hr.	—	1.5–2 hr.	

MONDAY

SESSION ONE

SUPPORTING **BIKE**
TECHNICAL Recovery, 20–45 min.

Main
20–45 min. very low stress
First and last 10 min. at fast rpm, in a small gear.
If you ride outside, practice some cornering and handling skills to refine control and comfort on the bike.

Scale for Time Trim as needed or skip if unable to complete.

Scale for Fatigue It may still be worth moving blood here, not for fitness, but to enhance recovery and adaptations.

SESSION TWO

PM OFF

TUESDAY

SESSION ONE

KEY **SWIM**
ENDURANCE Over-Distance, 3600–4700

Warm-Up 10 min. easy with mix of strokes

Pre-Main
100 smooth
2 × 75 build to fast
3 × 50 build to fast
4 × 25 fast
All with 15 sec. rest

Main
100 with toys, 200 swim at 80%
200 with toys, 400 swim at 80%
300 with toys, 600 swim at 80%
200 with toys, 800 swim at 80%
100 with toys, 1000 swim at 80% (for advanced swimmers)
All with 1 min. rest between intervals
Use snorkel and buoy for intervals with toys; add paddles for strength-endurance. In the solid swims, sight 3 times per lap.

Add-On 12 × 25 with paddles and fins, do as 4 rounds of: easy, MAX, MAX
Always 10 sec. rest

Scale for Time Trim Main set to finish at the 600 or 800 as needed.

Scale for Fatigue Trim the Main set to finish at 600.

CONTINUES…

TUESDAY CONTINUED
SESSION TWO

SUPPORTING **RUN**
ENDURANCE General Endurance, 50–80 min.

This is a recommended session.

Warm-Up 10 min. easy
Add dynamic warm-up if possible.

Main
40–70 min. low stress
Include some fartlek-style speed changes as 2–3 rounds of:
10-20-30-20-10 sec. of form-based speed pick-ups
1 min. easy running between efforts

Scale for Time Simple scale of duration as needed.

Scale for Fatigue Remove the speed play or skip if needed.

WEDNESDAY
SESSION ONE

KEY **RUN**
ENDURANCE General Endurance, 1–2 hr.

Main
1–2 hr.
Endurance-focused run on soft surface with variable terrain. Integrate walk breaks as needed to retain form and minimize global fatigue. If you are newer to training, this might be more hiking than running.

TREADMILL OPTION

Warm-Up 10 min. easy

Pre-Main 4 rounds of:
90 sec. walk at 5%,
3 min. run smooth Z2 at 1%,
30 sec. walk at 1%

Main
Smooth endurance running with 30 sec. at 3% grade every 3rd min. Walk breaks as needed.

Add-On 30–50 min. low-stress, MFP run in the evening. Keep effort down by consciously reducing leg speed or push off and practice the run/walk protocol.

Scale for Time Reduce duration as needed.

Scale for Fatigue Choose flatter terrain and integrate more walk breaks.

SESSION TWO

STRENGTH & CONDITIONING
30 min.

Scale for Time Be sure you hit at least 5–10 min. of mobility.

Scale for Fatigue This is a floating session that can occur any day.

WEEK
6
CONTINUED

SESSION ONE

SUPPORTING **SWIM**
ENDURANCE Short Intervals, 2900–3950

This is a recommended session.

Warm-Up 10 min. easy

Pre-Main 5–7 rounds (fins can be used):
50 at 70% with 10 sec. rest,
50 at 80% with 5–7 sec. rest,
50 at 90% with 3–5 sec. rest

Then, 2 rounds of:
2 × 25 fast,
50 easy, 50 fast,
2 × 25 easy
All with 15 sec. rest

Main
35–50 × 50 at 85% with 5–7 sec. rest
Choose a send-off interval and aim to leave on the same time each 50. Introduce sighting 3 times per lap without losing rhythm, tempo, or stroke.

Scale for Time Scale Pre-Main and Main sets as needed.

Scale for Fatigue Evolve Main set to focus on form over effort. Reduce effort to 70–75%.

SESSION TWO

SUPPORTING **BIKE**
TECHNICAL Activation, 1 hr.

Warm-Up 20 min. easy

Pre-Main
6 × 3 min. Z2
Build rpm by 1 min.: 80, 90, 100
30 sec. rest between intervals

Main
3 min. building effort by 45 sec. to Z3+
2 min. spin
2 min. building effort by 30 sec. to Z3
2 min. spin
1 min. building effort by 15 sec. to Z4
2 min. spin

5–10 min. Z1 spin

This is a feel-good ride to prepare for tomorrow's ride.

Scale for Time Trim Warm-Up to 10 min., then reduce Pre-Main to 3 × 3 min. Then hit Main set. Cut the final 5–10 min. spin.

Scale for Fatigue Keep all building efforts as a build to Z3.

SESSION ONE

KEY **BIKE**
END-OF-RANGE Strength-Endurance, 95 min.

Today is a double-day on the trainer. If you only have time for a single session, do this one.

Warm-Up 10 min. at >90 rpm

Pre-Main
1 min. Z2 at 60 rpm,
3 min. Z2 at 60 rpm,
5 min. Z2 at 60 rpm
All with 3 min. Z1 at >100 rpm

Main
5 × 8 min. at <60 rpm, progress as:
1 smooth, 2 strong, 3 very strong,
4 strong, 5 smooth
3 min. Z3 at >100 rpm between intervals

10 min. IM effort (no data) and smooth home

Scale for Time Scale duration as needed.

Scale for Fatigue Do 3–4 × 8 min. Z2 at rpm of choice for Main set.

SESSION TWO

SUPPORTING **BIKE**
TECHNICAL Prep, 1 hr.

Main
20 min. Z1 easy at choice rpm
20 min. Z2 smooth at choice rpm
20 min. Z3 steady at choice rpm

Scale for Time Scale to 15 min. or 10 min. for each step.

Scale for Fatigue Skip the session if fatigued.

SATURDAY

KEY **BIKE + RUN**
ENDURANCE Over-Distance, 3–6.5 hr.

Main
3–6 hr.
Riding tour on variable terrain with mostly endurance-focused effort. No need to chase power or stick to heart rate zones. Enjoy being outside and building resilience on the bike.

TRAINER OPTION

Warm-Up 30 min. smooth

Pre-Main
15 min. Z2
10 min. Z2/Z3
5 min. Z3

Main 1–2 rounds of:
6 min. build by 2 min. to Z3+,
10 min. Z3 steady state at <70 rpm,
4 min. build by 1 min. to Z3+,
8 min. Z2 (power) steady state at >90 rpm,
2 min. build by 30 sec. to Z3+,
6 min. Z3 steady state at choice rpm

RUN OFF THE BIKE

15–30 min. form-based smooth endurance running

Scale for Time Trim the Warm-Up to 15 min. easy ramp, then only do a single round of the Main set.

Scale for Fatigue Keep the entire ride at Z2 and don't go longer than 2 hr. on the trainer. Outside ride can be very easy, up to 3 hr.

PM OFF

SUNDAY

KEY **BIKE**
ENDURANCE General Endurance, 2–4 hr.

Main
2–4 hr.
Another interval-free touring ride outside in variable terrain. Only choose the trainer option if you are forced to. If you can only go long one day, prioritize Saturday's ride.

TRAINER OPTION

Warm-Up 30 min. stepper
Easy spin and gradually ramp to steady Z3 effort.

Main 55 min. stepper up:
10, 9, 8, 7, 6, 5, 4, 3, 2, 1 min.
All with 30 sec. rest between intervals
Begin with 10 min. Z1 and gradually ramp effort with each interval to finish with 1 min. at Z4.

Add-On 28 min. stepper down:
7, 6, 5, 4, 3, 2, 1 min.
Begin at steady Z3 and ramp down in effort to finish with 1 min. at Z1.

Scale for Time Reduce each stepper (both up and down) to 15 min. Do as 5, 4, 3, 2, 1 min. but retain the theme and progression in effort.

Scale for Fatigue Evolve to be a Z2 ride. Outside can be very easy, up to 3 hr. Don't go longer than 2 hr. on the trainer.

KEY **SWIM**
EVENT-SPECIFIC Race Simulation, 4400

Warm-Up 10 min. jog prior to swimming if possible

Main 2 rounds of ladder:
200 smooth with some little builds
1 min. float
200 take out (TO) effort, 400 race effort
50 TO effort, 200 race effort
50 TO effort, 100 race effort
50 TO effort, 50 race effort
50 TO effort, 100 race effort
50 TO effort, 200 race effort
Always 10 sec. rest
All race efforts at 85%
Then 1000 continuous with toys of choice. Hold smooth form.

Scale for Time Reduce Main set to 1 round of ladder.

Scale for Fatigue Reduce the race effort to 200, 100, 50, 100, 200, then do 600 continuous with toys. Only 1 round.

FOCUS We take a few days to clean out the endurance load of the last week or so. We can then transition to another round of strength-endurance training. I encourage you to split the week in half, with the first half focused on recuperation and the other half on strength-endurance work. We will prepare for the upcoming work by including some integrated efforts at high rpm.

WEEKLY OVERVIEW

	M	T	W	TH	F	SA	SU	TOTAL
S1	20–45 min.	40–90 min.	80–90 min.	45–60 min.	45–90 min.	110–155 min.	50–75 min.	10.5–15.2 hr.
S2	30 min.	60–80 min.	—	60–75 min.	30 min.	—	1–1.5 hr.	

MONDAY

SESSION ONE

SUPPORTING BIKE
TECHNICAL Recovery, 20–45 min.

Main
20–45 min. very low stress
First and last 10 min. at fast rpm in a small gear.

If you ride outside, practice cornering and bike handling skills to refine control and comfort on the bike.

Scale for Time Trim as needed or skip if unable to complete.

Scale for Fatigue It may still be worth fitting in the ride not for fitness, but to enhance recovery and adaptations.

SESSION TWO

STRENGTH & CONDITIONING
30 min.

Scale for Time Be sure you get in at least 5–10 min. of mobility work.

Scale for Fatigue This is a floating session that can occur any day.

TUESDAY

SESSION ONE

SUPPORTING SWIM
ENDURANCE Short Intervals, 2150–3200

This is a recommended session.

Warm-Up 10 min. easy

Pre-Main 5–7 rounds (fins can be used):
50 at 70% with 10 sec. rest,
50 at 80% with 5–7 sec. rest,
50 at 90% with 3–5 sec. rest

Then, 2 rounds of:
2 × 25 fast,
50 easy, 50 fast,
2 × 25 easy
All with 15 sec. rest

Main With paddles:
40–70 × 25 at 85–90% with 2–5 sec. rest

Scale for Time Trim first Pre-Main set to 3 rounds, trim second set to 1 round. Adjust Main set as needed.

Scale for Fatigue Reduce Main set to 20–40 × 25 at 80%, no paddles.

SESSION TWO

SUPPORTING RUN
ENDURANCE General Endurance, 60–80 min.

Warm-Up 10 min. easy
Add dynamic warm-up if possible.

Main
50–70 min. low stress
Every 4th min. or so check on form, posture, etc.
Aim for best MFP. Do not exceed Z2 effort.

Scale for Time Simple scale of duration as needed.

Scale for Fatigue Trim duration as needed.

WEDNESDAY

SESSION ONE

KEY **BIKE + RUN**
END-OF-RANGE High Cadence, 80–90 min.

Warm-Up As needed, include a few ramps to higher output so you can select work gear for Main set.

Main Up to 2 rounds of MAX sprints:
10 sec. MAX, 50 sec. easy,
20 sec. MAX, 40 sec. easy,
30 sec. MAX, 30 sec. easy,
40 sec. MAX, 20 sec. easy,
50 sec. MAX, 10 sec. easy,
60 sec. MAX,
10 sec. easy, 50 sec. MAX,
20 sec. easy, 40 sec. MAX,
30 sec. easy, 30 sec. MAX,
40 sec. easy, 20 sec. MAX,
50 sec. easy, 10 sec. MAX
7 min. easy spinning between rounds
Do MAX efforts as best effort at >90 rpm
Use the same gear for each work effort. Cadence decreases as set progresses. Shift from recovery gear 3 sec. before work starts. Begin each interval at MAX, a power decline is expected throughout each interval.

Cool-down 5-15 min. spin

RUN OFF THE BIKE

5 min. ramp to IM effort
5 min. form-based running
10 min. at IM effort
5 min. above IM effort
5 min. form-based running

Scale for Time Trim Main set to 1 round.

Scale for Fatigue Remove the MAX effort work and replace with an easy ride.

SESSION TWO

PM OFF

THURSDAY

SESSION ONE

KEY **SWIM**
INTERVALS Building, 2200

Warm-Up 10 min. easy

Pre-Main 2 rounds of:
2 × 25 MAX with paddles,
50 easy float with good form,
50 fast with paddles,
2 × 25 easy

Main
An exercise in pacing, increasing speed with effort.
Sight 3 times per lap.
8 × 100 as:
2 at 70%, 2 at 80%, 2 at 90%, 2 very strong
All with 30 sec. rest

8 × 75 as:
2 at 70%, 2 at 80%, 2 at 90%, 2 very strong
All with 20 sec. rest

8 × 50 as:
2 at 70%, 2 at 80%, 2 at 90%, 2 very strong
All with 10 sec. rest

Scale for Time Reduce repetitions in Main set from 8 to 4, maintaining pace and effort.

Scale for Fatigue Adjust the very strong efforts in the Main set to form-based short intervals, endurance and smooth.

SESSION TWO

SUPPORTING **BIKE**
TECHNICAL Activation, 60–75 min.

Warm-Up 30 min. smooth

Main 2–3 rounds of:
5 min. smooth,
2 min. spin higher rpm in a small gear,
3 min. steady,
2 min. spin higher rpm in a small gear,
1 min. strong,
2 min. spin higher rpm in a small gear

TRAINER OPTION

Warm-Up 10 min. spin

Pre-Main
5 × 3 min. smooth, ramp rpm by 1 min. to fast rpm

Then complete Main set detailed above.

Scale for Time Simple scale of duration as needed.

Scale for Fatigue Trim duration or skip if needed. Remove the neurological high-cadence work if needed.

FRIDAY

SUPPORTING **BIKE**
TECHNICAL Prep, 45–90 min.

This is a recommended session.

This is a feel-good ride, whatever that is for you: more, less, building intervals, spinning, etc. Be aware and look for patterns to better manage readiness. Here is a possible option, but do what works for you.

Main
45–90 min. smooth
Include 4 × 3 min., ramp by 1 min. to strong but not deep effort
3–4 min. Z2 riding between intervals

Scale for Time Adjust duration as needed.

Scale for Fatigue Remove the ramping effort, but moving the body will still help.

STRENGTH & CONDITIONING
30 min.

Scale for Time Be sure you get in at least 5–10 min. of mobility work.

Scale for Fatigue This is a floating session that can occur any day.

SATURDAY

KEY **BIKE + RUN**
END-OF-RANGE Building, 110–155 min.

Warm-Up 60 min.

Main
2–3 × 5 min. strong effort in aero position at 60 rpm
5 min. form-based endurance at choice rpm between intervals
10 min. smooth endurance

2–3 × 5 min. strong effort at >90 rpm
5 min. form-based endurance at choice rpm between intervals
10 min. smooth endurance

1–2 × 20 min. at IM effort/pace. Feel good with tidy form.
5 min. easy between intervals

Smooth endurance riding home

RUN OFF THE BIKE

5 min. quick ramp to IM goal pace
5 min. form-based running
10 min. above IM goal pace
5 min. easy cool-down

Scale for Time Scale duration and do 2 intervals of both low and high rpm for 5 min., but remove the 10 min. endurance intervals.

Scale for Fatigue Transition to a feel-good endurance ride with 3 × 6 min. smooth, build by 2 min. to strong but not deep effort.

PM OFF

SUNDAY

SESSION ONE

KEY **SWIM**
EVENT-SPECIFIC Pyramid, 2650

Warm-Up Smooth 10 min. light, then
400 pull smooth with choice of equipment at 70%

Main
Progressive building effort with medium-duration
swims: 1850 swim with variable pace. Always
20 sec. rest, followed by a form-based swim
interval.

200 steady at 85%, 150 form-based Z2 at 70%
150 strong at 90%, 150 form-based Z2 at 70%
100 very strong at 95%, 150 form-based Z2 at 70%
50 MAX with good, tidy hold on the water (no panic)
150 form-based Z2 at 70%, 100 very strong at 95%
150 form-based Z2 at 70%, 150 strong at 90%
150 form-based Z2 at 70%, 200 steady at 85%

400 pull smooth to finish

Scale for Time Reduce performance pyramid to be:
100, 75, 50, 75, 100, with 100 form-based swim
interval.

Scale for Fatigue Do about 1500–2000, very easy.
Mix it up with toys, etc. Feel good and move the
body.

SESSION TWO

SUPPORTING **RUN**
EVENT-SPECIFIC Building, 1–1.5 hr.

Warm-Up 10 min. easy

Main
50–80 min. low-stress endurance run on variable
terrain
Include 20 min. as:
5 min. at IM effort,
5 min. above IM effort,
10 min. at IM effort

Scale for Time Scale duration as needed. No more
fitness to be gained.

Scale for Fatigue Skip the run completely.

FOCUS The strength-endurance aspect of this week will feel familiar. It is a progression of Week 5. Now we include some high rpm and speed work. Globally, this week is very challenging, especially the weekend Key Run, as well as the endurance swim and end-of-range bike sessions.

WEEKLY OVERVIEW

	M	T	W	TH	F	SA	SU	TOTAL
S1	20–45 min.	45–60 min.	2–2.75 hr.	45–70 min.	45–60 min.	100–150 min.	2–4 hr.	9.4–11.3 hr.
S2	—	40–90 min.	30 min.	70–90 min.	30 min.	1–1.5 hr.	60–75 min.	

MONDAY

SESSION ONE

SUPPORTING BIKE
TECHNICAL Prep, 20–45 min.

Main
20–45 min. very low stress
First and last 10 min. at fast rpm, in a small gear. If you ride outside, practice some cornering and handling skills to refine control and comfort on the bike.

Scale for Time Trim as needed or skip if unable to complete.

Scale for Fatigue If your muscles are sore from last week, convert to a 30–45 min. flush/spin on the bike or a very easy 1–2 km swim.

SESSION TWO

PM OFF

TUESDAY

SESSION ONE

KEY SWIM
ENDURANCE Over-Distance, 3400

Warm-Up 5–10 min. easy with mix of strokes

Pre-Main 2 × 400 as:
75 smooth, 25 strong,
75 smooth, 25 very strong,
75 smooth, 25 MAX,
100 smooth
1 min. rest between intervals

Main
2000 straight swim, gradually build by 500 to 85%
1 min. rest
6 × 100 very strong with paddles
15 sec. rest between intervals

Scale for Time Scale the Pre-Main to only 1 × 400, then trim the Main set to 1000–1500 and 4 × 100 to finish.

Scale for Fatigue Remove the 100s at the end of the Main set and maintain smooth swimming for a straight 1000–1500 pull.

SESSION TWO

SUPPORTING RUN
ENDURANCE General Endurance, 40–90 min.

This is a recommended session.
Warm-Up 10 min. easy
Add dynamic warm-up if possible.

Main
30–80 min. low stress
Every 4th min. or so check on form, posture, etc. Aim for best MFP. Do not exceed Z2 effort.

Scale for Time Simple scale of duration as needed.

Scale for Fatigue Trim duration or skip if needed.

WEDNESDAY

KEY **BIKE + RUN**
END-OF-RANGE High Cadence, 2–2.75 hr.

Warm-Up 10 min. spin

Pre-Main
5 min. Z2 build rpm, 3 min. build Z1 to Z3/Z4,
3 min. Z2 build rpm, 3 min. build Z1 to Z3/Z4,
1 min. Z2 build rpm, 3 min. build Z1 to Z3/Z4

Main 3–5 rounds of:
2 min. Z3, 4 min. Z4 at >95 rpm,
30 sec. Z1, 2 min. Z2,
4 min. Z4 at <65 rpm, 30 sec. Z1,
2 min. Z2
5 min. Z2 between rounds

2 min. easy, then
5–8 min. at IM 70.3 effort without looking at the watch

RUN OFF THE BIKE

5 min. ramp to IM 70.3 effort, 2 min. easy
3 min. at 5–10 sec. per mile faster than IM 70.3 effort,
2 min. easy
3 min. at 10–15 sec. per mile faster than IM 70.3 effort,
2 min. easy
3 min. at 5–10 sec. per mile faster than IM 70.3 effort,
2 min. easy
Finish with 5–8 min. at feeling of IM 70.3 without looking at the watch
Smooth MFP to finish

Scale for Time Scale to 2–3 rounds of the Main set, then reduce the run to a 15 min. build to very strong.

Scale for Fatigue Maintain the Pre-Main but convert the Main set to 4 × 10 min. Z2, build rpm to fast on each. Remove all work from the brick run and convert to smooth 15 min. with good form.

STRENGTH & CONDITIONING
30 min.

Scale for Time Be sure you get in at least 5–10 min. of mobility work.

Scale for Fatigue This is a floating session that can occur any day.

THURSDAY

SUPPORTING **SWIM**
ENDURANCE Short Intervals, 2550–3550

This is a recommended session.

Warm-Up 10 min. easy

Pre-Main 5–7 rounds (fins can be used):
50 at 70% with 10 sec. rest,
50 at 80% with 5–7 sec. rest,
50 at 90% with 3–5 sec. rest

Then, 2 rounds of:
2 × 25 fast,
50 easy, 50 fast,
2 × 25 easy
All with 15 sec. rest

Main
20–30 × 50 at 85% with 5–7 sec. rest
Choose a send-off interval and aim to leave on the same time each 50. Introduce sighting 3 times per lap without losing rhythm, tempo, or stroke.

16–24 × 25 at 90–95% with only 3–5 sec. rest
Remove sighting to focus on keeping rhythm but increasing your tempo (without slipping off the hold/push of the water on each lap).

Scale for Time Scale Pre-Main and Main sets as needed.

Scale for Fatigue Maintain the session, but make the 50s all 80% and remove the 25s at the end. In the Pre-Main, skip the 2 rounds of 2 × 25, 50, 50, 2 × 25.

SUPPORTING **RUN**
TECHNICAL Activation, 70–90 min.

This is a recommended session.

Warm-Up 10 min. easy

Main
60–80 min. low-stress endurance run on variable terrain. If you are injury prone, then a softer surface is ideal.
Include 9 × 20 sec. blast (remain supple, yet fast) with 90 sec. easy form-based running between each. Take short 20–40 sec. walk breaks as needed to retain form.

Scale for Time Simply reduce time but retain the 9 × 20 sec. sharpeners.

Scale for Fatigue Begin very easy and scale for time but retain the 9 × 20 sec. sharpeners.

FRIDAY

SESSION ONE

SUPPORTING **BIKE**
TECHNICAL Prep, 45–60 min.

Main
45–60 min.
First and last 10 min. at >95 rpm with minimum power while retaining chain tension. Focus on posture and good pedaling.
Include 4-6 × 30 sec., build to Z5 effort (10 sec. at Z3, Z4, and Z5)
3–4 min. spin between each 30 sec. build

TRAINER OPTION

Warm-Up 10–20 min. Z1 spin

Pre-Main
5 × 90 sec. Z1 at very high rpm
30 sec. spin between intervals

Main 4–6 rounds of:
15 sec. build as 5 sec. at Z3, Z4, and Z5
3 min. Z1 spin between intervals

Steady and smooth ride home

Scale for Time Scale duration as needed.

Scale for Fatigue Remove the Z5 effort, but moving the body will still help. Do something that feels good.

SESSION TWO

STRENGTH & CONDITIONING
30 min.

Scale for Time Be sure you get in at least 5–10 min. of mobility work.

Scale for Fatigue This is a floating session that can occur any day.

SATURDAY

SESSION ONE

KEY **RUN**
INTERVALS Tempo, 100–150 min.

Warm-Up 10 min. easy

Pre-Main 1–2 rounds until you are ready to go:
3 min. smooth, 30 sec. easy,
2 min. steady, 30 sec. easy,
1 min. strong, 30 sec. easy

Main
2 × 30 min. at above IM effort, very much in control with fluid, smooth running
10 min. easy between intervals

Then 10 min. smooth form-based run home.

OPTIONAL PM RUN

20–40 min. very low stress
Include 10-20-30-20-10 sec. blasts with 90 sec. easy running between each effort.

Scale for Time Adjust the Main set to be 2 × 20 min. with 7 min. easy between intervals.

Scale for Fatigue Convert Main set to be 3 × 15 min. at above IM effort, and keep the recovery interval the same.

SESSION TWO

SUPPORTING **SWIM**
ENDURANCE Building, 3200–4500

Warm-Up 300–600, swim every 4th lap as non-free

Pre-Main Pull set with paddles, snorkel, and buoy:
200, 175, 150, 125, 100, 75, 50, 25
All with 10 sec. rest
Progress effort as you go to feel good.

Main 2–3 rounds of:
400, 300, 200, 100, progress effort to strong
1 min. rest between intervals

Scale for Time Start Pre-Main set at 100 and do just 1 round of Main set if needed.

Scale for Fatigue Convert Main set to smooth endurance effort. Nothing over 80%.

SUNDAY

SESSION ONE

KEY **BIKE**

ENDURANCE General Endurance, 2–4 hr.

Main

2–4 hr. endurance ride on variable terrain
Include 5 rounds of:
20 sec. MAX effort,
2 min. Z2/Z3,
5 min. Z1

TRAINER OPTION

Warm-Up 30 min. stepper (gradually ramp effort from very easy to steady over the duration)

Main 4 rounds of:
4 min. Z1/Z2 choice pedaling, 30 sec. Z1,
3 min. Z2 build rpm to fast, 30 sec. Z1,
2 min. Z2/3 choice pedaling, 30 sec. Z1,
1 min. Z3 build rpm to fast, 30 sec. Z1
For choice pedaling efforts, select an efficient cadence.

Add-On 20 min. Z2 choice pedaling, every 4th min. ramp rpm to MAX and hold

Scale for Time Reduce Warm-Up to 15 min. stepper. In Main set, reduce the number of rounds as needed.

Scale for Fatigue Reduce Warm-Up to 15 min. stepper. Do 2 rounds of Main set.

SESSION TWO

KEY **SWIM**

ENDURANCE Over-Distance, 3700

Main

100 toys, form and tech, 100 race pace,
200 toys, 200 race pace,
400 toys, 400 race pace,
200 toys, 800 race pace,
100 toys, 1000 smooth endurance,
200 race pace
All with 30 sec. rest

For intervals with toys start with snorkel, paddles, and fins and strip off a toy per set, then add buoy and band. The idea is to use the swim toys in the sequence that promotes best connection with the water for free swims.

Scale for Time Trim Main set to finish at 800.

Scale for Fatigue Trim the Main set to finish at 800.

FOCUS This is a heavy block of work focused on strength and endurance. A challenging end-of-range bike ride is the feature of the week. Think of this week as building-block sessions that will allow you to blossom in the mix of low- and high-rpm work as you progress toward your goal race.

WEEKLY OVERVIEW

	M	T	W	TH	F	SA	SU	TOTAL
S1	30–50 min.	1–1.5 hr.	45–90 min.	1–1.5 hr.	45–60 min.	160–200 min.	80–90 min.	12.75–
S2	—	50–80 min.	30 min.	75–100 min.	30 min.	—	100–130 min.	17.3 hr.

MONDAY

SESSION ONE

SUPPORTING **RUN**
TECHNICAL Recovery, 30–50 min.

Warm-Up 10 min. easy

Main
20–40 min. very low stress
Aim for best MFP. Control effort by adding leg speed, striding/bounding, activation, and practice the run/walk protocol.

Scale for Time Trim as needed or skip if unable to complete.

Scale for Fatigue If your muscles are sore from last week, convert to a 30–45 min. flush/spin on the bike or a very easy 1–2 km swim.

SESSION TWO

PM OFF

TUESDAY

SESSION ONE

KEY **SWIM**
INTERVALS Building, 3000–4650

Warm-Up 10 min. easy

Pre-Main 2–3 rounds with snorkel:
300 at 70%, focusing on hand entry in line with the shoulder, with 30 sec. rest,
3 × 50 form-based swimming, building tempo, effort, and stroke rate throughout each 50 with 10 sec. rest

Main 3–4 rounds of:
400 at 80%,
200 at 85%,
100 at 90%

Add-On 2 rounds of power:
4 × 25 MAX with paddles,
150 form-based swimming, feeling the connection

Scale for Time Trim Pre-Main set to a single round.

Scale for Fatigue Shift Main set to 2–3 rounds of 300, 200, 100 smooth endurance. Trim the Pre-Main to a single round.

SESSION TWO

SUPPORTING **RUN**
ENDURANCE General Endurance, 50–80 min.

Warm-Up 10 min. easy
Add dynamic warm-up if possible.

Main
40–70 min. low stress
Every 4th min. check on form, posture, etc. Aim for best MFP. Do not exceed Z2 effort.

Scale for Time Scale duration as needed.

Scale for Fatigue Trim duration or skip if needed.

WEDNESDAY

SESSION ONE

SUPPORTING **BIKE**
TECHNICAL Prep, 45–90 min.

This is a recommended session.

Main
45–90 min. low-stress optional ride
First and last 10 min. at >95 rpm with minimum power while retaining chain tension. Focus on posture and good pedaling.
Include 4–6 × 30 sec., build to Z5 effort (10 sec. at Z3, Z4, and Z5)
3–4 min. spin between each 30 sec. build

TRAINER OPTION

Warm-Up 5–10 min. Z1 spin

Pre-Main
5 × 90 sec. Z1 at very fast rpm
30 sec. spin between intervals

Main 2 rounds of:
20 min. IM effort Z2 to Z3,
5 min. Z3 at above IM
5 min. spin between rounds

Scale for Time Scale duration as needed.

Scale for Fatigue Scale Main set to 2 × 15 min. Z1 as 5 min. high rpm, 5 min. spin, 5 min. high rpm.

SESSION TWO

STRENGTH & CONDITIONING
30 min.

Scale for Time Be sure you get in at least 5–10 min. of mobility work.

Scale for Fatigue This is a floating session that can occur any day.

THURSDAY

SESSION ONE

SUPPORTING **SWIM**
ENDURANCE Over-Distance, 3300–4400

This is a recommended session.

Warm-Up 10 min. easy with mix of strokes

Pre-Main
100 smooth
2 × 75 build to fast
3 × 50 build to fast
4 × 25 fast
All with 15 sec. rest

Main
100 with toys, 200 swim at 80%
200 with toys, 400 swim at 80%
300 with toys, 600 swim at 80%
200 with toys, 800 swim at 80%
100 with toys, 1000 swim at 80% (for advanced swimmers)
All with 1 min. rest between intervals
In the solid swims, sight 3 times per lap.

Add-On 12 × 25 with paddles and fins, do as
4 rounds of: easy, MAX, MAX
Always 10 sec. rest

Scale for Time Remove the speed Add-On, and trim Main set to finish at the 600 or 800 as needed.

Scale for Fatigue Remove the speed Add-On at the end, and trim the Main set to the 600.

SESSION TWO

KEY **RUN**
INTERVALS Strength, 75–100 min.

Warm-Up 10–15 min. easy running

Pre-Main
3 × 2 min., build by 30 sec. to feel-good, strong running

Main
3 × 15–20 min. hilly endurance running, maintaining strong endurance effort (Z3) throughout
5 min. easy running between intervals

TREADMILL OPTION

Main 2–3 rounds at Z2 pace (IM), increasing effort with grades:
4 min. at 2%, 2 min. at 4%, 4 min. at 0%,
2 min. at 2%, 1 min. at 4%, 2 min. at 0%
2 min. walk breaks between intervals

Scale for Time Reduce the number of rounds, but retain the rhythm and intent, as well as duration of the intervals.

Scale for Fatigue Begin very easy and gradually ramp up effort, but convert to a feel-good endurance run if needed.

FRIDAY

SESSION ONE

SUPPORTING **BIKE**
TECHNICAL Prep, 45–60 min.

Main
45–60 min.
First and last 10 min. at >95 rpm with minimum power while retaining chain tension. Focus on posture and good pedaling.
Include 4–6 × 30 sec., build to Z5 (10 sec. at Z3, Z4, and Z5)
3–4 min. spin between each 30 sec. build

TRAINER OPTION

Warm-Up 10–20 min. Z1 spin

Pre-Main
5 × 90 sec. Z1 at very fast rpm
30 sec. spin between intervals

Main 4–6 rounds of:
15 sec. build as 5 sec. at Z3, Z4, and Z5
3 min. Z1 spin between intervals

Steady and smooth home

Scale for Time Scale duration as needed.

Scale for Fatigue Remove the Z5 effort work, but moving the body will help. Do something that feels good.

SESSION TWO

STRENGTH & CONDITIONING
30 min.

Scale for Time Be sure you get in at least 5–10 min. of mobility work.

Scale for Fatigue This is a floating session that can occur any day.

SATURDAY

SESSION ONE

KEY **BIKE + RUN**
END-OF-RANGE Strength-Endurance, 160–200 min.

Warm-Up 30–45 min. smooth

Pre-Main 1–2 rounds of:
3 min. Z2 steady, 30 sec. Z1,
2 min. Z3 steady, 1 min. Z1,
1 min. Z3/Z4, 90 sec. Z1

Main
5 × 10 min. hill reps on a 4–6% grade, all very strong, sustained effort
Odds: <65 rpm
Evens: holding >95 rpm
Spin down with at least 5–6 min. recovery between intervals

30–45 min. at IM effort with great posture and form home

RUN OFF THE BIKE

5 min. quick ramp to or above IM goal pace
5 min. at IM goal pace
5 min. smooth, form-focused endurance
10 min. above IM pace
5 min. smooth, form-focused endurance
10 min. above IM pace

Scale for Time Trim Warm-Up and shift the Main set to 2 × 30 min. IM effort with the last 10 min. of each above IM effort.

Scale for Fatigue Transition to a feel-good endurance ride.

SESSION TWO

PM OFF

SUNDAY

SESSION ONE

KEY **SWIM**

ENDURANCE Over-Distance, 4150–4450

Warm-Up 10 min. easy

Pre-Main 5–7 rounds (fins can be used):
50 at 70% with 10 sec. rest,
50 at 80% with 5–7 sec. rest,
50 at 90% with 3–5 sec. rest

Then, 2 rounds of:
2 × 25 fast,
50 easy, 50 fast,
2 × 25 easy
All with 15 sec. rest

Main
1500 straight with buoy, build by 500 to strong
1 min. rest
15 × 100 very strong with 10 sec. rest

Scale for Time Scale Pre-Main and Main sets as needed.

Scale for Fatigue Alter Main Set to: 3 × 400 smooth pull, then 16 × 50 Z2 with great form, with 10 sec. rest.

SESSION TWO

SUPPORTING **RUN**

ENDURANCE General Endurance, 100–130 min.

This is a recommended session.

Warm-Up 10 min. easy

Main
90–120 min. low-stress endurance run on variable terrain. If you are injury prone, a softer surface is ideal.
Take short 20–40 sec. walk breaks as needed to retain form.

Scale for Time Scale duration as needed.

Scale for Fatigue Include more walk breaks and keep the effort purely conversational. Make total run no more than 1 hr.

FOCUS Enjoy a little recuperation before ramping into a weekend of fast, high-intensity sessions. The weekend is a great opportunity to include a sprint- or Olympic-distance race, or even a 70.3. If so, make early next week easy. Test your fueling strategy in the race-simulation.

WEEKLY OVERVIEW

	M	T	W	TH	F	SA	SU	TOTAL
S1	20–45 min.	40–70 min.	70–80 min.	45–60 min.	45–90 min.	3–4 hr.	40–60 min.	10.8–15.3 hr.
S2	30 min.	60–80 min.	—	60–75 min.	—	—	1–1.5 hr.	

MONDAY

SESSION ONE

SUPPORTING **BIKE**
TECHNICAL Recovery, 20–45 min.

Main
20–45 min. very low stress
First and last 10 min. at high rpm in a small gear. Feel free to be on a trainer or outside.

If you ride outside, practice some cornering and bike handling skills to refine control and comfort on the bike.

Scale for Time Trim as needed or skip if unable to complete.

Scale for Fatigue It may still be worth moving your blood here, not for fitness, but rather to enhance recovery and adaptations.

SESSION TWO

STRENGTH & CONDITIONING
30 min.

Scale for Time Be sure you get in at least 5–10 min. of mobility work.

Scale for Fatigue This is a floating session that can occur any day.

TUESDAY

SESSION ONE

SUPPORTING **SWIM**
ENDURANCE Short Intervals, 2400–3800

This is a recommended session.

Warm-Up 10 min. easy

Pre-Main 5–7 rounds (fins can be used):
50 at 70% with 10 sec. rest,
50 at 80% with 5–7 sec. rest,
50 at 90% with 3–5 sec. rest

Then, 2 rounds of:
2 × 25 fast,
50 easy, 50 fast,
2 × 25 easy
All with 15 sec. rest

Main With paddles:
50–90 × 25 at 85–90% with 2–5 sec. rest between intervals

Scale for Time Reduce Warm-Up slightly and do fewer rounds in Pre-Main set.

Scale for Fatigue Shift Main set to 30 × 25 at 80% with 5 sec. rest, then 2 rounds of 8 × 25 (odds smooth, evens MAX with 10 sec. rest) with 50 easy between each 25.

SESSION TWO

SUPPORTING **RUN**
ENDURANCE General Endurance, 60–80 min.

Warm-Up 10 min. easy
Add dynamic warm-up if possible.

Main
50–70 min. low stress
Every 4th min. or so check on form, posture, etc. Aim for best MFP. Do not exceed Z2 effort.

Scale for Time Adjust duration as needed.

Scale for Fatigue Adjust duration or skip if needed.

WEDNESDAY

SESSION ONE

KEY BIKE + RUN
END-OF-RANGE High Cadence, 70–80 min.

Warm-Up As needed.

Main Up to 2 rounds of MAX sprints:
10 sec. MAX, 50 sec. easy,
20 sec. MAX, 40 sec. easy,
30 sec. MAX, 30 sec. easy,
40 sec. MAX, 50 sec. easy,
50 sec. MAX, 50 sec. easy,
60 sec. MAX,
10 sec. easy, 50 sec. MAX,
20 sec. easy, 40 sec. MAX,
30 sec. easy, 30 sec. MAX,
40 sec. easy, 20 sec. MAX,
50 sec. easy, 10 sec. MAX
7 min. easy spinning between rounds
Do MAX efforts as best effort at >90 rpm

Cool-down 5–15 min. spin

RUN OFF THE BIKE

5 min. ramp to IM effort
5 min. at IM effort
5 min. MFP
10 min. above IM effort
5 min. MFP

Scale for Time Scale Main set as needed.

Scale for Fatigue Remove the MAX sprint efforts and replace with an easy ride.

SESSION TWO

PM OFF

THURSDAY

SESSION ONE

KEY SWIM
INTERVALS Building, 2200

Warm-Up 10 min. easy

Pre-Main 2 rounds of:
2 × 25 MAX with paddles,
50 easy float with good form,
50 fast with paddles,
2 × 25 easy

Main
Practice pacing, increasing speed with effort.
Sight 3 times per lap.
8 × 100 as:
2 at 70%, 2 at 80%, 2 at 90%, 2 very strong
All with 30 sec. rest

8 × 75 as:
2 at 70%, 2 at 80%, 2 at 90%, 2 very strong
All with 20 sec. rest

8 × 50 as:
2 at 70%, 2 at 80%, 2 at 90%, 2 very strong
All with 10 sec. rest

Scale for Time Transition to 5 × 100, 5 × 75, 5 × 50, always 1 at 70%, 1 at 80%, 1 at 90%, 2 very strong.

Scale for Fatigue Adjust the very strong efforts in the Main set to form-based short intervals, endurance and smooth.

SESSION TWO

SUPPORTING BIKE
TECHNICAL Activation, 60–75 min.

Warm-Up 30 min. smooth

Main 2–3 rounds of:
5 min. smooth,
2 min. spin higher rpm in a small gear,
3 min. steady,
2 min. spin higher rpm in a small gear,
1 min. strong,
2 min. spin higher rpm in a small gear

TRAINER OPTION

Warm-Up 10 min. spin

Pre-Main
5 × 3 min. smooth, ramp rpm by 1 min. to fast rpm

Then complete Main set detailed above.

Scale for Time Simple scale of duration as needed.

Scale for Fatigue Trim duration or skip if needed. Remove the neurological high-cadence speed work if needed.

FRIDAY

SESSION ONE

SUPPORTING **BIKE**
TECHNICAL Prep, 45–90 min.

This is a recommended session.

This is a feel-good ride, whatever that is for you: more, less, building intervals, spinning, etc. Be aware and look for patterns to better manage readiness. Here is a possible option, but do what works for you.

Main
45–90 min. smooth
Include 4 × 3 min., ramp by 1 min. to strong but not deep effort
3–4 min. easy spin between intervals

Scale for Time Scale duration as needed.

Scale for Fatigue Remove the ramping effort, but moving the body will still help. Do something that feels good.

SESSION TWO

PM OFF

SATURDAY

SESSION ONE

KEY **BIKE** + **RUN**
END-OF-RANGE Building, 3–4 hr.

Warm-Up 60 min.

Main
2–3 × 5 min. strong effort in aero position at 60 rpm
5 min. form-based endurance at choice rpm between intervals
10 min. smooth endurance

2–3 × 5 min. strong effort at >90 rpm
5 min. form-based endurance at choice rpm between intervals
10 min. smooth endurance

1–2 × 20 min. at IM effort
Feel good with tidy form.
5 min. easy between intervals

Finish with smooth endurance ride home with good posture and pedaling.

RUN OFF THE BIKE

5 min. ramp to IM goal pace
5 min. at IM pace
5 min. above IM pace
5 min. at MFP
10 min. at IM goal pace

Scale for Time Scale duration and do 2 intervals of both low and high rpm for 5 min., but remove the 10 min. smooth endurance intervals.

Scale for Fatigue Transition to a feel-good endurance ride with 3 × 6 min. smooth, build by 2 min. to strong but not deep effort.

SESSION TWO

PM OFF

SUNDAY

SESSION ONE

KEY **SWIM**
EVENT-SPECIFIC Pyramid, 2300–3800

Warm-Up Smooth 10 min. light, then
400 pull smooth with choice of equipment at 70%

Main
Progressive building effort with medium-duration swims: 1500 swim with variable pace. Always 15 sec. rest.

150 steady at 85%, 100 form-based Z2 at 70%
125 strong at 90%, 100 form-based Z2 at 70%
100 very strong at 95%, 100 form-based Z2 at 70%
50 MAX with good, tidy hold on the water
(no panic)
100 form-based Z2 at 70%, 100 very strong at 95%
100 form-based Z2 at 70%, 125 strong at 90%
100 form-based Z2 at 70%, 150 steady at 85%
100 form-based Z2 at 70%

400 pull smooth with 2 min. rest, then repeat round if feeling very good

Scale for Time Reduce performance pyramid to be: 100, 75, 50, 75, 100, progressing as strong, very strong, MAX.

Scale for Fatigue Convert to 1500–2000 very easy. Mix it up with toys, etc. Do as you wish, but feel good and move the body.

SESSION TWO

SUPPORTING **RUN**
EVENT-SPECIFIC Intervals, 1–1.5 hr.

Warm-Up 10 min. easy

Main
50–80 min. low stress endurance run on variable terrain
Include 20 min. as:
5 min. form-based running,
10 min. IM race effort,
5 min. just above IM race effort

Scale for Time Scale duration as needed. No more fitness to be gained.

Scale for Fatigue Skip the run completely.

FOCUS We now finalize the preparation with a race-focused block of work and some open-water skills practice in the pool (sighting), as well as event-specific preparation on the bike and run. We have very little strength-endurance now, but enough to remind the body of the stressor. We move to faster and flatter riding and running. Simulate race fueling and hydration in the key sessions.

WEEKLY OVERVIEW

	M	T	W	TH	F	SA	SU	TOTAL
S1	40–60 min.	45–75 min.	1–1.5 hr.	45–70 min.	45–90 min.	45–75 min.	3.5–4 hr.	13.4– 18.8 hr.
S2	—	50–80 min.	30 min.	2–3 hr.	30 min.	85–110 min.	—	

MONDAY

SESSION ONE

SUPPORTING RUN
TECHNICAL Recovery, 40–60 min.

Warm-Up 10 min. easy

Main
30–50 min. very low stress
Aim for best MFP. Control effort by adding leg speed, striding/bounding, activation, and practice the run/walk protocol.

Scale for Time Trim as needed or skip if unable to complete.

Scale for Fatigue If your muscles are sore, convert to a 30–45 min. flush/spin on the bike or a very easy 1–2 km swim.

SESSION TWO

PM OFF

TUESDAY

SESSION ONE

KEY SWIM
ENDURANCE Building, 2400–3700

Warm-Up 600–800, swim every 4th lap as non-free

Main 12 × 150–200, do as 3 rounds of:
1 at 70% with 30 sec. rest,
1 at 80% with 20 sec. rest,
2 at 90–95% with 10 sec. rest

Add-On 20 × 25 with paddles (or parachute), do as 5 rounds of: 3 fast, 1 easy
Always 10 sec. rest

Scale for Time Adjust Main set to 12 × 100 and skip the Add-On.

Scale for Fatigue Drop Main set to 6 intervals and only build to 85% as 2 rounds of 1 at 70%, 1 at 80%, 1 at 85%.

SESSION TWO

SUPPORTING RUN
ENDURANCE General Endurance, 50–80 min.

Warm-Up 10 min. easy
Add dynamic warm-up if possible.

Main
40–70 min. MFP, smooth
Every 4th min. or so, check in on form, posture, etc. Do not exceed Z2. Control effort by adding leg speed, striding/bounding, activation, and practice the run/walk protocol.

Scale for Time Simple scale of duration as needed.

Scale for Fatigue Trim duration or skip if needed.

SESSION ONE

KEY **RUN**
INTERVALS Speed, 1–1.5 hr.

Warm-Up 10 min. easy

Pre-Main 1–2 rounds:
3 min. smooth, 30 sec. easy,
2 min. steady, 30 sec. easy,
1 min. strong, 30 sec. easy

Main
6–8 × 1 km at 10 sec. per mile faster than IM 70.3 goal pace
90 sec. rest between intervals

10 min. smooth form-based endurance home

OPTIONAL PM RUN

20–40 min. very low stress
Include 10-20-30-20-10 sec. blasts with 90 sec. easy running between each effort.

Scale for Time Maintain the 1 km intervals, but reduce the number of intervals as needed.

Scale for Fatigue Convert to a smooth and progressively building effort to finish feeling better than when you started.

SESSION TWO

STRENGTH & CONDITIONING
30 min.

Scale for Time Be sure you hit at least 5–10 min. of mobility.

Scale for Fatigue This is a floating session that can occur any day.

SESSION ONE

SUPPORTING **SWIM**
ENDURANCE Short Intervals, 1950–3150

This is a recommended session.

Warm-Up 10 min. easy

Pre-Main 5–7 rounds (fins can be used):
50 at 70% with 10 sec. rest,
50 at 80% with 5–7 sec. rest,
50 at 90% with 3–5 sec. rest

Then, 2 rounds of:
2 × 25 fast,
50 easy, 50 fast,
2 × 25 easy
All with 15 sec. rest

Main 20–30 × 50 at 85% with 5–7 sec. rest
Choose a send-off interval and aim to leave on the same time each 50. Introduce sighting 3 times per lap.

Add-On 16–24 × 25 at 90–95% with only 3–5 sec. rest. Remove sighting to focus on keeping rhythm but increase your tempo.

Scale for Time Scale Pre-Main and Main sets as needed.

Scale for Fatigue Maintain the session, but make the 50s all at 80% and remove the 25s at the end. Skip the rounds of 2 × 25, 50, 50, 2 × 25 in the Pre-Main set.

SESSION TWO

SUPPORTING **BIKE**
TECHNICAL Activation, 2–3 hr.

This is a recommended session.

Main
2–3 hr. endurance ride
Include 5 rounds of:
20 sec. MAX effort,
2 min. Z3 steady,
5 min. Z1 spin

TRAINER OPTION

Warm-Up 30 min. stepper, building easy to moderate

Main 5 rounds of:
20 sec. MAX effort,
2 min. Z3 steady,
5 min. Z1 spin

Add-On 15 min. Z2 smooth riding home

Scale for Time Scale the length, but maintain the restorative nature of the ride.

Scale for Fatigue Skip the ride if needed.

IRONMAN

RACE SPECIFIC

FRIDAY	SATURDAY

FRIDAY

SESSION ONE

SUPPORTING BIKE
TECHNICAL Prep, 45–90 min.

Main
45–90 min. smooth
Include 4 × 3 min., ramp by 1 min. to Z5 strong but
not deep effort
3–4 min. rest between intervals

Scale for Time Scale duration as needed.

Scale for Fatigue Remove the Z5 effort, but moving
the body will still help. Do something that feels
good.

SESSION TWO

STRENGTH & CONDITIONING
30 min.

Scale for Time Be sure you hit at least 5–10 min.
of mobility.

Scale for Fatigue This is a floating session that can
occur any day.

SATURDAY

SESSION ONE

KEY SWIM
ENDURANCE Building, 2550–3750

Warm-Up 10 min. easy

Pre-Main 2–3 rounds with snorkel:
300 at 70% with 30 sec. rest,
3 × 50 form-based swimming, building tempo,
effort, and stroke rate throughout
All with 10 sec. rest

Main 3–4 rounds of:
400 at 80%,
200 at 85%,
100 at 90%

Add-On 2 rounds of power:
4 × 25 MAX with paddles,
150 form-based swimming

Scale for Time Trim the Pre-Main set to a single
round and remove the Add-On power work.

Scale for Fatigue Trim the Pre-Main to a single
round. Shift Main set to 2-3 rounds of 300, 200,
100 smooth endurance. Remove the Add-On
power work.

SESSION TWO

SUPPORTING RUN
ENDURANCE General Endurance, 85–110 min.

Warm-Up 10 min. easy

Main
75–100 min. low-stress endurance run on variable
terrain
If you are injury prone, a softer surface is ideal.
Take short 20–40 sec. walk breaks as needed to
retain form.

Scale for Time Scale duration as needed. No more
fitness to be gained.

Scale for Fatigue Trim duration or skip if needed.

SUNDAY

KEY **BIKE** + **RUN**
EVENT-SPECIFIC Race Simulation, 3.5–4 hr.

Warm-Up 30–45 min. smooth

Pre-Main 1–2 rounds of:
3 min. Z2 steady, 30 sec. Z1, 2 min. Z3 steady,
1 min. Z1, 1 min. Z3/Z4, 90 sec. Z1

Main
20 min. steady endurance choice rpm (IM or so)
5 min. Z4 very strong as:
1 min. at 80 rpm,
1 min. at 90 rpm,
1 min. at 100+ rpm,
1 min. at 90 rpm,
1 min. at 80 rpm
5 min. spin

Then, 2 rounds of:
20 min. steady endurance choice rpm (IM or so)
5 min. Z4 very strong as:
1 min. at 70 rpm,
1 min. at 60 rpm,
1 min. at 50 rpm,
1 min. at 60 rpm,
1 min. at 70 rpm
5 min. spin

Then, 20 min. steady endurance choice rpm
(IM or so)
5 min. Z4 very strong as:
1 min. at 80 rpm,
1 min. at 90 rpm,
1 min. at 100+ rpm,
1 min. at 90 rpm,
1 min. at 80 rpm
5 min. spin

Endurance riding home

RUN OFF THE BIKE

5 min. ramp to at or above IM effort
Hold IM effort for 20 min.
5 min. above IM effort
5 min. easy cool-down

Scale for Time Trim Warm-Up and shift the Main
set to: 2 × 30 min. IM effort with the last 10 min.
of each above IM effort.

Scale for Fatigue Transition to a feel-good
endurance ride.

PM OFF

FOCUS Highlights include a hearty event-specific brick in the middle of the week and a weekend dominated with run preparation and an endurance ride. Don't forget to practice race-day fueling and hydration in the key sessions.

WEEKLY OVERVIEW

	M	T	W	TH	F	SA	SU	TOTAL
S1	20–45 min.	70–90 min.	135 min.	70–100 min.	45–60 min.	70–90 min.	2–4 hr.	15.2–20.5 hr.
S2	—	40–100 min.	30 min.	75 min.	30 min.	115 min.	1.5–2 hr.	

MONDAY

SESSION ONE

SUPPORTING BIKE
TECHNICAL Recovery, 20–45 min.

Main
20–45 min.
Very low stress ride on a trainer or outside with first and last 10 min. at fast rpm, in a small gear.

If you ride outside, practice cornering and bike handling skills to refine control and comfort on the bike.

Scale for Time Trim as needed or skip if unable to complete.

Scale for Fatigue It may still be worth fitting in the ride not for fitness, but to enhance recovery and adaptations.

SESSION TWO

PM OFF

TUESDAY

SESSION ONE

KEY SWIM
ENDURANCE Over-Distance, 4700

Warm-Up 5–10 min. easy with mix of strokes

Pre-Main 2 × 400 as:
75 smooth, 25 strong,
75 smooth, 25 very strong,
75 smooth, 25 MAX,
100 smooth
1 min. rest between intervals

Main
3000 straight swim, gradually build by 500 to 85%
1 min. rest
9 × 100 very strong, with paddles
15 sec. rest between intervals

Scale for Time Scale Pre-Main set to 1 × 400, then trim the Main set to 1500–2000 and 6 × 100 to finish.

Scale for Fatigue Remove the 100s at the end of the Main set and maintain smooth swimming for a straight 1000–1500 pull.

SESSION TWO

SUPPORTING RUN
ENDURANCE General Endurance, 40–100 min.

Warm-Up 10 min. easy
Add dynamic warm-up if possible.

Main
30–90 min.
Every 4th min. or so check on form, posture, etc.
Aim for best MFP. Do not exceed Z2 effort.

Scale for Time Adjust duration as needed.

Scale for Fatigue Trim duration or skip if needed.

WEDNESDAY

KEY **BIKE + RUN**
EVENT-SPECIFIC Intervals, 135 min.

Warm-Up 10 min. spin

Pre-Main
2 × 4 min. build to Z3/Z4, then spin easy

Main
4 × 8 min. Z3+ effort at <65 rpm
4 min. Z2 between intervals

Then, 5 min. Z1 into:
20 min. above IM goal effort at choice rpm

RUN OFF THE BIKE

This run forces you into goal pace, so aim to do so with great form and posture.
4 min. ramp to IM goal pace (or Z3/Z3+)
2 min. Z2 easy endurance

7 min. at 10-15 sec. per mile faster than IM 70.3 goal pace (or Z3/Z3+)
2 min. Z2 easy endurance

7 min. at 20 sec. per mile faster than IM 70.3 goal pace (or Z3+/Z4)
2 min. Z2 easy endurance

7 min. at 10-15 sec. per mile faster than IM 70.3 goal pace (or Z3/Z3+)
2 min. Z2 easy endurance

Finish with 10 min. at IM pace feel without looking at the watch.

Scale for Time Reduce the number of intervals in the Main set, but still aim to retain at least 7 min. of IM goal effort at the end with rpm of choice. The brick run becomes 5 min. ramp to 70.3, 5 min. above 70.3, 5 min. easy.

Scale for Fatigue Maintain the Pre-Main but convert the Main set to: 4 × 10 min. Z2, build rpm to fast on each. Remove all work from the brick run and convert to smooth 15 min. with good form.

STRENGTH & CONDITIONING
30 min.

Scale for Time Be sure you get in at least 5–10 min. of mobility work.

Scale for Fatigue This is a floating session that can occur any day.

THURSDAY

SUPPORTING **SWIM**
ENDURANCE Building, 3800–5300

Warm-Up 10 min. easy

Pre-Main 5–7 rounds (fins can be used):
50 at 70% with 10 sec. rest,
50 at 80% with 5–7 sec. rest,
50 at 90% with 3–5 sec. rest

Then, 2 rounds of:
2 × 25 fast,
50 easy, 50 fast,
2 × 25 easy
All with 15 sec. rest

Main 3 rounds of:
12–18 × 50 at 85% with 5–7 sec. rest
(paddles are OK if you can retain stroke rate),
10–14 × 25 at 90–95% with 3–5 sec. rest
100 easy with 45 sec. rest between rounds

Scale for Time Scale Pre-Main and Main sets by reducing the number of rounds or intervals within the rounds.

Scale for Fatigue Alter Main set to: 30–60 × 25, but only at 80%, no paddles.

KEY **RUN**
ENDURANCE General Endurance, 75 min.

Main 75 min. steady and smooth build as:
30 min. easy and low stress (likely Z2),
20 min. moderate effort (lower Z3),
15 min. moderately strong effort, just above IM effort (Z3),
10 min. strong (Z3+)

Scale for Time Scale the length of the run, but with similar pace/effort ramp, such as: 20, 15, 10, 5 min.

Scale for Fatigue Begin very easy and gradually ramp up in effort, but it can convert to a feel-good endurance run.

FRIDAY

SESSION ONE

SUPPORTING **BIKE**
TECHNICAL Prep, 45–60 min.

Main
45–60 min.
First and last 10 min. at >95 rpm with minimum power while retaining chain tension. Focus on posture and good pedaling.
Include 4–6 × 30 sec., build to Z5 effort in the last 10 sec. of each.
3–4 min. endurance riding between each 30 sec. build.

TRAINER OPTION

Warm-Up 10–20 min. Z1 easy

Pre-Main
5 × 90 sec. Z1 at very fast rpm
30 sec. spin between intervals

Main 4–6 rounds of:
15 sec. build as 5 sec. at Z3, Z4, Z5
3 min. Z1 spin between intervals

Finish with smooth endurance ride home.

Scale for Time Scale duration as needed.

Scale for Fatigue Remove the Z5 effort, but moving the body will still help. Do something that feels good.

SESSION TWO

STRENGTH & CONDITIONING
30 min.

Scale for Time Be sure you get in at least 5–10 min. of mobility work.

Scale for Fatigue This is a floating session that can occur any day.

SATURDAY

SESSION ONE

KEY **SWIM**
ENDURANCE Over-Distance, 4150–4450

Warm-Up 10 min. easy

Pre-Main 5–7 rounds (fins can be used):
50 at 70% with 10 sec. rest,
50 at 80% with 5–7 sec. rest,
50 at 90% with 3–5 sec. rest

Then, 2 rounds of:
2 × 25 fast,
50 easy, 50 fast,
2 × 25 easy
All with 15 sec. rest

Main
1500 straight with buoy, build by 500 to strong
1 min. rest
15 × 100 very strong with 10 sec. rest

Scale for Time Scale Pre-Main and Main sets as needed.

Scale for Fatigue Alter Main set to: 3 × 400 smooth pull, then 16 × 50 smooth with great form, with 10 sec. rest.

SESSION TWO

KEY **RUN**
INTERVALS Tempo, 115 min.

Warm-Up 10 min. easy

Pre-Main 1–2 rounds until you are ready to go:
3 min. smooth, 30 sec. easy,
2 min. steady, 30 sec. easy,
1 min. strong, 30 sec. easy

Main
2 × 30 min. at above IM effort, Z3 to Z3+, very much in control, with fluid and smooth running
10 min. easy between intervals

Then 10 min. smooth, form-based endurance home

Scale for Time Reduce the 2 × 30 min. efforts to 2 × 20 min.

Scale for Fatigue Convert to a smooth and progressively building effort to finish feeling better than when you started (no matter how weak the build is).

SUNDAY

SESSION ONE

SUPPORTING **BIKE**
ENDURANCE General Endurance, 2–4 hr.

This is a recommended session.

Main
2–4 hr. endurance ride on variable terrain
Include 5 rounds of:
20 sec. MAX effort,
2 min. Z2/Z3,
5 min. Z1

TRAINER OPTION

Warm-Up 30 min. stepper, gradually ramp effort from very easy to steady

Main 4 rounds of:
4 min. Z1/Z2 easy choice pedaling,
30 sec. Z1 easy,
3 min. Z2 smooth build rpm to fast,
30 sec. Z1 easy,
2 min. Z2/Z3 smooth choice pedaling,
30 sec. Z1 easy,
1 min. steady Z3 build rpm to fast,
30 sec. Z1 easy

Add-On 30 min. Z2 choice, no stronger than IM effort to finish

Scale for Time Reduce Warm-Up to 15 min. stepper. Reduce rounds in Main set as needed.

Scale for Fatigue Reduce the Warm-Up to a 15 min. stepper. Main set can be 2 rounds.

SESSION TWO

KEY **SWIM**
EVENT-SPECIFIC Race Simulation, 5400

Warm-Up 10 min. jog prior to swimming if possible

Main 2 rounds of ladder:
200 smooth with some little builds
1 min. float
200 take out (TO) effort, 400 race effort
50 TO effort, 200 race effort
50 TO effort, 100 race effort
50 TO effort, 50 race effort
50 TO effort, 100 race effort
50 TO effort, 200 race effort
Always 10 sec. rest
All race efforts at 85%

Then 1000 continuous with toys of choice. Hold smooth form.

Scale for Time Scale Main set to 1 round of ladder.

Scale for Fatigue Convert all efforts to a smooth form-based endurance session; nothing over 80%.

FOCUS A massive mental shift begins: You cannot gain any more fitness, and you must gain control over your program with confidence. It is all feel-good, smooth, sharpening work. You might feel flat in the coming days, but the mission is for you to do the work you are good at and enjoy it, without creating any deep fatigue or searching for validation. When in doubt, go less and go easier.

WEEKLY OVERVIEW

	M	T	W	TH	F	SA	SU	TOTAL
S1	20–45 min.	85–100 min.	45–60 min.	40–60 min.	45–90 min.	165–195 min.	50–75 min.	11.5–
S2	30 min.	—	60–80 min.	60–75 min.	30 min.	—	1–1.5 hr.	15.5 hr.

MONDAY

SESSION ONE

SUPPORTING **BIKE**
TECHNICAL Recovery, 20–45 min.

Main
20–45 min. very low stress
First and last 10 min. at high rpm in a small gear. Feel free to ride on a trainer or outside.

If you ride outside, practice cornering and bike handling skills to refine control and comfort on the bike.

Scale for Time Trim as needed or skip if unable to complete.

Scale for Fatigue It may still be worth fitting in the ride not for fitness, but to enhance recovery and adaptations.

SESSION TWO

STRENGTH & CONDITIONING
30 min.

Scale for Time Be sure you get in at least 5–10 min. of mobility work.

Scale for Fatigue This is a floating session that can occur any day.

TUESDAY

SESSION ONE

KEY **BIKE + RUN**
END-OF-RANGE High Cadence, 85–100 min.

Warm-Up As needed.

Main Up to 2 rounds of MAX sprints:
10 sec. MAX, 50 sec. easy,
20 sec. MAX, 40 sec. easy,
30 sec. MAX, 30 sec. easy,
40 sec. MAX, 20 sec. easy,
50 sec. MAX, 10 sec. easy,
60 sec. MAX,
10 sec. easy, 50 sec. MAX,
20 sec. easy, 40 sec. MAX,
30 sec. easy, 30 sec. MAX,
40 sec. easy, 20 sec. MAX,
50 sec. easy, 10 sec. MAX
7 min. easy spinning between rounds
Do MAX efforts as best effort at >90 rpm
Use the same gear for each work effort. Cadence decreases as set progresses. Shift from recovery gear 3 sec. before work starts.

Cool-down 5–15 min. spin

RUN OFF THE BIKE

5 min. ramp to IM feel
5 min. form-based running
10 min. at IM feel
5 min. above IM feel
5 min. form-based running

Scale for Time Reduce Warm-Up slightly, but this is a very short session as it is.

Scale for Fatigue Remove the MAX effort and replace it with an easy ride.

SESSION TWO

PM OFF

WEDNESDAY

SESSION ONE

SUPPORTING **SWIM**
ENDURANCE Short Intervals, 2150–2950

This is a recommended session.

Warm-Up 10 min. easy

Pre-Main 5–7 rounds (fins can be used):
50 at 70% with 10 sec. rest,
50 at 80% with 5–7 sec. rest,
50 at 90% with 3–5 sec. rest

Then, 2 rounds of:
2 × 25 fast,
50 easy, 50 fast,
2 × 25 easy
All with 15 sec. rest

Main With paddles:
40–60 × 25 at 85–90% with 2–5 sec. rest
between intervals

Scale for Time Scale Pre-Main and Main sets as
needed.

Scale for Fatigue Alter Main Set to: 20–40 × 25,
but only at 80% and no paddles.

SESSION TWO

SUPPORTING **RUN**
ENDURANCE General Endurance, 60–80 min.

Warm-Up 10 min. easy
Add dynamic warm-up if possible.

Main
50–70 min. low stress
Every 4th min. or so, check on form, posture, etc.
Aim for best MFP. Do not exceed Z2 effort.

Scale for Time Scale the duration as needed.

Scale for Fatigue Trim duration or skip if needed.

THURSDAY

SESSION ONE

KEY **SWIM**
ENDURANCE Over-Distance, 3400

Warm-Up 5–10 min. easy with mix of strokes

Pre-Main 2 × 400 as:
75 smooth, 25 strong,
75 smooth, 25 very strong,
75 smooth, 25 MAX,
100 smooth
Always 1 min. rest

Main
2000 straight swim gradually build by 500 to 85%
1 min. rest
6 × 100 very strong with 15 sec. rest with paddles
on to finish

Scale for Time Scale Pre-Main set to only 1 × 400,
then trim Main set to 1000–1500 and 4 × 100 to
finish.

Scale for Fatigue Remove the 100s at the end of
the Main set and maintain smooth swimming for a
straight 1000–1500 pull.

SESSION TWO

SUPPORTING **BIKE**
TECHNICAL Activation, 60–75 min.

Warm-Up 30 min. smooth

Main 2–3 rounds of:
5 min. smooth,
2 min. spin higher rpm in a small gear,
3 min. steady,
2 min. spin higher rpm in a small gear,
1 min. strong,
2 min. spin higher rpm in a small gear

TRAINER OPTION

Warm-Up 10 min. spin

Pre-Main
5 × 3 min. smooth, ramp rpm by 1 min. to fast rpm

Main 2–3 rounds of:
5 min. smooth,
2 min. spin higher rpm in a small gear,
3 min. steady,
2 min. spin higher rpm in a small gear,
1 min. strong,
2 min. spin higher rpm in a small gear

Scale for Time Scale the duration as needed.

Scale for Fatigue Trim duration or skip if needed.
Remove the neurological speed work if needed.

FRIDAY	SATURDAY

FRIDAY

SESSION ONE

SUPPORTING **BIKE**
TECHNICAL Prep, 45–90 min.

This is a feel-good ride, whatever that is for you: more, less, building intervals, spinning, etc. Be aware and look for patterns to better manage readiness. Here is a possible option, but do what works for you.

Main
45–90 min. smooth
Include 4 × 3 min., ramp by 1 min. to strong but not deep effort
3–4 min. Z2 riding between intervals

Scale for Time Scale duration as needed.

Scale for Fatigue Remove the ramping effort, but moving the body will still help. Do something that feels good.

SESSION TWO

STRENGTH & CONDITIONING
30 min.

Scale for Time Be sure you get in at least 5–10 min. of mobility work.

Scale for Fatigue This is a floating session that can occur any day.

SATURDAY

SESSION ONE

KEY **BIKE + RUN**
END-OF-RANGE Building, 165–195 min.

Warm-Up 60 min.

Main
2–3 × 5 min. strong effort at 60 rpm
5 min. form-based endurance at choice rpm between intervals
10 min. smooth endurance

2–3 × 5 min. strong effort at >90 rpm
5 min. form-based endurance at choice rpm between intervals
10 min. smooth endurance

20–30 min. at IM effort/pace. Feel good with tidy form.

Finish with smooth endurance riding home with good posture and pedaling.

RUN OFF THE BIKE

5 min. ramp to IM goal pace
5 min. at MFP
5 min. above IM goal pace
5 min. at MFP
5 min. at IM goal pace

Scale for Time Reduce to 90 min. to 2 hr. and only do 1 round of the Main set.

Scale for Fatigue Transition to a feel-good 1.5–2 hr. endurance ride; in the first and last 10 min. spin at high rpm.

SESSION TWO

PM OFF

SUNDAY

KEY **SWIM**
EVENT-SPECIFIC Pyramid, 2150–3900

Warm-Up Smooth 10 min. light, then 400 pull smooth with choice of equipment at 70%

Main
Progressive 1350 building effort with shorter swims and variable pace:
125 steady at 85%, 100 form-based Z2 at 70%
100 strong at 90%, 100 form-based Z2 at 70%
75 at very strong at 95%, 100 form-based Z2 at 70%
50 MAX with good, tidy hold on the water
(no panic)
100 form-based Z2 at 70%, 75 very strong at 95%
100 form-based Z2 at 70%, 100 strong at 90%
100 form-based Z2 at 70%, 125 steady at 85%
100 form-based Z2 at 70%
Always 15 sec. rest

400 pull smooth with 2 min. rest then repeat round if you're feeling very good.

Scale for Time Reduce the Main set to only 50 form-based Z2 between higher efforts.

Scale for Fatigue Go about 1500–2000, very easy. Mix it up with toys, etc. Swim as you wish, but feel good and move the body.

KEY **RUN**
EVENT-SPECIFIC Intervals, 1–1.5 hr.

Warm-Up 10 min. easy

Main
50–80 min. low stress endurance run on variable terrain
Include 20 min. as:
5 min. form-based running,
10 min. at IM race effort,
5 min. just above IM race effort

Scale for Time Scale duration as needed. No more fitness to be gained.

Scale for Fatigue Skip the run completely.

IRONMAN

RACE SPECIFIC

14

FOCUS No more worrying about "what if's." Let this week be the celebration. How you feel is irrelevent to race day performance, so set yourself up well by maintaining a clean set of eating habits, resting as much as possible, planning the race weekend experience, and getting excited. Let your race performance be an expression of your preparation.

WEEKLY OVERVIEW

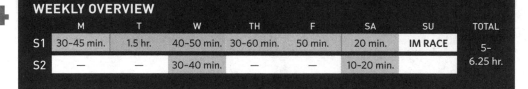

	M	T	W	TH	F	SA	SU	TOTAL
S1	30–45 min.	1.5 hr.	40–50 min.	30–60 min.	50 min.	20 min.	IM RACE	5–6.25 hr.
S2	—	—	30–40 min.	—	—	10–20 min.		

MONDAY

SESSION ONE

SUPPORTING BIKE
TECHNICAL Activation, 30–45 min.

Main
30–45 min. spin recuperation
First and last 10 min. high rpm in a small gear

TRAINER OPTION

Warm-Up 10 min. spin

Pre-Main
3 × 2 min. smooth, ramp 30 sec. at
75, 85, 95, 105 rpm
30 sec. break between intervals

Main
3 × 2 min., ramp by 30 sec. from easy to strong
2 min. spin very easy between intervals

Add-On 5 min. spin easy at higher rpm

Scale for Time Trim as needed or skip if unable to complete.

Scale for Fatigue If you're sore from last week, convert to a 30–45 min. flush/spin on the bike or very easy 1–2 km swim.

SESSION TWO

PM OFF

TUESDAY

SESSION ONE

KEY BIKE + RUN
TECHNICAL Prep, 1.5 hr.

Warm-Up 10 min. spin

Pre-Main
3 min. ramp Z1 to Z3/Z4
3 min. Z2 build rpm to fast
3 min. ramp Z1 to Z3/Z4
3 min. ramp Z2 build rpm to fast

Main
4 × 2 min. build by 30 sec. to Z4+
90 sec. Z1 spin between intervals
3 × 1 min. build by 20 sec. to Z5
90 sec. Z1 spin between intervals
2 × 30 sec. build by 10 sec. to Z5+
90 sec. Z1 spin between intervals

Then 10 min. smooth Z2

RUN OFF THE BIKE

5 min. ramp to IM effort
2 min. Z2 easy
2 min. IM effort
2 min. Z2 easy
2 min. build to above IM effort
2 min. Z2 easy
5 min. IM effort

10 min. smooth and floating

Scale for Time Cut Pre-Main to 2 × 3 min. Then Main is two rounds of each set.

Scale for Fatigue Remove the Main set but add a 15 min. build by 5 min. to the last 5 min. feeling steady and open.

SESSION TWO

PM OFF

WEDNESDAY

KEY **SWIM**
INTERVALS Building, 1700–2100

Warm-Up 10 min. smooth

Pre-Main
Pull 200, 175, 150, 125, 100, 75, 50, 25; progress to 80–85%

Main
8 × 100–150 build effort by 2 intervals to the last 2 being above race effort
Always 30 sec. rest

Scale for Time Reduce the Pre-Main set to begin at the 150. Drop to 6 Intervals in Main set as: 1 at 65%, 1 at 70%, 1 at 75%, 1 at 80%, 1 at 85%, 1 at 90%.

Scale for Fatigue Reduce the Pre-Main set to begin at the 150. Drop to 6 Intervals in the Main set and only build to 85%.

SUPPORTING **RUN**
TECHNICAL Activation, 30–40 min.

This is a recommended session.

Warm-Up 10 min. easy
Add dynamic warm-up if possible.

Main
20–30 min. low stress
Every 4th min. or so, check on form, posture, etc.
Aim for best MFP. Do not exceed Z2 effort.

Scale for Time Simple scale of duration as needed.

Scale for Fatigue Trim duration or skip if needed.

THURSDAY

SUPPORTING **BIKE**
TECHNICAL Recovery, 30–60 min.

This is a recommended session.

Main
30–60 min. smooth endurance
Nothing hard.

Add-On Do a 20–30 min. shake-out run if you travel today.

Scale for Time Scale as needed, but this may become a walk if time-crunched.

Scale for Fatigue Going for a walk and moving the blood is a good thing.

PM OFF

IRONMAN

RACE SPECIFIC

FRIDAY

SESSION ONE

SUPPORTING **BIKE + RUN**
TECHNICAL Prep, 50 min.

This is a recommended session.

Warm-Up 15 min. smooth

Pre-Main
3 × 3 min. build by 1 min. to Z3+/Z4

Main 8 min. as:
3 min. at IM effort,
2 min. at IM 70.3 effort,
3 min. at IM effort

Smooth home and feel good

RUN OFF THE BIKE

5 min. ramp to IM effort
10 min. at IM effort
5 min. at MFP

Scale for Time Scale duration as needed.

Scale for Fatigue Skip this session.

SESSION TWO

PM OFF

SATURDAY

SESSION ONE

KEY **SWIM**
TECHNICAL Prep, 20 min.

Open water session at the racecourse.

Main
10 min. to loosen up
4 × 2 min. build by 30 sec. to 90%

Then a few take-out efforts if you need to spark it up a touch.

Scale for Time Scale as needed; you are the boss to make yourself feel good for tomorrow.

Scale for Fatigue Not needed.

SESSION TWO

KEY **BIKE**
TECHNICAL Activation, 10–20 min.

Main
10–20 min. smooth easy endurance
Include 3 × 30–45 sec. ramp to strong but not deep effort
3–4 min. riding between intervals

Follow the pattern and theme of previous weeks and nail this ride. Note that this is your last chance to check out your equipment prior to racing your bike.

Scale for Time Not needed.

Scale for Fatigue Not needed.

SUNDAY

IRONMAN RACE DAY

Ironman 70.3-Distance Race-Prep Program

IRONMAN 70.3 Overview of Key Workouts in the Race-Prep Phase

WEEK TYPE	M	T	W	TH
WEEK 1 — BUILD		KEY SWIM #1 Endurance, Building	KEY BIKE #1 End-of-Range, Strength-Endurance (low rpm)	KEY RUN #1 Intervals, Tempo
WEEK 2 — BUILD		KEY SWIM #1 Endurance, Short Intervals	KEY BIKE #1 + RUN End-of-Range, Strength-Endurance (low rpm)	Supporting Swim Endurance, Short Intervals
WEEK 3 — STRENGTH-ENDURANCE		KEY BIKE #1 End-of-Range, Strength- Endurance (low rpm)	KEY SWIM #1 Technical, Form	KEY RUN #1 Technical, Prep
WEEK 4 — STRENGTH-ENDURANCE		KEY SWIM #1 Endurance, Building	KEY BIKE #1 End-of-Range, High Cadence	KEY SWIM #2 Event-Specific, Threshold
WEEK 5 — TRANSITION to Endurance		KEY BIKE #1 + RUN End-of-Range, High Cadence (max sprints)	Supporting Swim Technical, Form	KEY SWIM #1 Event-Specific, Pyramid
WEEK 6 — ENDURANCE		KEY SWIM #1 Endurance, Over-Distance	KEY RUN #3, *continues weekend work* General Endurance (1–2 hr.) + Optional Evening Run	Supporting Swim Endurance, Short Intervals
WEEK 7 — TRANSITION		KEY BIKE #1 + RUN End-of-Range, High Cadence (max sprints)	Supporting Swim Endurance, Short Intervals	KEY SWIM #1 Intervals, Building
WEEK 8 — EVENT-SPECIFIC		KEY SWIM #1 Endurance, Building	KEY BIKE #1 + RUN End-of-Range, High Cadence (high/low rpm)	KEY RUN #1 Technical, Prep
WEEK 9 — EVENT-SPECIFIC		KEY SWIM #1 Endurance, Short Intervals	Supporting Bike Technical, Prep	KEY RUN #1 Intervals, Strength
WEEK 10 — TRANSITION		KEY BIKE #1 + RUN End-of-Range, High Cadence (max sprints)	Supporting Swim Endurance, Short Intervals	KEY SWIM #1 Intervals, Building
WEEK 11 — EVENT-SPECIFIC		KEY SWIM #1 Endurance, Building	KEY RUN #1 Intervals, Speed + Optional Evening Run	Easier Supporting Sessions (Swim, Bike)
WEEK 12 — EVENT-SPECIFIC		KEY SWIM #1 Endurance, Short Intervals	KEY BIKE #1 + RUN Event-Specific, Simulation	KEY RUN #1 Intervals, Tempo
WEEK 13 — TRANSITION		KEY BIKE #1 + RUN End-of-Range, High- Cadence (max sprints)	Supporting Swim Endurance, Short Intervals	KEY SWIM #1 Intervals, Building
WEEK 14 — RACE		KEY BIKE #1 + RUN Technical, Prep	KEY SWIM #1 Endurance, Building Supporting Run Technical, Prep	Easier Supporting Sessions (Swim, Bike)

F	SA	SU	TOTAL TIME (HR.)
	KEY BIKE #2 + RUN Event-Specific, Intervals	KEY SWIM #2 Event-Specific, Threshold	6.2–7.1
	KEY RUN #1 Intervals, Tempo	KEY BIKE #2 + RUN General Endurance (2.5–4.5 hr.)	7.25–10.2
	KEY BIKE #2 + RUN Event-Specific, Simulation	KEY SWIM #2 Endurance, Over-Distance KEY RUN #2 Intervals, Strength	7.6–9.6
	KEY RUN #1 Intervals, Strength	KEY BIKE #2 General Endurance (2–4 hr.)	6.2–9.2
	KEY RUN #1 General Endurance (75–100 min.)	KEY RUN #2 General Endurance (75–100 min.)	4.75–7.2
Double trainer ride	KEY BIKE #1 + RUN Endurance, Over-Distance Riding Tour (3.25–5.5 hr.)	KEY BIKE #2 General Endurance Riding Tour (2–4 hr.)	8–14.2
	KEY BIKE #2 + RUN End-of-Range, Building	KEY SWIM #2 Event-Specific, Pyramid KEY RUN #1 Event-Specific, Building	6.6–9.6
	KEY RUN #2 Intervals, Strength	KEY SWIM #2 Technical, Speed and Power	5.75–8
	KEY BIKE #1 + RUN End-of-Range, Strength- Endurance (high/low rpm)	KEY SWIM #2 Event-Specific, Threshold	6.3–9.1
	KEY BIKE #2 + RUN End-of-Range, Building	KEY SWIM #2 Event-Specific, Pyramid	5.3–7.1
	KEY BIKE #1 + RUN Event-Specific, Simulation (rpm mix)	KEY SWIM #2 Endurance, Building	8.25–11.4
	KEY RUN #2 Intervals, Speed KEY SWIM #2 Event-Specific, Threshold	Supporting Bike General Endurance (2–4 hr.)	5.75–7.9
	KEY BIKE #2 + RUN End-of-Range, Building	KEY SWIM #2 Event-Specific, Pyramid	5.6–7.1
Supporting Bike + Run Technical, Prep	KEY SWIM #2 Technical, Prep KEY BIKE #2 Technical, Activation	IRONMAN 70.3 RACE	3.3–4.3

FOCUS This is a building week to prepare you for the challenging strength-endurance work ahead. The key sessions are similar to preseason training—building blocks with a touch of speed and intensity.

WEEKLY OVERVIEW

	M	T	W	TH	F	SA	SU	TOTAL
S1	50 min.	45–60 min.	80 min.	45–60 min.	45–60 min.	2–2.5 hr.	50–60 min.	10.8–
S2	—	40–60 min.	30 min.	75 min.	—	30 min.	70–90 min.	13.4 hr.

MONDAY

SESSION ONE

SUPPORTING **BIKE**
TECHNICAL Activation, 50 min.

This is an optional session.

Warm-Up 10 min. easy spin

Pre-Main
10 min. ramp effort from Z1 to Z3

Main 3 rounds of:
2 min. Z1 ramp rpm to fast, 30 sec. easy,
90 sec. Z2 ramp rpm to fast, 1 min. easy,
1 min. Z3 ramp rpm to fast, 90 sec. easy,
30 sec. Z4 ramp rpm to fast, 2 min. easy

Scale for Time Trim as needed or skip if unable to complete.

Scale for Fatigue If you are very sore, you can maintain all the rpm builds in the Main set as Z1 to Z2 and keep low power/effort.

SESSION TWO

PM OFF

TUESDAY

SESSION ONE

KEY **SWIM**
ENDURANCE Building, 1800–3350

Warm-Up 5–10 min. easy with mix of strokes

Pre-Main 3–6 rounds with paddles and fins:
50 at 75%,
50 at 85%,
50 at 95%
Always 10 sec. rest

Main
9 × 150–250
Increase effort/pace every 2 intervals:
1 and 2 at 65%, 3 and 4 at 75%, 5 and 6 at 85%,
7 and 8 at 95%, 9 at MAX
Always 30 sec. rest

Add-On 200 cool-down

Scale for Time Drop Main set to 6 intervals: 1 at 65%, 1 at 75%, 1 at 85%, 1 at 95%, 2 at best effort.

Scale for Fatigue Drop Main set to 6 intervals and only build to 85%.

SESSION TWO

SUPPORTING **RUN**
ENDURANCE General Endurance, 40–60 min.

Warm-Up 10 min. easy
Add dynamic warm-up if possible.

Main
30–50 min.
Every 4th min. or so, check on form, posture, etc.
Aim for best MFP (minimal form pace). Do not exceed Z2 effort.

Scale for Time Scale duration as needed.

Scale for Fatigue Trim duration or skip if needed.

WEDNESDAY

KEY **BIKE**
END-OF-RANGE Strength-Endurance, 80 min.

Warm-Up 10 min. easy spin

Pre-Main 2 rounds of:
4 min. Z2 build rpm to fast,
3 min. build effort Z1 to Z3/Z4,
2 min. Z2 build rpm to fast,
1 min. build effort Z1 to Z3/Z4

Main 3 rounds Z3/Z4 at low rpm, progress as:
3 min. at 65 rpm,
2 min. at 55 rpm,
1 min. at 45 rpm,
2 min. at 55 rpm,
3 min. at 65 rpm
5 min. Z1 between rounds

Scale for Time Cut the 4 min. interval from the Pre-Main set and trim the number of intervals in the Main set.

Scale for Fatigue Maintain the Pre-Main set but convert the Main set to 4 × 10 min. Z2 build rpm to fast on each.

STRENGTH & CONDITIONING
30 min.

Scale for Time Be sure you hit at least 5–10 min of mobility.

Scale for Fatigue This is a floating session that can occur any day.

THURSDAY

SUPPORTING **SWIM**
ENDURANCE Short Intervals, 2450–3300

Warm-Up 300–600 with non-free on every 4th lap

Pre-Main Pull set with paddles, snorkel, and buoy:
200, 175, 150, 125, 100, 75, 50, 25
All with 10 sec. rest
Progress effort as you go to feel good.

Main
25–30 × 50 at 85% effort with 5–7 sec. rest
Choose a send-off interval and aim to leave on the same time each 50.

Add-On 12 × 25 with paddles, do as 3 rounds of:
1 easy form, 2 building effort to fast, 3 and 4 fast
Always 15 sec. rest

Scale for Time Reduce the number of 50s you complete with good form and rhythm.

Scale for Fatigue Reduce Main set to 20 × 50 at 80% and complete with good form and rhythm.

KEY **RUN**
INTERVALS Tempo, 75 min.

Main
75 min. steady and smooth build as:
30 min. Z2 easy and low stress,
20 min. Z2/Z3 moderate effort,
15 min. Z3 strong,
10 min. Z3/Z4 very strong

Scale for Time Scale the length of the run with similar effort ramp: 20 min., 15 min., 10 min., 5 min.

Scale for Fatigue Begin very easy and do a gradual ramp in effort, but can convert to a feel-good endurance run.

IRONMAN 70.3

RACE SPECIFIC

FRIDAY

SESSION ONE

SUPPORTING **BIKE**
TECHNICAL Prep, 45–60 min.

This is an optional session.

Main
45–90 min.
First and last 10 min. at >95 rpm with minimum power to maintain chain tension.
Include 4–6 × 30 sec. build as 10 sec. at Z3, Z4, and Z5
3–4 min. spin between each 30 sec. build

TRAINER OPTION

Warm-Up 5–10 min. Z1 spin

Pre-Main
5 × 90 sec. Z1 at very fast rpm
30 sec. spin between intervals

Main 3–5 rounds of:
30 sec. build as 10 sec. at Z3, Z4, and Z5,
2 min. Z3 steady and smooth riding (aiming to settle post Z5 effort)
2 min. Z1 spin easy between rounds

Scale for Time Scale duration as needed.

Scale for Fatigue Remove the Z5 work, but moving the body will help. Do something that feels good.

SESSION TWO

PM OFF

SATURDAY

SESSION ONE

KEY **BIKE + RUN**
EVENT-SPECIFIC Intervals, 2–2.5 hr.

Warm-Up 30–45 min. smooth

Pre-Main
6 min. as 4 × 90 sec. in Z1, Z2, Z3, Z4 to open the engine

Main 6 rounds of:
2 min. Z3 moderate,
2 min. Z3/Z4 strong,
2 min. Z4 very strong
4 min. spin between rounds
Odd rounds: <75 rpm
Even rounds: >90 rpm

Add-On 15 min. smooth home with good form

RUN OFF THE BIKE

3 min. ramp to Z3, 3 min. MFP
1 min. Z4, 3 min. MFP
1 min. Z4, 3 min. MFP
1 min. Z5, 3 min. MFP
1 min. Z4, 3 min. MFP
1 min. Z4

Scale for Time Trim Warm-Up to 15–20 min. and do just 4 rounds of Main set.

Scale for Fatigue Transition to a feel-good endurance ride.

SESSION TWO

STRENGTH & CONDITIONING
30 min.

Scale for Time Be sure you hit at least 5–10 min. of mobility.

Scale for Fatigue This is a floating session that can occur any day.

SUNDAY

KEY **SWIM**
EVENT-SPECIFIC Threshold, 2400–2700

Warm-Up 10 min. easy with mix of strokes

Pre-Main
100 smooth
2 × 75 build to fast
3 × 50 build to fast
4 × 25 fast
All with 15 sec. rest

Main With paddles and buoy:
100 at 70% with 20 sec. rest
100 at 80% with 10 sec. rest
1 × 100 at 90–95% with 5 sec. rest

100 at 70% with 20 sec. rest
100 at 80% with 10 sec. rest
2 × 100 at 90–95% with 5 sec. rest

100 at 70% with 20 sec. rest
100 at 80% with 10 sec. rest
3 × 100 at 90–95% with 5 sec. rest

100 at 70% with 20 sec. rest
100 at 80% with 10 sec. rest
4 × 100 at 90–95% with 5 sec. rest

100 easy to finish

Add-On 12 × 25 with paddles and fins, swim as
4 rounds of: easy, MAX, MAX
Always 10 sec. rest

Scale for Time Finish the Main set at 3 × 100 and
skip the Add-On 25s.

Scale for Fatigue Maintain the rhythm and intent,
but scale intensity for hard 100s to 80–85% effort.

SUPPORTING **RUN**
ENDURANCE General Endurance, 70–90 min.

This is a recommended session.

Warm-Up 10 min. easy

Main
60–80 min.
MFP run on variable terrain. If you are injury-prone,
a softer surface is ideal.
Take short 20–40 sec. walk breaks as needed to
retain form and manage heart rate.
For capable runners, control overall pace with
inclusion of downhill leg speed and form-based
activation: bench strides, bounding, challenging
terrain, etc.

Scale for Time Reduce duration as needed, but it is
important to get this run in.

Scale for Fatigue Include more walk breaks and
keep the effort conversational. Make total run no
more than 60 min.

IRONMAN 70.3

RACE SPECIFIC

WEEKLY OVERVIEW

	M	T	W	TH	F	SA	SU	TOTAL
S1	50 min.	1–1.5 hr.	95 min.	45–70 min.	45–90 min.	1–1.5 hr.	2.5–4.5 hr.	11.25–
S2	—	40–60 min.	30 min.	—	30 min.	70–85 min.	—	14.8 hr.

MONDAY

SESSION ONE

SUPPORTING BIKE
TECHNICAL Activation, 50 min.

This is an optional session.
Warm-Up 10 min. easy spin
Pre-Main
10 min. ramp effort from Z1 to Z3
Main 3 rounds of:
2 min. Z1 ramp rpm to fast, 30 sec. easy,
90 sec. Z2 ramp rpm to fast, 1 min. easy,
1 min. Z3 ramp rpm to fast, 90 sec. easy,
30 sec. Z4 ramp rpm to fast, 2 min. easy

Scale for Time Trim as needed or skip if unable to complete.

Scale for Fatigue If you are very sore you can maintain all the rpm builds in the Main set as Z1 to Z2 and keep it low power/effort.

SESSION TWO

PM OFF

TUESDAY

SESSION ONE

KEY SWIM
ENDURANCE Short Intervals, 3500–4100

Warm-Up 5–10 min. easy with mix of strokes

Pre-Main 2 rounds with buoy and snorkel:
200 at 70%,
2 × 100 at 75%,
2 × 50 at 80%,
2 × 25 at 90%
All with 10 sec. rest

Main
12 × 25 at 90% with great tempo and rhythm
with 2–3 sec. rest right into:
6 × 50 with 10 sec. rest

12 × 25 at 90% with great tempo and rhythm
with 2–3 sec. rest right into:
3 × 100 with 20 sec. rest

12 × 25 at 90% with great tempo and rhythm
with 2–3 sec. rest right into:
2 × 150 with 30 sec. rest

12 × 25 at 90% with great tempo and rhythm
with 2–3 sec. rest right into:
300 straight swimming

Maintain rhythm and form of the 25s on longer distances.

Add-On Up to 3 rounds with paddles (parachute or ankle strap OK):
2 × 25 MAX with 20 sec. rest, 50 easy float
50 MAX with 30 sec. rest, 2 × 25 easy

Scale for Time Trim Pre-Main to a single round. Start Main set at second 12 × 25 set (right into 3 × 100). Then trim the 25s if needed.

Scale for Fatigue Trim Pre-Main to one round, then complete Main set through the end of the 100s.

CONTINUES...

TUESDAY CONTINUED

SUPPORTING RUN
ENDURANCE General Endurance, 40–60 min.

Warm-Up 10 min. easy
Add dynamic warm-up if possible.

Main
30–50 min.
Aim for best MFP. Every 4th min. or so check in on form, posture, etc. Do not exceed Z2 effort.

Keep the effort down by adding leg speed, striding/bounding, and activation; also practice the run/walk protocol.

Scale for Time Simple scale of duration as needed.

Scale for Fatigue Trim duration or skip if needed.

WEDNESDAY

KEY BIKE + RUN
END-OF-RANGE Strength-Endurance, 95 min.

Warm-Up 10 min. easy spin

Pre-Main 2 rounds of:
4 min. Z2 build rpm to fast,
3 min. build effort Z1 to Z3/Z4,
2 min. Z2 build rpm to fast,
1 min. build effort Z1 to Z3/Z4

Main 3 rounds at <65 rpm, progress as:
1 min. Z2/Z3 smooth,
1 min. Z3 moderate,
2 min. Z3 strong,
2 min. Z4 very strong,
2 min. Z3 strong,
1 min. Z3 moderate,
1 min. Z2/Z3 smooth
5 min. Z1 spin between rounds

RUN OFF THE BIKE

3 min. ramp to IM 70.3 effort
3 min. Z2 smooth, 1 min. Z4
3 min. Z2 smooth, 1 min. Z4+
3 min. Z2 smooth, 1 min. Z5
3 min. Z2 smooth, 1 min. Z4+
3 min. Z2 smooth, 1 min. Z4
Then easy home.

Scale for Time Cut the 4 min. from the Pre-Main set rounds, and trim the number of intervals in the Main set.

Scale for Fatigue Maintain the Pre-Main set but convert the Main set to 4 × 10 min. Z2 build rpm to fast on each. Remove all work from the Run and convert to smooth 15 min. with good form.

STRENGTH & CONDITIONING
30 min.

Scale for Time Be sure you hit at least 5–10 min. of mobility.

Scale for Fatigue This is a floating session that can occur any day.

THURSDAY

SESSION ONE

SUPPORTING **SWIM**
ENDURANCE Short Intervals, 2700–3800

This is a recommended session.

Warm-Up 300–600, swim every 4th lap as non-free

Pre-Main Pull set with paddles, snorkel, and buoy:
200, 175, 150, 125, 100, 75, 50, 25
All with 10 sec. rest
Progress effort as you go to feel good.

Main
30–40 × 50 with 5–7 sec. rest
Choose a send-off interval and aim to leave on the same time each 50. Always swim at 85% effort with heightened focus on rhythm and intent of the session.

Add-On 12 × 25 with paddles, swim as 3 rounds of:
1 easy form, 2 building effort to fast, 3 and 4 fast
All with 15 sec. rest

Scale for Time Reduce the number of 50s you complete with good form and rhythm.

Scale for Fatigue Skip the Add-On session and reduce the Pre-Main set to begin at the 150. You can still complete the Main set, but with a focus on form rather than hitting 85% (reduce to 70–75% effort).

SESSION TWO

PM OFF

FRIDAY

SESSION ONE

SUPPORTING **BIKE**
TECHNICAL Prep, 45–90 min.

This is an optional session.

Main
45–90 min.
First and last 10 min. at >95 rpm with minimum power while retaining chain tension. Focus on posture and good pedaling.
Include 4–6 × 30 sec. build to Z5 effort (10 sec. at Z3, Z4, and Z5)
3–4 min. spin between each 30 sec. build

TRAINER OPTION

Warm-Up 5–10 min. Z1 easy

Pre-Main
5 × 90 sec. Z1 at very fast rpm
30 sec. spin between intervals

Main 3–5 rounds of:
30 sec. build to Z5 effort (10 sec. at Z3, Z4, and Z5),
2 min. Z3 steady and smooth riding
2 min. Z1 spin between intervals

Add-On 5 × 90 sec. Z1 at very fast rpm,
30 sec. spin between intervals

Scale for Time Scale duration as needed.

Scale for Fatigue Remove the Z5 effort work. Do something that feels good.

SESSION TWO

STRENGTH & CONDITIONING
30 min.

Scale for Time Be sure you hit at least 5–10 min. of mobility.

Scale for Fatigue This is a floating session that can occur any day.

SATURDAY

SUPPORTING SWIM
ENDURANCE Over-Distance, 3300–3600

Warm-Up 10 min. easy with mix of strokes

Pre-Main
100 smooth
2 × 75 build to fast
3 × 50 build to fast
4 × 25 fast
All with 15 sec. rest

Main
100 with toys, 200 swim at 80%,
200 with toys, 400 swim at 80%,
300 with toys, 600 swim at 80%,
200 with toys, 800 swim at 80%
All with 1 min. rest
Toys are snorkel and buoy to help retain form.
In the solid swims, sight 3 times per lap.

Add-On 12 × 25 with paddles and fins, do as
4 rounds of: easy, MAX, MAX
All with 10 sec. rest

Scale for Time Remove the speed Add-On, as well
as trim the Main set to finish at the 600 as needed.

Scale for Fatigue Remove the additional speed at
the end, and trim the Main set to the 600.

KEY RUN
INTERVALS Tempo, 70–85 min.

Warm-Up 10 min. at MFP

Pre-Main
3 × 2 min., build by 30 sec. to strong
30 sec. rest between intervals

Main
2 × 15 min. sustained Z3+, strong but sustainable
10 min. at MFP between intervals

Add-On 10–15 min. easy endurance running at
the end

Scale for Time Remove any additional endurance
running and scale Warm-Up as needed.

Scale for Fatigue Transfer into a variable trail run
up to 75 min. with walk breaks on the steep grades.

SUNDAY

KEY BIKE + RUN
ENDURANCE General Endurance, 2.5–4.5 hr.

Main
2–4 hr.
After at least 30 min. build in with variation as
terrain allows:
5 × 5 min. strong effort at <65 rpm
5 min. Z1 spin between intervals

TRAINER OPTION

Warm-Up 30 min., build from Z1 to Z3

Pre-Main 2 rounds:
2 min. Z2/Z3, 30 sec. easy,
90 sec. Z3, 30 sec. easy,
1 min. Z3/Z4, 30 sec. easy

Main
5 × 4 min. Z3 at <65 rpm
4 min. Z1 spin at fast rpm between intervals

Add-On 15 min. build by 5 min. (5 min. at Z2,
Z2/Z3, and Z3)

RUN OFF THE BIKE

20–30 min. with good form at smooth to moderate
(steady) effort

Scale for Time Trim Warm-Up and do 1 round of
Pre-Main set. Change Main set to 3 × 6 min. at low
rpm, then 15 min. form-based run.

Scale for Fatigue Transition to a feel-good
endurance ride.

PM OFF

IRONMAN 70.3

RACE SPECIFIC

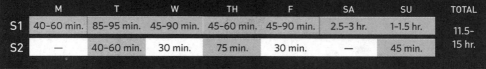

WEEK

3

FOCUS These are building block sessions that mix low- and high-rpm work as you evolve your fitness and progress toward the main race. A challenging low-rpm bike ride is the main feature of this strength-endurance week.

WEEKLY OVERVIEW

	M	T	W	TH	F	SA	SU	TOTAL
S1	40–60 min.	85–95 min.	45–90 min.	45–60 min.	45–90 min.	2.5–3 hr.	1–1.5 hr.	11.5–
S2	—	40–60 min.	30 min.	75 min.	30 min.	—	45 min.	15 hr.

MONDAY

SESSION ONE

SUPPORTING RUN
ENDURANCE General Endurance, 40–60 min.

Warm-Up 10 min. easy
Add dynamic warm-up if possible.

Main
30–50 min. smooth
Focus on form and posture. No more than Z2 effort.

MFP running with walk breaks as needed to retain the ability to run with form and maintain a conversational and endurance-focused performance.

Scale for Time Trim as needed or skip if unable to complete.

Scale for Fatigue If your muscles are sore from last week, convert to a 30–45 min. flush/spin on the bike or a very easy 1–2 km swim.

SESSION TWO

PM OFF

TUESDAY

SESSION ONE

KEY BIKE
END-OF-RANGE Strength-Endurance, 85–95 min.

Warm-Up 10 min. easy spin

Pre-Main 1–2 rounds of:
3 min. Z2 steady, 30 sec. Z1,
2 min. Z3 steady, 1 min. Z1,
1 min. Z3/Z4, 90 sec. Z1

Main
8 min. steady endurance at choice rpm,
5 min. spin

Then 5 × 5 min. Z4 very strong:
5 min. at 50 rpm, 5 min. at 60 rpm, 5 min. at 70 rpm,
5 min. at 60 rpm, 5 min. at 50 rpm
4 min. Z1 spin between intervals

Finish with 8 min. Z3 steady state at choice rpm

Scale for Time Trim the Pre-Main to one round and do 4 × 5 min. in the Main (alternating between 50 rpm and 70 rpm). Trim the 8 min. endurance intervals to 6 min.

Scale for Fatigue Maintain the Pre-Main set but change the Main to: 5 min. Z3, 5 min. Z2 ramp to fast, 5 min. Z3, 5 min. Z2 ramp to fast, 5 min. Z3. Remove the 8 min. endurance intervals.

SESSION TWO

SUPPORTING RUN
TECHNICAL Recovery, 40–60 min.

This is an optional session.

Warm-Up 10 min. easy
Add dynamic warm-up if possible.

Main
30–50 min.
Every 4th min. or so check in on form, posture, etc.
Do not exceed Z2 effort.

Scale for Time Simple scale of duration as needed.

Scale for Fatigue Trim duration or skip if needed.

WEDNESDAY

SESSION ONE

KEY SWIM
TECHNICAL Form, 2400–4450

Warm-Up 10 min. easy

Pre-Main Up to 2 rounds with snorkel:
300 at 70% with 30 sec. rest,
3 × 50 form-based swimming, building tempo,
effort, and stroke rate throughout
All with 10 sec. rest

Main With paddles (and ankle-strap for advanced swimmers):
15–30 × 100 at 80%, keep stroke rate up, swim every 5th 100 very strong (Z4)
All with 10 sec. rest

Add-On 2 rounds of power:
4 × 25 MAX with paddles,
150 form-based swimming

Scale for Time Trim Pre-Main to one round and reduce the number of 100s if needed.

Scale for Fatigue Trim Pre-Main to one round. Use fins for Main set and trim to 10–20 × 100.

SESSION TWO

STRENGTH & CONDITIONING
30 min.

Scale for Time Be sure you get at least 5–10 min. of mobility.

Scale for Fatigue This is a floating session that can occur any day.

THURSDAY

SESSION ONE

SUPPORTING SWIM
ENDURANCE Short Intervals, 2150–3200

This is an optional session.

Warm-Up 10 min. easy

Pre-Main 5-7 rounds with fins:
50 at 70% with 10 sec. rest,
50 at 80% with 5–7 sec. rest,
50 at 90% with 3–5 sec. rest

Then, 2 rounds of:
2 × 25 fast, 50 easy,
50 fast, 2 × 25 easy
All with 15 sec. rest

Main With paddles:
40–70 × 25 at 85–90% with only 2–5 sec. rest between intervals

Scale for Time Scale Pre-Main and Main as needed.

Scale for Fatigue Cut Main set to 20–40 × 25 at 80%, without paddles.

SESSION TWO

KEY RUN
TECHNICAL Prep, 75 min.

Main
75 min. steady and smooth build as:
30 min. Z2 easy and low stress,
20 min. Z2/Z3 moderate effort,
15 min. Z3 strong,
10 min. Z3/Z4 very strong

Scale for Time Scale the length of the run with similar effort ramp: 20 min., 15 min., 10 min., 5 min.

Scale for Fatigue Begin very easy and do a gradual ramp in effort, but can convert to a feel-good endurance run.

IRONMAN 70.3

RACE SPECIFIC

FRIDAY

SESSION ONE

SUPPORTING **BIKE**
TECHNICAL Prep, 45–90 min.

Main
45–90 min.
First and last 10 min. at >95 rpm with minimum power to maintain chain tension. Focus on posture and good pedaling.
Include 4–6 × 30 sec. build as 10 sec. at Z3, Z4, and Z5
3–4 min. between each 30 sec. build

Steady endurance, smooth home

TRAINER OPTION

Warm-Up 5–10 min. Z1 spin

Pre-Main
5 × 90 sec. Z1 at very fast rpm
30 sec. spin between intervals

Main 3–5 rounds of:
30 sec. build as 10 sec. at Z3, Z4, and Z5,
2 min. Z3 steady and smooth riding
2 min. Z1 spin between rounds

Add-On 5 × 90 sec. Z1 at very fast rpm,
30 sec. spin between intervals

Scale for Time Scale duration as needed.

Scale for Fatigue Remove the Z5 effort work.
Do something that feels good.

SESSION TWO

STRENGTH & CONDITIONING
30 min.

Scale for Time Be sure you get at least 5–10 min. of mobility.

Scale for Fatigue This is a floating session that can occur any day.

SATURDAY

SESSION ONE

KEY **BIKE + RUN**
EVENT-SPECIFIC Race Simulation, 2.5–3 hr.

Warm-Up 30–45 min. smooth

Pre-Main
6 min. build to open the engine as 90 sec.
at Z1, Z2, Z3, Z4

Main
6 × 8 min.
Build effort every 2 intervals as:
2 just under IM 70.3 race effort,
2 right at IM 70.3 race effort,
2 above IM 70.3 race effort
4 min. spin between intervals

Add-On 15 min. smooth home with good form

RUN OFF THE BIKE

6 × 4 min.
Build effort every 2 intervals to very strong on the last 2.
2 min. easy running between intervals

Scale for Time Trim Warm-Up and shift the Main set to: 1 under, 2 at, 1 above race effort, on both the bike and the run.

Scale for Fatigue Transition to a feel-good endurance ride.

SESSION TWO

PM OFF

SUNDAY

KEY **SWIM**
ENDURANCE Over-Distance, 3300–4700

Warm-Up 10 min. easy with mix of strokes

Pre-Main
100 smooth
2 × 75 build to fast
3 × 50 build to fast
4 × 25 fast
All with 15 sec. rest

Main With paddles (add ankle strap for advanced swimmers):
100 with toys, 200 at 80%,
200 with toys, 400 at 80%,
300 with toys, 600 at 80%,
200 with toys, 800 at 80%
100 with toys, 1000 at 80% (for advanced swimmers)
All with 1 min. rest between intervals
In the solid swims, sight 3 times per lap.

Add-On 12 × 25 with paddles and fins, do as
4 rounds of: easy, MAX, MAX
Always 10 sec. rest

Scale for Time Remove the speed Add-On, and trim the Main set to finish at the 600 or 800 as needed.

Scale for Fatigue Finish the Main set at the 600.

KEY **RUN**
INTERVALS Strength, 45 min.

Warm-Up 5–10 min. easy

Pre-Main Prep with feel-good builds, up to 2 rounds of:
40 sec. moderate, 30 sec. easy,
30 sec. strong, 30 sec. easy,
20 sec. strong, 30 sec. easy,
10 sec. very strong, 30 sec. easy

Main 4 loops of hill running:
3 min. flat and smooth, MFP
90 sec. at 4% grade, very strong and sustained powerful running
30 sec. MAX at 6–10%, driving off the toes, arms pumping behind, eyes up
2 min. downhill on shallow grade (2–4%), pick up leg speed but not hard
If you cannot find a loop, run on the treadmill. Use 1% for flat and 0% for downhill.

Scale for Time Trim Warm-Up and do just 3 loops of hill running in the Main set.

Scale for Fatigue Begin easy and gradually ramp effort. Convert to a feel-good endurance run on rolling hills if needed.

IRONMAN 70.3

RACE SPECIFIC

303

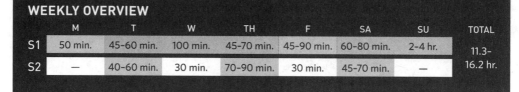

FOCUS Strength-endurance work is very challenging, especially Saturday's Key Run where you are asked to maintain great form and posture while running very hard uphill. Midweek highlights include the strong, end-of-range ride and the beginning of event-specific swimming.

WEEKLY OVERVIEW

	M	T	W	TH	F	SA	SU	TOTAL
S1	50 min.	45–60 min.	100 min.	45–70 min.	45–90 min.	60–80 min.	2–4 hr.	11.3–16.2 hr.
S2	—	40–60 min.	30 min.	70–90 min.	30 min.	45–70 min.	—	

MONDAY

SESSION ONE

SUPPORTING **BIKE**
TECHNICAL Activation, 50 min.

This is an optional session.

Warm-Up 10 min. easy spin

Pre-Main
10 min. ramp effort from Z1 to Z3

Main 3 rounds of:
2 min. Z1 ramp rpm to fast, 30 sec. easy,
90 sec. Z2 ramp rpm to fast, 1 min. easy,
1 min. Z3 ramp rpm to fast, 90 sec. easy,
30 sec. Z4 ramp rpm to fast, 2 min. easy

Scale for Time Trim as needed or skip if unable to complete.

Scale for Fatigue If you are very sore maintain the rpm builds in the Main set, but keep it low power/effort, Z1/Z2.

SESSION TWO

PM OFF

TUESDAY

SESSION ONE

KEY **SWIM**
ENDURANCE Building, 1800–3350

Warm-Up 5–10 min. easy with mix of strokes

Pre-Main 3–6 rounds with paddles and fins:
50 at 75%,
50 at 85%,
50 at 95%
All with 10 sec. rest

Main
9 × 150–250, progress every 2 intervals as:
2 at 65%, 2 at 75%, 2 at 85%, 2 at 95%, and last one at MAX
As effort increases, the pace should, too.
Always 30 sec. rest

Option to add paddles for this strength-focused set. Advanced swimmers can add an ankle strap.

Add-On 200 cool-down

Scale for Time Drop Main set to 5 intervals: 1 at 65%, 1 at 75%, 1 at 85%, 1 at 95%, 1 at MAX.

Scale for Fatigue Drop to 6 intervals in Main set, only building to 85%.

SESSION TWO

SUPPORTING **RUN**
ENDURANCE General Endurance, 40–60 min.

Warm-Up 10 min. easy
Add dynamic warm-up if possible.

Main
30–50 min. low stress
Every 4th min. or so, check in on form, posture, etc.
Aim for best MFP. Do not exceed Z2 effort.

Scale for Time Simple scale of duration as needed.

Scale for Fatigue Trim duration or skip if needed.

WEDNESDAY

KEY **BIKE**
END-OF-RANGE High Cadence, 100 min.

Warm-Up 10 min. easy spin

Pre-Main
2 × 4 min.
2 × 3 min.
2 × 2 min.
2 × 1 min.
Set 1: Z2 build rpm to fast,
Set 2: build effort Z1 to Z3/Z4

Main 5 rounds Z3+ to Z4 always do as:
4 min. at <50 rpm,
1 min. at >95 rpm,
4 min. at <50 rpm,
1 min. at >95 rpm
4 min. Z1 spin between rounds

Scale for Time Cut the 4 min. interval from the Pre-Main set and trim the number of rounds in the Main set.

Scale for Fatigue Maintain the Pre-Main set but convert the Main set to 4 rounds Z2 build rpm to fast on each.

STRENGTH & CONDITIONING
30 min.

Scale for Time Ensure you hit at least 5–10 min. of mobility

Scale for Fatigue This is a floating session that can occur any day.

THURSDAY

KEY **SWIM**
EVENT-SPECIFIC Threshold, 3100–3400

Warm-Up 10 min. easy with mix of strokes

Pre-Main
100 smooth
2 × 75 build to fast
3 × 50 build to fast
4 × 25 fast
All with 15 sec. rest

Main With paddles and buoy:
100 at 70% with 20 sec. rest
100 at 80% with 10 sec. rest
1 × 100 at 90–95% with 5 sec. rest

100 at 70% with 20 sec. rest
100 at 80% with 10 sec. rest
2 × 100 at 90–95% with 5 sec. rest

100 at 70% with 20 sec. rest
100 at 80% with 10 sec. rest
3 × 100 at 90–95% with 5 sec. rest

100 at 70% with 20 sec. rest
100 at 80% with 10 sec. rest
4 × 100 at 90–95% with 5 sec. rest

100 at 70% with 20 sec. rest
100 at 80% with 10 sec. rest
5 × 100 at 90–95% with 5 sec. rest

100 easy to finish

Add-On 12 × 25 with paddles and fins, do as
4 rounds of: easy, MAX, MAX
Always 10 sec. rest

Scale for Time End Main set at 4 × 100.

Scale for Fatigue End Main set at 4 × 100. Build efforts to 70%, 75%, and 80%. Keep the fast 25s at the end.

SUPPORTING **RUN**
TECHNICAL Activation, 70–90 min.

Warm-Up 10 min. easy

Main
60-80 low stress endurance run on variable terrain.
If you are injury prone, a softer surface is ideal.
Include 9 × 20 sec. blasts with 90 sec. form-based running between intervals.
Take short 20–40 sec. walk breaks as needed to retain form.

Scale for Time Simply reduce time but retain the 9 × 20 sec. sharpeners.

Scale for Fatigue Begin very easy and try to fit in 20 sec. blasts, but can convert to a feel-good endurance run if needed.

FRIDAY

SESSION ONE

SUPPORTING **BIKE**
TECHNICAL Prep, 45–90 min.

This is an optional session.

Main
45–90 min.
First and last 10 min. at >95 rpm with minimum power while retaining chain tension. Focus on posture and good pedaling.
Include 4–6 × 30 sec. build as 10 sec. at Z3, Z4, and Z5
3–4 min. spin between each 30 sec. build

TRAINER OPTION

Warm-Up 5–10 min. Z1 spin

Pre-Main
5 × 90 sec. Z1 at very fast rpm
30 sec. spin between intervals

Main 4–6 rounds of:
30 sec. build as 10 sec. at Z3, Z4, Z5
3 min. Z1 spin between intervals

Steady and smooth home

Add-On 5 × 90 sec. Z1 at very fast rpm,
30 sec. spin between intervals

Scale for Time Trim duration as needed.

Scale for Fatigue Remove the Z5 effort from Main set, building as Z2, Z3, Z4. Moving the body will help. Do something that feels good.

SESSION TWO

STRENGTH & CONDITIONING
30 min.

Scale for Time Ensure you hit at least 5–10 min. of mobility.

Scale for Fatigue This is a floating session that can occur any day.

SATURDAY

SESSION ONE

KEY **RUN**
INTERVALS Strength, 60–80 min.

Warm-Up 10–15 min. easy and smooth

Pre-Main Up to 3 rounds, until you feel ready for work:
90 sec. smooth, 30 sec. easy,
1 min. steady, 30 sec. easy,
30 sec. strong, 30 sec. easy

Main 3 loops of hill running:
3–4 min. flat with great form at smooth endurance (Z2/Z3)
3 min. sustained hill at very strong sustained effort with great form (bounding)
30 sec. MAX effort on steeper grade (5-8%) to finish hill
3 min. downhill running on shallow grade (3-5%), pick up feet and float down with fast foot speed
No breaks. This will be very tough. If you cannot find a loop, run on the treadmill. Use 1% for flat and 0% for downhill.

Following the loops:
3 × 4 min. Z3 tempo with 2 min. easy between intervals

Scale for Time Trim Warm-Up and skip the 3 × 4 min. of the Main set. The hills are the meat and potatoes today.

Scale for Fatigue Do a 50–75 min. feel-good endurance run over rolling terrain.

CONTINUES...

SATURDAY CONTINUED

SUPPORTING **SWIM**
ENDURANCE Short Intervals, 2950–4050

Warm-Up 300–600, swim every 4th lap as non-free

Pre-Main Pull set with paddles, snorkel, and buoy:
200, 175, 150, 125, 100, 75, 50, 25
All with 10 sec. rest
Progress effort as you go to feel good.

Main
35–45 × 50 at 85% with 5–7 sec. rest
Choose a send-off interval and aim to leave on the same tight time each 50. Strong push-off and streamlines on every wall.
Paddles are OK if you can retain stroke rate.

Add-On 12 × 25 with paddles, do as 3 rounds of:
1 easy form, 2 build effort to fast, 3 and 4 fast
Always 15 sec. rest

Scale for Time Reduce the number of 50s you complete with good form and rhythm.

Scale for Fatigue Reduce the Warm-Up and begin Pre-Main set at 150. Complete the Main set (without paddles), and focus on form over hitting 85% (reduce to 70–75% effort).

SUNDAY

KEY **BIKE**
ENDURANCE General Endurance, 2–4 hr.

Main
2–4 hr.
Endurance ride on variable terrain

TRAINER OPTION

Warm-Up 30 min. stepper, building very easy to steady

Main Up to 4 rounds of:
4 min. Z1/Z2 choice pedaling,
30 sec. Z1 easy,
3 min. Z2 smooth build rpm to fast,
30 sec. Z1 easy,
2 min. Z2/Z3 smooth choice pedaling,
30 sec. Z1 easy,
1 min. Z3 steady build rpm to fast,
30 sec. Z1 easy

Add-On 20 min. Z2 choice with every 4th min. ramp rpm to MAX

Scale for Time Reduce Warm-Up to 15 min. stepper. Reduce rounds in the Main set as needed. Remove the final 20 min.

Scale for Fatigue Reduce the Warm-Up to a 15 min. stepper. Main can be 2 rounds.

PM OFF

IRONMAN 70.3

RACE SPECIFIC

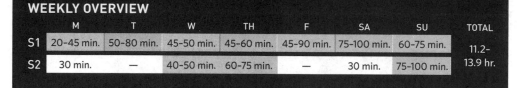

WEEK

5

FOCUS We remove some of the muscular-loading strength and endurance work early in the week and freshen up. At the end of the week we begin 8 days focused on endurance with an endurance run weekend. The goal is 3 longer endurance runs over 5 days to build resilience before the upcoming block of work.

WEEKLY OVERVIEW

	M	T	W	TH	F	SA	SU	TOTAL
S1	20–45 min.	50–80 min.	45–50 min.	45–60 min.	45–90 min.	75–100 min.	60–75 min.	11.2–
S2	30 min.	—	40–50 min.	60–75 min.	—	30 min.	75–100 min.	13.9 hr.

MONDAY

SESSION ONE

SUPPORTING BIKE
TECHNICAL Recovery, 20–45 min.

This is an optional session.

Main
20–45 min.
Very low stress with first and last 10 min. at fast rpm, in a small gear.
If you ride outside, practice cornering and handling skills to refine control and comfort on the bike.

Scale for Time Trim as needed or take a rest day.

Scale for Fatigue It may still be worth fitting in the ride not for fitness, but to enhance recovery and adaptations.

SESSION TWO

STRENGTH & CONDITIONING
30 min.

Scale for Time Be sure you get in at least 5–10 min. of mobility work.

Scale for Fatigue This is a floating session that can occur any day.

TUESDAY

SESSION ONE

KEY BIKE + RUN
END-OF-RANGE High Cadence, 50–80 min.

Warm-Up As needed, include a few ramps to higher output so you can select work gear for Main set.

Main Up to 2 rounds of MAX sprints:
10 sec. MAX, 50 sec. easy,
20 sec. MAX, 40 sec. easy,
30 sec. MAX, 30 sec. easy,
40 sec. MAX, 20 sec. easy,
50 sec. MAX, 10 sec. easy,
60 sec. MAX,
10 sec. easy, 50 sec. MAX,
20 sec. easy, 40 sec. MAX,
30 sec. easy, 30 sec. MAX,
40 sec. easy, 20 sec. MAX,
50 sec. easy, 10 sec. MAX
7 min. easy spinning between rounds
Do MAX efforts as best effort at >90 rpm
Use the same gear for each work effort. Cadence decreases as set progresses. Shift from recovery gear 3 sec. before work starts.

Cool-down 5–15 min. spin

RUN OFF THE BIKE

5 min. ramp to IM 70.3 effort
5 min. form-based running
5 min. at IM 70.3 effort
5 min. form-based running

Scale for Time Trim MAX sprints to 1 round.

Scale for Fatigue Remove the MAX sprint efforts and replace with an easy ride.

SESSION TWO

PM OFF

WEDNESDAY

SUPPORTING **SWIM**
TECHNICAL Form, 2450–2850

This is a recommended session.

Warm-Up 10 min. easy

Pre-Main 15 × 50 with fins and snorkel, do as
5 rounds of:
25 kick on back, 25 free at 70% effort,
25 kick on back, 25 free at 80% effort,
25 kick on back, 25 free at 90% effort
Always 10 sec. rest

Main With buoy (no paddles, as we want to retain
stroke rate):
100, 150, 200, 250, 300, 250, 200, 150, 100
All with 45 sec. rest
The first 25 of every swim is fast sighting 3 times
per lap. The rest of the swim is smooth, endurance-
focused swimming at 70%.

Add-On 400 with fins, alternate kick-swim by 25

Scale for Time Drop intervals in the Main set to
100, 150, 200, 200, 150, 100.

Scale for Fatigue Drop intervals in the Main set to
100, 150, 200, 200, 150, 100

SUPPORTING **RUN**
ENDURANCE General Endurance, 40–50 min.

Warm-Up 10 min. easy
Add dynamic warm-up if possible.

Main
30–40 min. low stress
Every 4th min. or so check on form, posture, etc.
Aim for best MFP. Do not exceed Z2 effort.

Scale for Time Adjust duration as needed.

Scale for Fatigue Adjust duration or skip if needed.

THURSDAY

KEY **SWIM**
EVENT-SPECIFIC Pyramid, 2650

Warm-Up Smooth 10 min. light, then
400 pull smooth with choice of equipment at 70%

Main
Progressive building effort with medium-duration
swims: 1850 swim with variable pace. Always 20
sec. rest, followed by a form-based swim interval.

200 steady at 85%, 150 form-based Z2 at 70%
150 strong at 90%, 150 form-based Z2 at 70%
100 very strong at 95%, 150 form-based Z2 at 70%
50 MAX with good, tidy hold on the water
(no panic)
150 form-based Z2 at 70%, 100 very strong at 95%,
150 form-based Z2 at 70%, 150 strong at 90%,
150 form-based Z2 at 70%, 200 steady at 85%

400 pull smooth to finish

Scale for Time Reduce form-based swim interval
to 100. Reduce performance pyramid to be: 125,
100, 75, 50, 75, 100, 125.

Scale for Fatigue Evolve to an endurance interval
session with all intervals at 70–80%.

SUPPORTING **BIKE**
ENDURANCE General Endurance, 60–75 min.

This is an optional session.

Warm-Up 30 min. smooth

Main 2–3 rounds of:
5 min. smooth,
2 min. spin higher rpm in a small gear,
3 min. steady,
2 min. spin higher rpm in a small gear,
1 min. strong,
2 min. spin higher rpm in a small gear

TRAINER OPTION

Warm-Up 10 min. spin

Pre-Main
5 × 3 min. smooth, ramp rpm by 1 min. to fast rpm

Then complete Main set detailed above.

Scale for Time Simple scale of duration as needed.

Scale for Fatigue Trim duration or skip if needed.
Remove the neurological high-cadence work if
needed.

IRONMAN 70.3 RACE SPECIFIC

FRIDAY

SESSION ONE

SUPPORTING **BIKE**
TECHNICAL Prep, 45–90 min.

This is a feel-good ride, whatever that is for you: more, less, building intervals, spinning, etc. Be aware and look for patterns to better manage readiness. Here is a possible option, but do what works for you.

Main
45–90 min. smooth
Include 4 × 3 min., ramp by 1 min. to strong but not deep effort.
3–4 min. Z2 riding between intervals

Scale for Time Adjust duration as needed.

Scale for Fatigue Remove the ramping effort, but moving the body will still help.

SESSION TWO

PM OFF

SATURDAY

SESSION ONE

KEY **RUN**
ENDURANCE General Endurance, 75–100 min.

Main
75–100 min.
This is the first of 3 endurance runs in 5 days, focused on building muscular endurance, so harder is not better.

Retain form under fatigue. Hills are good. Very steep grades are also fine, but just hike these sections with great form. Finish pleasantly fatigued, but without soreness.

OPTIONAL PM RUN

Add a second run in the evening, 30-50 min. low stress and focused on resiliency. All easy endurance; walk breaks are OK.

Scale for Time Trim to 1 hr. and do PM run.

Scale for Fatigue This is all feel-good work today, so you are under no pressure to run hard.

SESSION TWO

STRENGTH & CONDITIONING
30 min.

Scale for Time Be sure you get in at least 5–10 min. of mobility work.

Scale for Fatigue This is a floating session that can occur any day.

SUNDAY

SUPPORTING **SWIM**
EVENT-SPECIFIC Pyramid, 3050–3750

Warm-Up 300–600, swim every 4th lap as non-free

Pre-Main 15 × 50 with fins and snorkel (to help flush the legs), do as 5 rounds of:
50 at 70% effort,
50 at 80% effort,
50 at 90% effort
Always 10 sec. rest

Main With buoy (no paddles, as we want to retain stroke rate):
100, 150, 200, 250, 300,
300, 250, 200, 150, 100
All with 45 sec. rest
The first 25 of every swim is fast sighting 3 times per lap. The rest of the swim is smooth, endurance-focused swimming at 70%.

Add-On 400 with fins, alternate kick-swim by 25

Scale for Time Reduce the Main set pyramid to a distance that allows completion within time available.

Scale for Fatigue Convert to a Warm-Up of 500 easy, then Main is 1000 with buoy and snorkel.

KEY **RUN**
ENDURANCE General Endurance, 75–100 min.

Main
75–100 min.
Hills are great. Variable terrain and a soft surface is optimal. Walk breaks are OK as needed to retain form under fatigue. Finish pleasantly fatigued, but without soreness.

Very steep grades are fine in this run; just hike these sections with great form.

Scale for Time Simple scale of duration.

Scale for Fatigue This is all feel-good work today, so you are under no pressure to run hard.

IRONMAN 70.3

RACE SPECIFIC

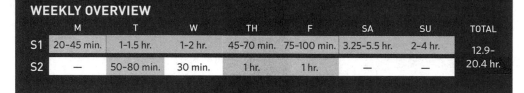

WEEK

6

FOCUS We retain the endurance focus, while integrating some strength-endurance work into the load. We have one endurance run remaining, then we transition to a weekend focused on riding to bank some miles and resilience. For the time-starved athlete, the trainer option can be used to sneak in some miles.

WEEKLY OVERVIEW

	M	T	W	TH	F	SA	SU	TOTAL
S1	20–45 min.	1–1.5 hr.	1–2 hr.	45–70 min.	75–100 min.	3.25–5.5 hr.	2–4 hr.	12.9–
S2	—	50–80 min.	30 min.	1 hr.	1 hr.	—	—	20.4 hr.

MONDAY

SESSION ONE

SUPPORTING **BIKE**
TECHNICAL Recovery, 20–45 min.

This is an optional session.

Main
20–45 min. very low stress
First and last 10 min. at fast rpm, in a small gear.
If you ride outside, practice some cornering and handling skills to refine control and comfort on the bike.

Scale for Time Trim as needed or skip if unable to complete.

Scale for Fatigue It may still be worth moving blood here, not for fitness, but to enhance recovery and adaptations.

SESSION TWO

PM OFF

TUESDAY

SESSION ONE

KEY **SWIM**
ENDURANCE Over-Distance, 3300–4700

Warm-Up 10 min. easy with mix of strokes

Pre-Main
100 smooth
2 × 75 build to fast
3 × 50 build to fast
4 × 25 fast
All with 15 sec. rest

Main
100 with toys, 200 swim at 80%
200 with toys, 400 swim at 80%
300 with toys, 600 swim at 80%
200 with toys, 800 swim at 80%
100 with toys, 1000 swim at 80% (for advanced swimmers)
All with 1 min. rest between intervals.
Use snorkel and buoy for intervals with toys; add paddles for strength-endurance. In the solid swims, sight 3 times per lap.

Add-On 12 × 25 with paddles and fins, do as
4 rounds of: easy, MAX, MAX
Always 10 sec. rest

Scale for Time Trim Main set to finish at the 600 or 800 as needed.

Scale for Fatigue Trim the Main set to finish at 600.

CONTINUES...

TUESDAY CONTINUED

SESSION TWO

SUPPORTING **RUN**
ENDURANCE General Endurance, 50–80 min.

Warm-Up 10 min. easy
Add dynamic warm-up if possible.

Main
40–70 min. low stress
Include some fartlek-style speed changes as 2–3 rounds of:
10-20-30-20-10 sec. of form-based speed pick-ups
1 min. easy running between efforts

Scale for Time Simple scale of duration as needed.

Scale for Fatigue Remove the speed play or skip if needed.

WEDNESDAY

SESSION ONE

KEY **RUN**
ENDURANCE General Endurance, 1–2 hr.

Main
1–2 hr.
Endurance-focused run on soft surface with variable terrain. Integrate walk breaks as needed to retain form and minimize global fatigue. If you are newer to training, this might be more hiking than running.

TREADMILL OPTION

Warm-Up 10 min. easy

Pre-Main 4 rounds of:
90 sec. walk at 5%,
3 min. run smooth Z2 at 1%,
30 sec. walk at 1%

Main
Smooth endurance running with 30 sec. at 3% grade every 3rd min. Walk breaks as needed.

OPTIONAL PM RUN

30–50 min. low-stress, MFP
Keep effort down by consciously reducing leg speed or push off and practice the run/walk protocol.

Scale for Time Reduce duration as needed.

Scale for Fatigue Choose flatter terrain and integrate more walk breaks.

SESSION TWO

STRENGTH & CONDITIONING
30 min.

Scale for Time Be sure you hit at least 5–10 min. of mobility.

Scale for Fatigue This is a floating session that can occur any day.

THURSDAY

SESSION ONE

SUPPORTING **SWIM**
ENDURANCE Short Intervals, 2900–3950

This is a recommended session.

Warm-Up 10 min. easy

Pre-Main 5–7 rounds (fins can be used):
50 at 70% with 10 sec. rest,
50 at 80% with 5–7 sec. rest,
50 at 90% with 3–5 sec. rest

Then, 2 rounds of:
2 × 25 fast,
50 easy, 50 fast,
2 × 25 easy
All with 15 sec. rest

Main
35–50 × 50 at 85% with 5–7 sec. rest
Choose a send-off interval and aim to leave on the
same time for each 50. Introduce sighting 3 times
per lap without losing rhythm, tempo, or stroke.

Scale for Time Scale Pre-Main and Main sets as
needed.

Scale for Fatigue Evolve Main set to focus on form
over effort. Reduce effort to 70-75%.

SESSION TWO

SUPPORTING **BIKE**
TECHNICAL Activation, 1 hr.

This is an optional session.

Warm-Up 20 min. easy

Pre-Main
6 × 3 min. Z2
Build rpm by 1 min.: 80, 90, 100
30 sec. rest between intervals

Main
4 min. building effort by 1 min. to Z3
2 min. spin
3 min. building effort by 1 min. to Z3+
2 min. spin
2 min. building effort by 1 min. to Z4
2 min. spin
1 min. building effort by 1 min. to Z4+
2 min. spin

5–10 min. Z1 spin

This is a feel-good ride to prepare for tomorrow's
ride.

Scale for Time Trim Warm-Up to 10 min., then
reduce Pre-Main to 3 × 3 min. Then hit Main set.
Cut the final 5–10 min. spin.

Scale for Fatigue Keep all building efforts as a
build to Z3.

FRIDAY

SESSION ONE

SUPPORTING **BIKE**
END-OF-RANGE Strength-Endurance, 75–100 min.

Today is a double-day on the trainer. If you only
have time for a single session, do this one.

Warm-Up 5–10 min. Z1 spin

Pre-Main
6 min. build Z1 to Z3
5 min. Z2 smooth build rpm to fast
4 min. build Z1 to Z3
3 min. Z2 smooth build rpm to fast
2 min. build Z1 to Z3
1 min. Z2 smooth build rpm to fast

Main 5 rounds of:
1 min. Z3+ at 75 rpm,
1 min. Z3+ at 55–65 rpm,
2 min. Z3+ at 45–55 rpm,
1 min. Z3+ at 55–65 rpm,
1 min. Z3+ at 75 rpm
4 min. Z2 at choice rpm between rounds

Add-On 15 min. Z3 steady state form-based
endurance

Scale for Time Scale duration as needed.

Scale for Fatigue Reduce the Main set efforts to Z2
and build the pyramid from 75 to 95 rpm.

SESSION TWO

SUPPORTING **BIKE**
TECHNICAL Prep, 1 hr.

Main
20 min. Z1 easy at choice rpm
20 min. Z2 smooth at choice rpm
20 min. Z3 steady at choice rpm

Scale for Time Scale to 15 min. or 10 min. for each
step.

Scale for Fatigue Skip the session if fatigued.

SATURDAY

KEY **BIKE** + **RUN**
ENDURANCE Over-Distance, 3.25–5.5 hr.

Main
3–5 hr.
Riding tour on variable terrain with mostly endurance-focused effort. No need to chase power or stick to heart rate zones. Enjoy being outside and building resilience on the bike.

TRAINER OPTION

Warm-Up 30 min. smooth

Pre-Main
15 min. Z2
10 min. Z2/Z3
5 min. Z3

Main 1–2 rounds of:
6 min. build by 2 min. to Z3+,
10 min. Z3 steady state at <70 rpm,
4 min. build by 1 min. to Z3+,
8 min. Z2 (power) steady state at >90 rpm,
2 min. build by 30 sec. to Z3+,
6 min. Z3 steady state at choice rpm

RUN OFF THE BIKE

15–30 min. form-based smooth endurance running

Scale for Time Trim the Warm-Up to 15 min. easy ramp, then only do a single round of the Main set.

Scale for Fatigue Keep the entire ride at Z2 and don't go longer than 2 hr. on the trainer. Outside ride can be very easy, up to 3 hr.

PM OFF

SUNDAY

KEY **BIKE**
ENDURANCE General Endurance, 2–4 hr.

Main
2–4 hr.
Another interval-free touring ride outside in variable terrain. Only choose the trainer option if you are forced to. If you can only go long one day, prioritize Saturday's ride.

TRAINER OPTION

Warm-Up 30 min. stepper
Easy spin and gradually ramp to steady Z3 effort.

Main 55 min. stepper up:
10, 9, 8, 7, 6, 5, 4, 3, 2, 1 min.
All with 30 sec. rest between intervals
Begin with 10 min. Z1 and gradually ramp effort with each interval to finish with 1 min. at Z4.

Add-On 28 min. stepper down:
7, 6, 5, 4, 3, 2, 1 min.
Begin at steady Z3 and ramp down in effort to finish with 1 min. at Z1.

Scale for Time Reduce each stepper (both up and down) to 15 min. Do as 5, 4, 3, 2, 1 min. but retain the theme and progression in effort.

Scale for Fatigue Evolve to be a Z2 ride. Outside can be very easy, up to 3 hr. Don't go longer than 2 hr. on the trainer.

PM OFF

FOCUS We take a few days to clean out the endurance load of the last week or so. We can then transition to another round of strength-endurance training. I encourage you to split the week in half, with the first half focused on recuperation and the other half on strength-endurance work. We will prepare for the upcoming strength-endurance work by including some integrated efforts at high rpm.

WEEKLY OVERVIEW

	M	T	W	TH	F	SA	SU	TOTAL
S1	40-60 min.	50-80 min.	40-60 min.	45-60 min.	45-90 min.	2.5-3.75 hr.	50-60 min.	10.6-
S2	30 min.	—	40-60 min.	60-75 min.	30 min.	—	1-1.5 hr.	15.3 hr.

MONDAY

SESSION ONE

SUPPORTING RUN
ENDURANCE General Endurance, 40–60 min.

Warm-Up 10 min. easy

Main
30–50 min. very low stress
Aim for best MFP. Control effort by adding leg speed, striding/bounding, activation, and practice the run/walk protocol.

Scale for Time Trim as needed or skip if unable to complete.

Scale for Fatigue If your muscles are sore, convert to a 30–45 min. flush/spin on the bike or a very easy 1–2 km swim.

SESSION TWO

STRENGTH & CONDITIONING
30 min.

Scale for Time Be sure you get in at least 5–10 min. of mobility work.

Scale for Fatigue This is a floating session that can occur any day.

TUESDAY

SESSION ONE

KEY BIKE + RUN
END-OF-RANGE High Cadence, 50–80 min.

Warm-Up As needed, include a few ramps to higher output so you can select work gear for Main set.

Main Up to 2 rounds of MAX sprints:
10 sec. MAX, 50 sec. easy,
20 sec. MAX, 40 sec. easy,
30 sec. MAX, 30 sec. easy,
40 sec. MAX, 20 sec. easy,
50 sec. MAX, 10 sec. easy,
60 sec. MAX,
10 sec. easy, 50 sec. MAX,
20 sec. easy, 40 sec. MAX,
30 sec. easy, 30 sec. MAX,
40 sec. easy, 20 sec. MAX,
50 sec. easy, 10 sec. MAX
7 min. easy spinning between rounds
Do MAX efforts as best effort at >90 rpm
Use the same gear for each work effort. Cadence decreases as set progresses. Shift from recovery gear 3 sec. before work starts. Begin each interval at MAX, a power decline is expected throughout each interval.

Cool-down 5-15 min. spin

RUN OFF THE BIKE

5 min. ramp to IM 70.3 effort
5 min. form-based running
5 min. at IM 70.3 effort
5 min. form-based running

Scale for Time Trim Main set to 1 round.

Scale for Fatigue Remove the MAX effort work and replace with an easy ride.

SESSION TWO

PM OFF

WEDNESDAY

SUPPORTING **SWIM**
ENDURANCE Short Intervals, 2150–3200

This is a recommended session.

Warm-Up 10 min. easy

Pre-Main 5–7 rounds (fins can be used):
50 at 70% with 10 sec. rest,
50 at 80% with 5–7 sec. rest,
50 at 90% with 3–5 sec. rest

Then, 2 rounds of:
2 × 25 fast,
50 easy, 50 fast,
2 × 25 easy
All with 15 sec. rest

Main With paddles:
40–70 × 25 at 85–90% with 2–5 sec. rest

Scale for Time Trim first Pre-Main set to 3 rounds, trim second set to 1 round. Adjust Main set as needed.

Scale for Fatigue Reduce Main set to 20–40 × 25 at 80%, no paddles.

SUPPORTING **RUN**
ENDURANCE General Endurance, 40–60 min.

Warm-Up 10 min. easy
Add dynamic warm-up if possible.

Main
30–50 min. low stress
Every 4th min. or so check on form, posture, etc. Aim for best MFP. Do not exceed Z2 effort.

Scale for Time Simple scale of duration as needed.

Scale for Fatigue Trim duration as needed.

THURSDAY

KEY **SWIM**
INTERVALS Building, 2200

Warm-Up 10 min. easy

Pre-Main 2 rounds of:
2 × 25 MAX with paddles,
50 easy float with good form,
50 fast with paddles,
2 × 25 easy

Main
An exercise in pacing, increasing speed with effort. Sight 3 times per lap.
8 × 100 as:
2 at 70%, 2 at 80%, 2 at 90%, 2 very strong
All with 30 sec. rest

8 × 75 as:
2 at 70%, 2 at 80%, 2 at 90%, 2 very strong
All with 20 sec. rest

8 × 50 as:
2 at 70%, 2 at 80%, 2 at 90%, 2 very strong
All with 10 sec. rest

Scale for Time Reduce repetitions in Main set from 8 to 4, maintaining pace and effort.

Scale for Fatigue Adjust the very strong efforts in the Main set to form-based short intervals, endurance and smooth.

SUPPORTING **BIKE**
TECHNICAL Activation, 60–75 min.

This is an optional session.

Warm-Up 30 min. smooth

Main 2–3 rounds of:
5 min. smooth,
2 min. spin higher rpm in a small gear,
3 min. steady,
2 min. spin higher rpm in a small gear,
1 min. strong,
2 min. spin higher rpm in a small gear

TRAINER OPTION

Warm-Up 10 min. spin

Pre-Main
5 × 3 min. smooth, ramp rpm by 1 min. to fast rpm

Then complete Main set detailed above.

Scale for Time Simple scale of duration as needed.

Scale for Fatigue Trim duration or skip if needed. Remove the neurological high-cadence work if needed.

FRIDAY

SESSION ONE

SUPPORTING **BIKE**
TECHNICAL Prep, 45–90 min.

This is a feel-good ride, whatever that is for you: more, less, building intervals, spinning, etc. Be aware and look for patterns to better manage readiness. Here is a possible option, but do what works for you.

Main
45–90 min. smooth
Include 4 × 3 min., ramp by 1 min. to strong but not deep effort
3–4 min. Z2 riding between intervals

Scale for Time Adjust duration as needed.

Scale for Fatigue Remove the ramping effort, but moving the body will still help.

SESSION TWO

STRENGTH & CONDITIONING
30 min.

Scale for Time Be sure you get in at least 5–10 min. of mobility work.

Scale for Fatigue This is a floating session that can occur any day.

SATURDAY

SESSION ONE

KEY **BIKE + RUN**
END-OF-RANGE Building, 2.5–3.75 hr.

Warm-Up 30-60 min.

Main
2–3 × 5 min. strong effort in aero position at 60 rpm
5 min. form-based endurance at choice rpm between intervals
10 min. smooth endurance

2–3 × 5 min. strong effort at >90 rpm
5 min. form-based endurance at choice rpm between intervals
10 min. smooth endurance

1–2 × 20 min. at IM effort/pace. Feel good with tidy form.
5 min. easy between intervals

Smooth endurance riding home

RUN OFF THE BIKE

5 min. quick ramp to IM 70.3 goal pace
5 min. form-based running
10 min. above IM 70.3 goal pace
5 min. easy cool-down

Scale for Time Scale duration and do 2 intervals of both low and high rpm for 5 min., but remove the 10 min. endurance intervals.

Scale for Fatigue Transition to a feel-good endurance ride with 3 × 6 min. smooth, build by 2 min. to strong but not deep.

SESSION TWO

PM OFF

SUNDAY

KEY **SWIM**
EVENT-SPECIFIC Pyramid, 2650

Warm-Up Smooth 10 min. light, then
400 pull smooth with choice of equipment at 70%

Main
Progressive building effort with medium-duration
swims: 1850 swim with variable pace. Always
20 sec. rest, followed by a form-based swim
interval.
200 steady at 85%, 150 form-based Z2 at 70%
150 strong at 90%, 150 form-based Z2 at 70%
100 very strong at 95%, 150 form-based Z2 at 70%
50 MAX with good, tidy hold on the water (no panic)
150 form-based Z2 at 70%, 100 very strong at 95%
150 form-based Z2 at 70%, 150 strong at 90%
150 form-based Z2 at 70%, 200 steady at 85%

400 pull smooth to finish

Scale for Time Reduce performance pyramid to be:
100, 75, 50, 75, 100, with 100 form-based swim
interval.

Scale for Fatigue Do about 1500–2000, very easy.
Mix it up with toys, etc. Feel good and move the
body.

KEY **RUN**
EVENT-SPECIFIC Building, 1–1.5 hr.

Warm-Up 10 min. easy

Main
50–80 min. low-stress endurance run on variable
terrain
Include 20 min. as:
5 min. at IM 70.3 effort,
5 min. above IM 70.3 effort,
10 min. at IM 70.3 effort

Scale for Time Scale duration as needed. No more
fitness to be gained.

Scale for Fatigue Skip the run completely.

IRONMAN 70.3

RACE SPECIFIC

FOCUS The strength-endurance aspect of this week will feel familiar. It is a progression of Week 5. Now we include some high rpm and speed work. Globally, this week is very challenging, especially the weekend key run, as well as the technical swim and end-of-range bike sessions.

WEEKLY OVERVIEW

	M	T	W	TH	F	SA	SU	TOTAL
S1	30–50 min.	45–70 min.	120–160 min.	45–70 min.	45–90 min.	1–1.5 hr.	50–70 min.	10.6–
S2	—	40–60 min.	30 min.	70–90 min.	—	30 min.	70–90 min.	15 hr.

MONDAY

SESSION ONE

SUPPORTING **RUN**
TECHNICAL Recovery, 30–50 min.

This is an optional session.

Warm-Up 10 min. easy

Main
20–40 min. very low stress
Aim for best MFP. Control effort by adding leg speed, striding/bounding, activation, and practice the run/walk protocol.

Scale for Time Trim as needed or skip if unable to complete.

Scale for Fatigue If your muscles are sore from last week, convert to a 30–45 min. flush/spin on the bike or a very easy 1–2 km swim.

SESSION TWO

PM OFF

TUESDAY

SESSION ONE

KEY **SWIM**
ENDURANCE Building, 2250–3800

Warm-Up 5–10 min. easy with mix of strokes

Pre-Main 3–6 rounds with paddles and fins:
50 at 75%,
50 at 85%,
50 at 95%
Always 10 sec. rest

Main
9 × 200–300
Increase effort/pace every 2 intervals:
1 and 2 at 65%, 3 and 4 at 75%, 5 and 6 at 85%,
7 and 8 at 95%, 9 at MAX
Always 30 sec. rest

Add-On 200 cool-down

Scale for Time Drop Main set to 6 intervals: 1 at 65%, 1 at 75%, 1 at 85%, 1 at 95%, 2 at best effort.

Scale for Fatigue Drop Main set to 6 intervals and only build to 85%.

SESSION TWO

SUPPORTING **RUN**
ENDURANCE General Endurance, 40–60 min.

Warm-Up 10 min. easy
Add dynamic warm-up if possible.

Main
30–50 min. low stress
Every 4th min. or so check on form, posture, etc.
Aim for best MFP. Do not exceed Z2 effort.

Scale for Time Simple scale of duration as needed.

Scale for Fatigue Trim duration or skip if needed.

WEDNESDAY

KEY **BIKE + RUN**
END-OF-RANGE High Cadence, 120–160 min.

Warm-Up 10 min. spin

Pre-Main 2 rounds of:
4 min. Z2 build rpm to fast,
3 min. build effort Z1 to Z3/Z4,
2 min. Z2 build rpm to fast,
1 min. build effort Z1 to Z3/Z4

Main 3–5 rounds of:
2 min. Z3, 4 min. Z4 at >95 rpm,
30 sec. Z1, 2 min. Z2,
4 min. Z4 at <65 rpm, 30 sec. Z1,
2 min. Z2
5 min. Z2 between rounds

RUN OFF THE BIKE

4 min. ramp to IM 70.3 effort, 2 min. easy
2 min. at 5–10 sec. per mile faster than IM 70.3
effort, 2 min. easy
2 min. at 10–15 sec. per mile faster than IM 70.3
effort, 2 min. easy
2 min. at 15–20 sec. per mile faster than IM 70.3
effort, 2 min. easy
2 min. at 10–15 sec. per mile faster than IM 70.3
effort, 2 min. easy
2 min. at 5–10 sec. per mile faster than IM 70.3
effort, 2 min. easy
Finish with 5–8 min. at feeling of IM 70.3 without
looking at the watch

Scale for Time Scale to 2–3 rounds of the Main
set, then reduce the run to a 15 min. build to very
strong.

Scale for Fatigue Maintain the Pre-Main but
convert the Main set to: 4 × 10 min. Z2, build rpm
to fast on each. Remove all work from the brick run
and convert to smooth 15 min. with good form.

STRENGTH & CONDITIONING
30 min.

Scale for Time Be sure you get in at least 5–10
min. of mobility work.

Scale for Fatigue This is a floating session that can
occur any day.

THURSDAY

SUPPORTING **SWIM**
ENDURANCE Short Intervals, 2550–3550

This is an optional session.

Warm-Up 10 min. easy

Pre-Main 5–7 rounds (fins can be used):
50 at 70% with 10 sec. rest,
50 at 80% with 5–7 sec. rest,
50 at 90% with 3–5 sec. rest

Then, 2 rounds of:
2 × 25 fast,
50 easy, 50 fast,
2 × 25 easy
All with 15 sec. rest

Main
20–30 × 50 at 85% with 5–7 sec. rest
Choose a send-off interval and aim to leave on the
same time each 50. Introduce sighting 3 times per
lap without losing rhythm, tempo, or stroke.

16–24 × 25 at 90–95% with only 3–5 sec. rest
Remove sighting to focus on keeping rhythm but
increasing your tempo (without slipping off the
hold/push of the water on each lap).

Scale for Time Scale Pre-Main and Main sets as
needed.

Scale for Fatigue Maintain the session, but make
the 50s all 80% and remove the 25s at the end. In
the Pre-Main, skip the second set of work.

KEY **RUN**
TECHNICAL Prep, 70–90 min.

Warm-Up 10 min. easy

Main
60–80 min. low-stress endurance run on variable
terrain. If you are injury prone, then a softer surface
is ideal.
Include 9 × 20 sec. blast (remain supple, yet fast)
with 90 sec. easy form-based running between
each.
Take short 20–40 sec. walk breaks as needed to
retain form.

Scale for Time Simply reduce time but retain the
9 × 20 sec. sharpeners.

Scale for Fatigue Begin very easy and scale for
time but retain the 9 × 20 sec. sharpeners.

IRONMAN 70.3 RACE SPECIFIC

FRIDAY

SESSION ONE

SUPPORTING BIKE
TECHNICAL Prep, 45–90 min.

Main
45–90 min.
First and last 10 min. at >95 rpm with minimum power while retaining chain tension. Focus on posture and good pedaling.
Include 4–6 × 30 sec., build to Z5 effort (10 sec. at Z3, Z4, and Z5)
3–4 min. spin between each 30 sec. build

TRAINER OPTION

Warm-Up 5–10 min. Z1 spin

Pre-Main
5 × 90 sec. Z1 at very high rpm
30 sec. spin between intervals

Main 4–6 rounds of:
30 sec. build as 10 sec. at Z3, Z4, and Z5
3 min. Z1 spin between intervals

Add-On 5 × 90 sec. Z1 at very fast rpm,
30 sec. spin between intervals

Scale for Time Scale duration as needed.

Scale for Fatigue Remove the Z5 effort, but moving the body will still help. Do something that feels good.

SESSION TWO

PM OFF

SATURDAY

SESSION ONE

KEY RUN
INTERVALS Strength, 1–1.5 hr.

Warm-Up 10–15 min. easy and smooth

Pre-Main Up to 3 rounds, until you feel ready for work:
90 sec. smooth, 30 sec. easy,
1 min. steady, 30 sec. easy,
30 sec. strong, 30 sec. easy

Main 3 loops of hill running:
3–4 min. flat with great form at smooth endurance (Z2/Z3)
3 min. sustained hill at very strong sustained effort with great form (bounding)
30 sec. MAX effort on steeper grade (5–8%) to finish hill
3 min. downhill running on shallow grade (3–5%), pick up feet and float down with fast foot speed
No breaks. This will be very tough. If you cannot find a loop, run on the treadmill. Use 1% for flat and 0% for downhill.

Following the loops:
15–30 min. Z3 tempo, form-based running

Scale for Time Trim Warm-Up and skip the tempo run at the end. The hills are the meat and potatoes today.

Scale for Fatigue Do a 50–75 min. feel-good endurance run over rolling terrain.

SESSION TWO

STRENGTH & CONDITIONING
30 min.

Scale for Time Be sure you get in at least 5–10 min. of mobility work.

Scale for Fatigue This is a floating session that can occur any day.

SUNDAY

KEY **SWIM**
TECHNICAL Speed and Power, 2450–3500

Warm-Up 300–600, swim every 4th lap as non-free

Pre-Main Pull set with paddles, snorkel, and buoy:
200, 175, 150, 125, 100, 75, 50, 25
All with 10 sec. rest
Progress effort as you go to feel good.

Main 2–4 rounds of:
4 × 25 MAX effort (with paddles and ankle strap or paddles and parachute),
20–30 sec. rest between intervals
150 smooth at 70% with paddles
1 min. rest between rounds

Then, do 15–20 × 50 at 80–85% with 5 sec. rest

Scale for Time Trim the Pre-Main to start at 150 and reduce the number of rounds in the Main set.

Scale for Fatigue Skip the 4 × 25 MAX effort in the Main set and reduce the 50s to 75–80%.

SUPPORTING **RUN**
ENDURANCE General Endurance, 70–90 min.

This is a recommended session

Warm-Up 10 min. easy

Main 60–80 min. form-based on variable terrain
If you are injury prone, a softer surface is ideal.
Take short 20–40 sec. walk breaks as needed to retain form.

Scale for Time Reduce Main set to 30–50 min.

Scale for Fatigue Reduce Main set to 30–50 min.

FOCUS This is a heavy block of work focused on strength and endurance. A challenging end-of-range bike ride is the feature of the week. Think of this week as building-block sessions that will allow you to blossom in the mix of low- and high-rpm work as you progress toward your goal race.

WEEKLY OVERVIEW

	M	T	W	TH	F	SA	SU	TOTAL
S1	30–50 min.	45–90 min.	45–90 min.	1–1.5 hr.	60–75 min.	160–205 min.	1–1.5 hr.	11.8–21.6 hr.
S2	—	40–60 min.	30 min.	70 min.	30 min.	—	80–120 min.	

MONDAY

SESSION ONE

SUPPORTING **RUN**
TECHNICAL Recovery, 30–50 min.

This is an optional session.
Warm-Up 10 min. easy

Main
20–40 min. very low stress
Aim for best MFP. Control effort by adding leg speed, striding/bounding, activation, and practice the run/walk protocol.

Scale for Time Trim as needed or skip if unable to complete.

Scale for Fatigue If your muscles are sore from last week, convert to a 30–45 min. flush/spin on the bike or a very easy 1–2 km swim.

SESSION TWO

PM OFF

TUESDAY

SESSION ONE

KEY **SWIM**
ENDURANCE Short Intervals, 2150–3600

Warm-Up 10 min. easy

Pre-Main 2–3 rounds with snorkel:
300 at 70%, focusing on hand entry in line with the shoulder, with 30 sec. rest,
3 × 50 form-based swimming, building tempo, effort, and stroke rate throughout each 50 with 10 sec. rest

Main
50–70 × 25 at 85–90% with 2–3 sec. rest
Good rhythm and tempo throughout. If you lose tempo, then add an extra 15–20 sec. rest and reset form.

Add-On 2 rounds of power:
4 × 25 MAX with paddles,
150 form-based swimming, feeling the connection

Scale for Time Trim Pre-Main set to a single round, remove the Add-On power, and trim the number of 25s if needed.

Scale for Fatigue Remove the Add-On power work. Make every 5th 25 easy backstroke with 15 sec. rest. Trim Pre-Main to a single round.

SESSION TWO

SUPPORTING **RUN**
ENDURANCE General Endurance, 40–60 min.

Warm-Up 10 min. easy
Add dynamic warm-up if possible.

Main
30–50 min. low stress
Every 4th min. check on form, posture, etc. Aim for best MFP. Do not exceed Z2 effort.

Scale for Time Scale duration as needed.

Scale for Fatigue Trim duration or skip if needed.

WEDNESDAY

SUPPORTING **BIKE**
TECHNICAL Prep, 45–90 min.

This is a recommended session.

Main
45–90 min. low-stress optional ride
First and last 10 min. at >95 rpm with minimum power while retaining chain tension. Focus on posture and good pedaling.
Include 4–6 × 30 sec. build as 10 sec. at Z3, Z4, and Z5
3–4 min. spin between each 30 sec. build

TRAINER OPTION

Warm-Up 5–10 min. Z1 spin

Pre-Main
5 × 90 sec. Z1 at very fast rpm
30 sec. spin between intervals

Main 4–6 rounds of:
30 sec. build as 10 sec. at Z3, Z4, and Z5
3 min. Z1 spin between each 30 sec. build

Add-On 5 × 90 sec. Z1 at very fast rpm,
30 sec. spin between intervals

Scale for Time Scale duration as needed.

Scale for Fatigue Remove the Z5 effort, but moving the body will help. Do something that feels good.

STRENGTH & CONDITIONING
30 min.

Scale for Time Be sure you get in at least 5–10 min. of mobility work.

Scale for Fatigue This is a floating session that can occur any day.

THURSDAY

SUPPORTING **SWIM**
ENDURANCE Over-Distance, 3300–4700

Warm-Up 10 min. easy with mix of strokes

Pre-Main
100 smooth
2 × 75 build to fast
3 × 50 build to fast
4 × 25 fast
All with 15 sec. rest

Main
100 with toys, 200 swim at 80%
200 with toys, 400 swim at 80%
300 with toys, 600 swim at 80%
200 with toys, 800 swim at 80%
100 with toys, 1000 swim at 80% (for advanced swimmers)
All with 1 min. rest between intervals
In the solid swims, sight 3 times per lap.

Add-On 12 × 25 with paddles and fins, do as
4 rounds of: easy, MAX, MAX
Always 10 sec. rest

Scale for Time Remove the speed Add-On, and trim Main set to finish at the 600 or 800 as needed.

Scale for Fatigue Remove the speed Add-On at the end, and trim the Main set to the 600.

KEY **RUN**
INTERVALS Strength, 70 min.

Warm-Up 10–15 min. easy running

Pre-Main
3 × 2 min., build by 30 sec. to feel-good, strong running

Main 3 rounds of:
2 × 3 min. strong, sustained effort up a 4% grade, form-based floating downhill with fast feet
30 sec. rest at the bottom of the hill
Following the second interval:
6 min. at goal IM 70.3 pace on the flats
4–5 min. easy endurance running

Scale for Time Reduce the number of rounds, but retain the rhythm and intent as well as duration of the intervals.

Scale for Fatigue Begin very easy and do a gradual ramp in effort, but can convert to a feel-good endurance run.

IRONMAN 70.3 RACE SPECIFIC

FRIDAY

SUPPORTING BIKE
TECHNICAL Activation, 60–75 min.

This is an optional session.

Warm-Up 30 min. smooth

Main 2–3 rounds of:
5 min. smooth,
2 min. spin higher rpm in a small gear,
3 min. steady,
2 min. spin higher rpm in a small gear,
1 min. strong,
2 min. spin higher rpm in a small gear

TRAINER OPTION

Warm-Up 10 min. spin

Pre-Main
5 × 3 min. smooth, ramp rpm by 1 min. to fast rpm

Then complete Main set detailed above.

Scale for Time Simple scale of duration as needed.

Scale for Fatigue Trim duration or skip if needed. Remove the neurological high-cadence work if needed.

STRENGTH & CONDITIONING
30 min.

Scale for Time Be sure you get in at least 5–10 min. of mobility work.

Scale for Fatigue This is a floating session that can occur any day.

SATURDAY

KEY BIKE + RUN
END-OF-RANGE Strength-Endurance, 160–205 min.

Warm-Up 30–45 min. smooth

Pre-Main 1–2 rounds of:
3 min. Z2 steady, 30 sec. Z1,
2 min. Z3 steady, 1 min. Z1,
1 min. Z3/Z4, 90 sec. Z1

Main
6 × 8–10 min. hill reps on a 4–6% grade, all very strong, sustained effort
Odd sets: <65 rpm
Even sets: holding >95 rpm
Spin down with at least 5–6 min. recovery between intervals

Endurance ride home until the last 10 min. at Z3+ or goal IM 70.3 effort

RUN OFF THE BIKE

5 min. quick ramp to or above IM 70.3 goal pace
5 min. at IM 70.3 goal pace
5 min. smooth, form-focused endurance
10 min. at IM 70.3 goal pace
5 min. easy cool-down

Scale for Time Reduce riding time but retain hill work.

Scale for Fatigue Choose a hilly 2–3 hr. endurance ride. Do a smooth building 20 min. run to Z3.

PM OFF

SUNDAY

KEY **SWIM**

EVENT-SPECIFIC Threshold, 3500–4550

Warm-Up 10 min. easy

Pre-Main 5-7 rounds (fins can be used):
50 at 70% with 10 sec. rest,
50 at 80% with 5-7 sec. rest,
50 at 90% with 3-5 sec. rest

Then, 2 rounds of:
2 × 25 fast,
50 easy, 50 fast,
2 × 25 easy
All with 15 sec. rest

Main
3-5 × 150 fast, right into 125 on the same send-off
300 pull smooth into 1 min. rest

3-5 × 125 fast, right into 100 on the same send-off
300 pull smooth into 1 min. rest

3-5 × 100 fast, right into 75 on the same send-off
300 pull smooth cool-down

Swim easy to finish

Scale for Time Scale Pre-Main and Main sets as needed.

Scale for Fatigue Alter Main set to: 3 rounds of 200 smooth at 70%, 150 build by 50-85%, 50 fast at 95%, all with 15-20 sec. rest.

SUPPORTING **RUN**

ENDURANCE General Endurance, 80–120 min.

This is a recommended session.

Warm-Up 10 min. easy

Main
70–110 min. low-stress endurance run on variable terrain. If you are injury prone, a softer surface is ideal.
Take short 20–40 sec. walk breaks as needed to retain form.

Scale for Time Scale duration as needed.

Scale for Fatigue Include more walk breaks and keep the effort purely conversational. Make total run no more than 1 hr.

IRONMAN 70.3

RACE SPECIFIC

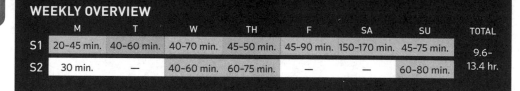

FOCUS Enjoy a little recuperation before ramping into a weekend of fast, high-intensity sessions. The weekend is a great opportunity to include a sprint- or Olympic-distance race, or even a 70.3. If so, make early next week easy. Test your fueling strategy in the race-simulation.

WEEKLY OVERVIEW

	M	T	W	TH	F	SA	SU	TOTAL
S1	20–45 min.	40–60 min.	40–70 min.	45–50 min.	45–90 min.	150–170 min.	45–75 min.	9.6–
S2	30 min.	—	40–60 min.	60–75 min.	—	—	60–80 min.	13.4 hr.

MONDAY

SESSION ONE

SUPPORTING **BIKE**
TECHNICAL Recovery, 20–45 min.

This is an optional session.

Main
20–45 min. very low stress
First and last 10 min. at high rpm in a small gear.
Feel free to be on a trainer or outside.

If you ride outside, practice some cornering and bike handling skills to refine control and comfort on the bike.

Scale for Time Trim as needed or skip if unable to complete.

Scale for Fatigue It may still be worth moving your blood here, not for fitness, but rather to enhance recovery and adaptations.

SESSION TWO

STRENGTH & CONDITIONING
30 min.

Scale for Time Be sure you get in at least 5–10 min. of mobility work.

Scale for Fatigue This is a floating session that can occur any day.

TUESDAY

SESSION ONE

KEY **BIKE + RUN**
END-OF-RANGE High Cadence, 40–60 min.

Warm-Up As needed.

Main Up to 2 rounds of MAX sprints:
10 sec. MAX, 50 sec. easy,
20 sec. MAX, 40 sec. easy,
30 sec. MAX, 30 sec. easy,
40 sec. MAX, 50 sec. easy,
50 sec. MAX, 50 sec. easy,
60 sec. MAX,
10 sec. easy, 50 sec. MAX,
20 sec. easy, 40 sec. MAX,
30 sec. easy, 30 sec. MAX,
40 sec. easy, 20 sec. MAX,
50 sec. easy, 10 sec. MAX
7 min. easy spinning between rounds
Do MAX efforts as best effort at >90 rpm

Cool-down 5–15 min. spin

RUN OFF THE BIKE

5 min. ramp to IM 70.3 effort
5 min. form-based running
5 min. at IM 70.3 effort
5 min. form-based running

Scale for Time Scale Main set as needed.

Scale for Fatigue Remove the MAX sprint efforts and replace with an easy ride.

SESSION TWO

PM OFF

WEDNESDAY

SUPPORTING **SWIM**
ENDURANCE Short Intervals, 2400–3800 min.

This is a recommended session.

Warm-Up 10 min. easy

Pre-Main 5–7 rounds (fins can be used):
50 at 70% with 10 sec. rest,
50 at 80% with 5–7 sec. rest,
50 at 90% with 3–5 sec. rest

Then, 2 rounds of:
2 × 25 fast,
50 easy, 50 fast,
2 × 25 easy
All with 15 sec. rest

Main With paddles:
50–90 × 25 at 85–90% with 2–5 sec. rest
between intervals

Scale for Time Reduce Warm-Up slightly and do
fewer rounds in Pre-Main set.

Scale for Fatigue Shift Main set to 30 × 25 at 80%
with 5 sec. rest, then 2 rounds of 8 × 25 (odds
smooth, evens MAX with 10 sec. rest) with 50 easy
between each 25.

SUPPORTING **RUN**
ENDURANCE General Endurance, 40–60 min.

Warm-Up 10 min. easy
Add dynamic warm-up if possible.

Main
30–50 min. low stress
Every 4th min. or so check on form, posture, etc.
Aim for best MFP. Do not exceed Z2 effort.

Scale for Time Adjust duration as needed.

Scale for Fatigue Adjust duration or skip if needed.

THURSDAY

KEY **SWIM**
INTERVALS Building, 2200

Warm-Up 10 min. easy

Pre-Main 2 rounds of:
2 × 25 MAX with paddles,
50 easy float with good form,
50 fast with paddles,
2 × 25 easy

Main
Practice pacing, increasing speed with effort.
Sight 3 times per lap.
8 × 100 as:
2 at 70%, 2 at 80%, 2 at 90%, 2 very strong
All with 30 sec. rest

8 × 75 as:
2 at 70%, 2 at 80%, 2 at 90%, 2 very strong
All with 20 sec. rest

8 × 50 as:
2 at 70%, 2 at 80%, 2 at 90%, 2 very strong
All with 10 sec. rest

Scale for Time Transition to 5 × 100, 5 × 75,
5 × 50, always 1 at 70%, 1 at 80%, 1 at 90%,
2 very strong.

Scale for Fatigue Adjust the very strong efforts
in the Main set to form-based short intervals,
endurance and smooth.

SUPPORTING **BIKE**
ENDURANCE General Endurance, 60–75 min.

This is an optional session.

Warm-Up 30 min. smooth

Main 2–3 rounds of:
5 min. smooth,
2 min. spin higher rpm in a small gear,
3 min. steady,
2 min. spin higher rpm in a small gear,
1 min. strong,
2 min. spin higher rpm in a small gear

TRAINER OPTION

Warm-Up 10 min. spin

Pre-Main
5 × 3 min. smooth, ramp rpm by 1 min. to fast rpm

Then complete Main set detailed above.

Scale for Time Simple scale of duration as needed.

Scale for Fatigue Trim duration or skip if needed.
Remove the neurological high-cadence speed work
if needed.

FRIDAY

SUPPORTING **BIKE**
TECHNICAL Prep, 45–90 min.

This is a feel-good ride, whatever that is for you: more, less, building intervals, spinning, etc. Be aware and look for patterns to better manage readiness. Here is a possible option, but do what works for you.

Main
45–90 min. smooth
Include 4 × 3 min., ramp by 1 min. to strong but not deep effort
3–4 min. easy spin between intervals

Scale for Time Scale duration as needed.

Scale for Fatigue Remove the ramping effort, but moving the body will still help. Do something that feels good.

PM OFF

SATURDAY

KEY **BIKE + RUN**
END-OF-RANGE Building, 150–170 min.

Warm-Up 60 min.

Main
2–3 × 5 min. strong effort in aero position at 60 rpm
5 min. form-based endurance at choice rpm between intervals
10 min. smooth endurance

2–3 × 5 min. strong effort at >90 rpm
5 min. form-based endurance at choice rpm between intervals
10 min. smooth endurance

10 min. at IM 70.3 goal pace
Feel good with tidy form.

Finish with smooth endurance ride home with good posture and pedaling.

RUN OFF THE BIKE

5 min. ramp to IM 70.3 goal pace
5 min. IM 70.3 goal pace
5 min. easy cool-down

Scale for Time Scale duration and do 2 intervals of both low and high rpm for 5 min., but remove the 10 min. smooth endurance intervals.

Scale for Fatigue Transition to a feel-good endurance ride with 3 × 6 min. smooth, build by 2 min. to strong but not deep effort.

PM OFF

SUNDAY

KEY **SWIM**
EVENT-SPECIFIC Pyramid, 2300–4200

Warm-Up Smooth 10 min. light, then
400 pull smooth with choice of equipment at 70%

Main
Progressive building effort with medium-duration swims: 1500 swim with variable pace. Always 15 sec. rest.

150 steady at 85%, 100 form-based Z2 at 70%
125 strong at 90%, 100 form-based Z2 at 70%
100 very strong at 95%, 100 form-based Z2 at 70%
50 MAX with good, tidy hold on the water
(no panic)
100 form-based Z2 at 70%, 100 very strong at 95%
100 form-based Z2 at 70%, 125 strong at 90%
100 form-based Z2 at 70%, 150 steady at 85%
100 form-based Z2 at 70%

400 pull smooth with 2 min. rest, then repeat round if feeling very good

Scale for Time Reduce performance pyramid to be: 100, 75, 50, 75, 100, progressing as strong, very strong, MAX.

Scale for Fatigue Convert to 1500–2000 very easy. Mix it up with toys, etc. Do as you wish, but feel good and move the body.

SUPPORTING **RUN**
ENDURANCE General Endurance, 60–80 min.

This is a recommended session.

Warm-Up 10 min. easy

Main
50–70 min. low stress endurance run on variable terrain
Include up to 2 rounds of fartlek-style builds as:
45-30-15 sec. with 90 sec. easy between

Scale for Time Scale duration as needed. No more fitness to be gained.

Scale for Fatigue Skip the run completely.

IRONMAN 70.3

RACE SPECIFIC

FOCUS We now finalize the preparation with a race-focused block of work and some open-water skills practice in the pool (sighting), as well as event-specific preparation on the bike and run. We have very little strength-endurance now, but enough to remind the body of the stressor. We move to faster and flatter riding and running. Simulate race fueling and hydration in the key sessions.

WEEKLY OVERVIEW

	M	T	W	TH	F	SA	SU	TOTAL
S1	40–60 min.	45–70 min.	1–1.5 hr.	45–70 min.	45–90 min.	150–175 min.	75–100 min.	12.6–
S2	—	50–80 min.	30 min.	2–3 hr.	30 min.	—	70–90 min.	18.4 hr.

MONDAY

SESSION ONE

SUPPORTING RUN
TECHNICAL Recovery, 40–60 min.

Warm-Up 10 min. easy

Main
30–50 min. very low stress
Aim for best MFP. Control effort by adding leg speed, striding/bounding, activation, and practice the run/walk protocol.

Scale for Time Trim as needed or skip if unable to complete.

Scale for Fatigue If your muscles are sore, convert to a 30–45 min. flush/spin on the bike or a very easy 1–2 km swim.

SESSION TWO

PM OFF

TUESDAY

SESSION ONE

KEY SWIM
ENDURANCE Building, 2400–3700

Warm-Up 600–800, swim every 4th lap as non-free

Main 12 × 150–200, do as 3 rounds of:
1 at 70% with 30 sec. rest,
1 at 80% with 20 sec. rest,
2 at 90–95% with 10 sec. rest

Add-On 20 × 25 with paddles (or parachute), do as 5 rounds of: 3 fast, 1 easy
Always 10 sec. rest

Scale for Time Adjust Main set to 12 × 100 and skip the Add-On.

Scale for Fatigue Drop Main set to 6 intervals and only build to 85% as 2 rounds of 1 at 70%, 1 at 80%, 1 at 85%.

SESSION TWO

SUPPORTING RUN
ENDURANCE General Endurance, 50–80 min.

Warm-Up 10 min. easy
Add dynamic warm-up if possible.

Main
40–70 min. MFP, smooth.
Every 4th min. or so, check in on form, posture, etc. Do not exceed Z2.
Control effort by adding leg speed, striding/bounding, activation, and practice the run/walk protocol.

Scale for Time Simple scale of duration as needed.

Scale for Fatigue Trim duration or skip if needed.

WEDNESDAY

KEY **RUN**
INTERVALS Speed, 1–1.5 hr.

Warm-Up 10 min. easy

Pre-Main 1–2 rounds:
3 min. smooth, 30 sec. easy,
2 min. steady, 30 sec. easy,
1 min. strong, 30 sec. easy

Main
6–8 × 1 km at 10 sec. per mile faster than IM 70.3
goal pace
90 sec. rest between intervals

10 min. smooth form-based endurance home

OPTIONAL PM RUN
20–40 min. very low stress
Include 10-20-30-20-10 sec. blasts with 90 sec.
easy between each effort.

Scale for Time Maintain the 1 km intervals, but
reduce the number of intervals as needed.

Scale for Fatigue Convert to a smooth and
progressively building effort to finish feeling better
than when you started.

STRENGTH & CONDITIONING
30 min.

Scale for Time Be sure you hit at least 5–10 min.
of mobility.

Scale for Fatigue This is a floating session that can
occur any day.

THURSDAY

SUPPORTING **SWIM**
ENDURANCE Short Intervals, 2550–3550

This is a recommended session.

Warm-Up 10 min. easy

Pre-Main 5–7 rounds (fins can be used):
50 at 70% with 10 sec. rest,
50 at 80% with 5–7 sec. rest,
50 at 90% with 3–5 sec. rest

Then, 2 rounds of:
2 × 25 fast,
50 easy, 50 fast,
2 × 25 easy
All with 15 sec. rest

Main 20–30 × 50 at 85% with 5–7 sec. rest
Choose a send-off interval and aim to leave on
the same time each 50. Introduce sighting 3 times
per lap.

Add-On 16–24 × 25 at 90–95% with only 3–5 sec.
rest. Remove sighting to focus on keeping rhythm
but increase your tempo.

Scale for Time Scale Pre-Main and Main sets
as needed.

Scale for Fatigue Maintain the session, but make
the 50s all at 80% and remove the 25s at the end.
Skip the rounds of 2 × 25, 50, 50, 2 × 25 in the
Pre-Main set.

SUPPORTING **BIKE**
TECHNICAL Activation, 2–3 hr.

This is a recommended session.

Warm-Up 10 min. easy

Main
2–3 hr. endurance ride
Include 5 rounds of:
20 sec. MAX effort,
2 min. Z3 steady,
5 min. Z1 spin

TRAINER OPTION
Warm-Up 30 min. stepper, building easy to
moderate

Main 5 rounds of:
20 sec. MAX effort,
2 min. Z3 steady,
5 min. Z1 spin

Add-On 15 min. Z2 smooth

Scale for Time Scale the length, but maintain the
restorative nature of the ride.

Scale for Fatigue Skip the ride if needed.

IRONMAN 70.3 RACE SPECIFIC

FRIDAY

SESSION ONE

SUPPORTING BIKE
TECHNICAL Prep, 45–90 min.

This is an optional session.

Main
45–90 min. smooth
Include 4 × 3 min., ramp by 1 min. to Z5 strong but not deep effort
3–4 min. rest between intervals

Scale for Time Scale duration as needed.

Scale for Fatigue Remove the Z5 effort, but moving the body will still help. Do something that feels good.

SESSION TWO

STRENGTH & CONDITIONING
30 min.

Scale for Time Be sure you hit at least 5–10 min. of mobility.

Scale for Fatigue This is a floating session that can occur any day.

SATURDAY

SESSION ONE

KEY BIKE + RUN
EVENT-SPECIFIC Race Simulation, 150–175 min.

Warm-Up 30–45 min. smooth

Pre-Main 1–2 rounds of:
3 min. Z2 steady, 30 sec. Z1,
2 min. Z3 steady, 1 min. Z1,
1 min. Z3/Z4, 90 sec. Z1

Main
10 min. steady endurance choice rpm (Z3 or so)
5 min. Z4 very strong as:
1 min. at 80 rpm,
1 min. at 90 rpm,
1 min. at 100+ rpm,
1 min. at 90 rpm,
1 min. at 80 rpm
5 min. spin

Then, 2 rounds of:
10 min. steady endurance choice rpm (Z3 or so)
5 min. Z4 very strong as:
1 min. at 70 rpm,
1 min. at 60 rpm,
1 min. at 50 rpm,
1 min. at 60 rpm,
1 min. at 70 rpm
5 min. spin

Then, 10 min. steady endurance choice rpm
5 min. Z4 very strong as:
1 min. at 80 rpm,
1 min. at 90 rpm,
1 min. at 100+ rpm,
1 min. at 90 rpm,
1 min. at 80 rpm
5 min. spin

Endurance riding home

RUN OFF THE BIKE

5 min. ramp to at or above IM 70.3 effort
5 min. at IM 70.3 effort
5 min. smooth endurance
10 min. at IM 70.3 effort
5 min. easy cool-down

Scale for Time Trim Warm-Up and shift the Main set to: 2 × 30 min. IM effort with the last 10 min. of each interval above IM effort.

Scale for Fatigue Transition to a feel-good endurance ride.

SESSION TWO

PM OFF

SUNDAY

KEY **SWIM**
ENDURANCE Building, 3900–5100

Warm-Up 10 min. easy

Pre-Main 3 × 500 as:
1 straight swim smooth,
1 with every 3rd 25 fast,
1 with every other 25 fast

Main 2-3 rounds, sighting 3 times per lap:
400 at 80-85% with 30 sec. rest,
4 × 100 at 85-90% with 10 sec. rest,
200 at 80-85% with 30 sec. rest,
4 × 50 at 90-95% with 5 sec. rest

Scale for Time Reduce the Pre-Main set to
3 × 300. Reduce the Main set to: 300, 3 × 100, 150,
3 × 100 and do as many rounds as possible.

Scale for Fatigue Reduce the Pre-Main set to
3 × 300. Convert the Main set to 400, 300, 200,
100, with 1 min. rest between intervals. Progress to
strong on the 100, then done.

SUPPORTING **RUN**
ENDURANCE General Endurance, 70–90 min.

Warm-Up 10 min. easy

Main
60–80 min. low-stress endurance run on variable
terrain. If you are injury prone, a softer surface is
ideal.
Take short 20–40 sec. walk breaks as needed to
retain form.

Scale for Time Scale duration as needed.

Scale for Fatigue Include more walk breaks and
keep the effort purely conversational. Make total
run no more than 1 hr.

IRONMAN 70.3

RACE SPECIFIC

FOCUS Highlights include a hearty event-specific brick in the middle of the week and a weekend dominated with run preparation and an endurance ride. Don't forget to practice race-day fueling and hydration in the key sessions.

WEEKLY OVERVIEW

	M	T	W	TH	F	SA	SU	TOTAL
S1	20–45 min.	40–70 min.	100–140 min.	1–1.5 hr.	45–90 min.	1–1.5 hr.	2–4 hr.	11.7–
S2	—	50–80 min.	30 min.	75 min.	30 min.	70–100 min.	—	18 hr.

MONDAY

SESSION ONE

SUPPORTING **BIKE**
TECHNICAL Recovery, 20–45 min.

Main
20–45 min.
Very low stress ride on a trainer or outside with first and last 10 min. at fast rpm, in a small gear.

If you ride outside, practice cornering and bike handling skills to refine control and comfort on the bike.

Scale for Time Trim as needed or skip if unable to complete.

Scale for Fatigue It may still be worth fitting in the ride not for fitness, but to enhance recovery and adaptations.

SESSION TWO

PM OFF

TUESDAY

SESSION ONE

KEY **SWIM** .
ENDURANCE Short Intervals, 2150–3600

Warm-Up 10 min. easy

Pre-Main 2–3 rounds with snorkel:
300 snorkel with focus on hand entry in line with the shoulder at 70% with 30 sec. rest,
3 × 50 form-based swimming building tempo, effort, and stroke rate throughout each 50
10 sec. rest between intervals

Main
50–70 × 25 at 85–90% with 2–3 sec. rest
Good rhythm and tempo throughout. If you lose tempo, add an extra 15–20 sec. rest and reset form.

Add-On 2 rounds of power:
4 × 25 MAX with paddles,
150 form-based swimming

Scale for Time Trim the Pre-Main set to a single round, and trim the number of 25s.

Scale for Fatigue Trim the Pre-Main set to a single round. Remove the Add-On power work. Make every 5th 25 easy backstroke with 15 sec. rest.

SESSION TWO

SUPPORTING **RUN**
ENDURANCE General Endurance, 50–80 min.

Warm-Up 10 min. easy
Add dynamic warm-up if possible.

Main
40–70 min.
Every 4th min. or so check on form, posture, etc.
Aim for best MFP. Do not exceed Z2 effort.

Scale for Time Adjust duration as needed.

Scale for Fatigue Trim duration or skip if needed.

WEDNESDAY

KEY BIKE + RUN
EVENT-SPECIFIC Race Simulation, 100–140 min.

Warm-Up 10 min. spin

Pre-Main
2 × 4 min. build to Z3/Z4, then spin easy

Main 2–4 rounds of:
2 min. Z3,
4 min. Z3+ to Z4 at >95 rpm,
1 min. Z1, 2 min. Z2,
4 min. Z3+ to Z4 at <70 rpm,
1 min. Z1, 2 min. Z2

Then, 5 min. Z1 into:
15 min. IM 70.3 goal effort (Z3 to Z3+) at choice rpm

RUN OFF THE BIKE

This run forces you into goal pace, so aim to do so with great form and posture.
4 min. ramp to IM 70.3 goal pace (or Z3 to Z3+)
2 min. Z2 easy endurance
2 min. at 5–10 sec. per mile faster than IM 70.3 goal pace (or Z4)
2 min. Z2 easy endurance
2 min. at 10–15 sec. per mile faster than IM 70.3 goal pace (or Z4+)
2 min. Z2 easy endurance
2 min. at 15–20 sec. per mile faster than IM 70.3 goal pace (or Z5)
2 min. Z2 easy endurance
2 min. at 10–15 sec. per mile faster than IM 70.3 goal pace (or Z4+)
2 min. Z2 easy endurance
2 min. at 5–10 sec. per mile faster than IM 70.3 goal pace (or Z4)
2 min. Z2 easy endurance
Finish with 5–8 min. at IM 70.3 pace feel without looking at the watch.

Scale for Time Reduce the number of rounds in the Main set, but still aim to retain at least 7 min. of IM 70.3 work at the end with rpm of choice. The brick run becomes 5 min. ramp to 70.3, 5 min. above IM 70.3, 5 min. easy.

Scale for Fatigue Convert the Main set to: 4 × 10 min. Z2, build rpm to fast on each. Remove all work from the brick run and convert to smooth 15 min. with good form.

STRENGTH & CONDITIONING
30 min.

Scale for Time Be sure you get in at least 5–10 min. of mobility work.

Scale for Fatigue This is a floating session that can occur any day.

THURSDAY

SUPPORTING SWIM
ENDURANCE Building, 2750–5200

This is an optional session.

Warm-Up 10 min. easy

Pre-Main 3–5 rounds (fins can be used):
50 at 70% with 10 sec. rest,
50 at 80% with 5–7 sec. rest,
50 at 90% with 3–5 sec. rest

Then, 2 rounds of:
2 × 25 fast,
50 easy, 50 fast,
2 × 25 easy
All with 15 sec. rest

Main 2–3 rounds of:
12–18 × 50 at 85% with 5–7 sec. rest
(paddles are OK if you can retain stroke rate),
10–14 × 25 at 90–95% with 3–5 sec. rest
100 easy with 45 sec. rest between rounds

Scale for Time Scale Pre-Main and Main sets by reducing the number of rounds or intervals within the rounds.

Scale for Fatigue Alter Main set to: 30–60 × 25, but only at 80%, no paddles.

KEY RUN
INTERVALS Tempo, 75 min.

Main 75 min. steady and smooth build as:
30 min. easy and low stress (likely Z2),
20 min. moderate effort (lower Z3),
15 min. moderately strong effort, just above IM effort (Z3),
10 min. strong (Z3+)

Scale for Time Scale the length of the run, but with similar pace/effort ramp, such as: 20, 15, 10, 5 min.

Scale for Fatigue Begin very easy and gradually ramp up in effort, but it can convert to a feel-good endurance run.

IRONMAN 70.3

RACE SPECIFIC

FRIDAY	SATURDAY

FRIDAY

SESSION ONE

SUPPORTING **BIKE**
TECHNICAL Prep, 45–90 min.

This is an optional session.

Main
45–90 min.
First and last 10 min. at >95 rpm with minimum power while retaining chain tension. Focus on posture and good pedaling.
Include 4–6 × 30 sec., build to Z5 effort in the last 10 sec. of each.
3–4 min. endurance riding between each 30 sec. build.

TRAINER OPTION

Warm-Up 10–20 min. Z1 easy

Pre-Main
5 × 90 sec. Z1 at very fast rpm
30 sec. spin between intervals

Main 4–6 rounds of:
30 sec. build as 10 sec. at Z3, Z4, Z5
3 min. Z1 spin between intervals

Add-On 5 × 90 sec. Z1 at very fast rpm,
30 sec. spin between intervals

Scale for Time Scale duration as needed.

Scale for Fatigue Remove the Z5 effort, but moving the body will still help. Do something that feels good.

SESSION TWO

STRENGTH & CONDITIONING
30 min.

Scale for Time Be sure you get in at least 5–10 min. of mobility work.

Scale for Fatigue This is a floating session that can occur any day.

SATURDAY

SESSION ONE

KEY **RUN**
INTERVALS Speed, 1–1.5 hr.

Warm-Up 10 min. easy

Pre-Main 1–2 rounds until you are ready to go:
3 min. smooth, 30 sec. easy,
2 min. steady, 30 sec. easy,
1 min. strong, 30 sec. easy

Main
6–8 × 1 km at 10 sec. per mile faster than IM 70.3 goal pace (or Z3+)
2 min. recovery between intervals

Then 10 min. smooth, form-based endurance home

OPTIONAL PM RUN

20–40 min. very low stress
Include 10-20-30-20-10 sec. blasts with 90 sec. easy between each blast.

Scale for Time Maintain the 1 km intervals, but reduce the number of intervals as needed.

Scale for Fatigue Convert to a smooth and progressively building effort to finish feeling better than when you started (no matter how weak the build is).

SESSION TWO

KEY **SWIM**
EVENT-SPECIFIC Threshold, 4650–6000

Warm-Up 10 min. easy

Pre-Main 5–7 rounds (fins can be used):
50 at 70% with 10 sec. rest,
50 at 80% with 5–7 sec. rest,
50 at 90% with 3–5 sec. rest

Then, 2 rounds of:
2 × 25 fast,
50 easy, 50 fast,
2 × 25 easy
All with 15 sec. rest

Main
3–5 × 150 fast, right into 125 on the same send-off
300 pull smooth into 1 min. rest

3–5 × 125 fast, right into 100 on the same send-off
300 pull smooth into 1 min. rest

3–5 × 100 fast, right into 75 on the same send-off
300 pull smooth cool-down

Swim easy to finish

Scale for Time Scale Pre-Main and Main as needed.

Scale for Fatigue Alter Main set to 3 rounds of 200 smooth at 70%, 150 build by 50–85%, 50 fast at 95%, all with 15–20 sec. rest.

SUNDAY

SUPPORTING **BIKE**
ENDURANCE General Endurance, 2–4 hr.

This is a recommended session.

Main
2–4 hr. endurance ride on variable terrain
Include 5 rounds of:
20 sec. MAX effort,
2 min. Z2/Z3,
5 min. Z1

TRAINER OPTION

Warm-Up 30 min. stepper, gradually ramp effort
from very easy to steady

Main 4 rounds of:
4 min. Z1/Z2 easy choice pedaling,
30 sec. Z1 easy,
3 min. Z2 smooth build rpm to fast,
30 sec. Z1 easy,
2 min. Z2/Z3 smooth choice pedaling,
30 sec. Z1 easy,
1 min. steady Z3 build rpm to fast,
30 sec. Z1 easy

Add-On 20 min. Z2 choice with every 4th min.
ramp rpm to MAX

Scale for Time Reduce Warm-Up to 15 min.
stepper. Reduce rounds in Main set as needed.

Scale for Fatigue Reduce the Warm-Up to a
15 min. stepper. Main set can be 2 rounds. Remove
the Add-On.

PM OFF

FOCUS A massive mental shift begins: You cannot gain any more fitness, and you must gain control over your program with confidence. It is all feel-good, smooth, sharpening work. You might feel flat in the coming days, but the mission is for you to do the work you are good at and enjoy it, without creating any deep fatigue nor searching for validation. When in doubt, go less and go easier.

WEEKLY OVERVIEW

	M	T	W	TH	F	SA	SU	TOTAL
S1	20–45 min.	50–75 min.	45–60 min.	45–50 min.	45–90 min.	145–165 min.	50–75 min.	9.8–
S2	30 min.	—	40–50 min.	60–75 min.	—	—	60–80 min.	13.25 hr.

MONDAY

SESSION ONE

SUPPORTING BIKE
TECHNICAL Recovery, 20–45 min.

Main
20–45 min. very low stress
First and last 10 min. at high rpm in a small gear. Feel free to ride on a trainer or outside.

If you ride outside, practice cornering and bike handling skills to refine control and comfort on the bike.

Scale for Time Trim as needed or skip if unable to complete.

Scale for Fatigue It may still be worth fitting in the ride not for fitness, but to enhance recovery and adaptations.

SESSION TWO

STRENGTH & CONDITIONING
30 min.

Scale for Time Be sure you get in at least 5–10 min. of mobility work.

Scale for Fatigue This is a floating session that can occur any day.

TUESDAY

SESSION ONE

KEY BIKE + RUN
END-OF-RANGE High Cadence, 50–75 min.

Warm-Up As needed.

Main Up to 2 rounds of MAX sprints:
10 sec. MAX, 50 sec. easy,
20 sec. MAX, 40 sec. easy,
30 sec. MAX, 30 sec. easy,
40 sec. MAX, 20 sec. easy,
50 sec. MAX, 10 sec. easy,
60 sec. MAX,
10 sec. easy, 50 sec. MAX,
20 sec. easy, 40 sec. MAX,
30 sec. easy, 30 sec. MAX,
40 sec. easy, 20 sec. MAX,
50 sec. easy, 10 sec. MAX
7 min. easy spinning between rounds
Do MAX efforts as best effort at >90 rpm
Use the same gear for each work effort. Cadence decreases as set progresses. Shift from recovery gear 3 sec. before work starts.

Cool-down 5–15 min. spin

RUN OFF THE BIKE

5 min. ramp to IM 70.3 feel
5 min. form-based running
5 min. at IM 70.3 feel
5 min. form-based running

Scale for Time Reduce Warm-Up slightly, but this is a very short session as it is.

Scale for Fatigue Remove the MAX effort and replace it with an easy ride.

SESSION TWO

PM OFF

WEDNESDAY

SUPPORTING **SWIM**
ENDURANCE Short Intervals, 2150–2950

This is a recommended session.

Warm-Up 10 min. easy

Pre-Main 5-7 rounds (fins can be used):
50 at 70% with 10 sec. rest,
50 at 80% with 5–7 sec. rest,
50 at 90% with 3–5 sec. rest

Then, 2 rounds of:
2 × 25 fast,
50 easy, 50 fast,
2 × 25 easy
All with 15 sec. rest

Main With paddles:
40–60 × 25 at 85–90% with 2–5 sec. rest
between intervals

Scale for Time Scale Pre-Main and Main sets as
needed.

Scale for Fatigue Alter Main Set to: 20–40 × 25,
but only at 80% and no paddles.

SUPPORTING **RUN**
TECHNICAL Recovery, 40–50 min.

Warm-Up 10 min. easy
Add dynamic warm-up if possible.

Main
30–40 min. low stress
Every 4th min. or so, check on form, posture, etc.
Aim for best MFP. Do not exceed Z2 effort.

Scale for Time Scale the duration as needed.

Scale for Fatigue Trim duration or skip if needed.

THURSDAY

KEY **SWIM**
INTERVALS Building, 2200

Warm-Up 10 min. easy

Pre-Main 2 rounds of:
2 × 25 MAX with paddles,
50 easy float with good form,
50 fast with paddles,
2 × 25 easy

Main
An exercise in pacing, increasing speed with effort.
Sight 3 times per lap.
8 × 100 as:
2 at 70%, 2 at 80%, 2 at 90%, 2 very strong
All with 30 sec. rest

8 × 75 as:
2 at 70%, 2 at 80%, 2 at 90%, 2 very strong
All with 20 sec. rest

8 × 50 as:
2 at 70%, 2 at 80%, 2 at 90%, 2 very strong
All with 10 sec. rest

Scale for Time Reduce repetitions in Main set from
8 to 4, maintaining pace and effort.

Scale for Fatigue Adjust the very strong efforts
in the Main set to form-based short intervals,
endurance and smooth.

SUPPORTING **BIKE**
ENDURANCE General Endurance, 60–75 min.

Warm-Up 30 min. smooth

Main 2–3 rounds of:
5 min. smooth,
2 min. spin higher rpm in a small gear,
3 min. steady,
2 min. spin higher rpm in a small gear,
1 min. strong,
2 min. spin higher rpm in a small gear

TRAINER OPTION

Warm-Up 10 min. spin

Pre-Main
5 × 3 min. smooth, ramp rpm by 1 min. to fast rpm

Then complete Main set detailed above.

Scale for Time Scale the duration as needed.

Scale for Fatigue Trim duration or skip if needed.
Remove the neurological speed work if needed.

FRIDAY	SATURDAY
SESSION ONE	**SESSION ONE**

FRIDAY

SESSION ONE

SUPPORTING **BIKE**
TECHNICAL Prep, 45–90 min.

This is a feel-good ride, whatever that is for you: more, less, building intervals, spinning, etc. Be aware and look for patterns to better manage readiness. Here is a possible option, but do what works for you.

Main
45–90 min. smooth
Include 4 × 3 min., ramp by 1 min. to strong but not deep effort
3–4 min. Z2 riding between intervals

Scale for Time Scale duration as needed.

Scale for Fatigue Remove the ramping effort, but moving the body will still help. Do something that feels good.

SESSION TWO

PM OFF

SATURDAY

SESSION ONE

KEY **BIKE + RUN**
END-OF-RANGE Building, 145–165 min.

Warm-Up 60 min.

Main
2–3 × 5 min. strong effort at 60 rpm
5 min. form-based endurance at choice rpm between intervals
10 min. smooth endurance

2–3 × 5 min. strong effort at >90 rpm
5 min. form-based endurance at choice rpm between intervals
10 min. smooth endurance

Then, 10 min. at IM 70.3 effort/pace. Feel good with tidy form. Finish with smooth endurance riding home with good posture and pedaling.

RUN OFF THE BIKE

5 min. ramp to IM 70.3 goal pace
5 min. at IM 70.3 goal pace
5 min. easy cool-down

Scale for Time Reduce to 1.5–2 hr.: do 25–45 min. Warm-Up and only do 1 round of the Main set.

Scale for Fatigue Transition to a feel-good 1.5–2 hr. endurance ride; in the first and last 10 min. spin at high rpm.

SESSION TWO

PM OFF

SUNDAY

KEY **SWIM**
EVENT-SPECIFIC Pyramid, 2000–3550

Warm-Up Smooth 10 min. light, then 400 pull smooth with choice of equipment at 70%

Main
Progressive 1175 building effort with shorter swims and variable pace:
100 steady at 85%, 100 form-based Z2 at 70%
75 strong at 90%, 100 form-based Z2 at 70%
50 at very strong at 95%, 100 form-based Z2 at 70%
25 MAX with good, tidy hold on the water (no panic)
100 form-based Z2 at 70%, 50 very strong at 95%
100 form-based Z2 at 70%, 75 strong at 90%
100 form-based Z2 at 70%, 100 steady at 85%
100 form-based Z2 at 70%
Always 15 sec. rest

400 pull smooth with 2 min. rest then repeat round if you're feeling very good.

Swim easy to finish

Scale for Time Reduce the Main set to only 50 form-based Z2 between higher efforts.

Scale for Fatigue Go about 1500–2000, very easy. Mix it up with toys, etc. Swim as you wish, but feel good and move the body.

SUPPORTING **RUN**
ENDURANCE General Endurance, 60–80 min.

This is a recommended session.

Warm-Up 10 min. easy

Main
50–70 min. low-stress endurance run on variable terrain
Include up to 2 rounds of fartlek-style builds:
45-30-15 sec. fast with 90 sec. easy between

Scale for Time Scale duration as needed. No more fitness to be gained.

Scale for Fatigue Skip the run completely.

IRONMAN 70.3

RACE SPECIFIC

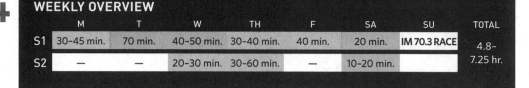

WEEK 14

FOCUS No more worrying about "what if's." Let this week be the celebration. How you feel is irrelevent to race day performance, so set yourself up well by maintaining a clean set of eating habits, resting as much as possible, planning the race weekend experience, and getting excited. Let your race performance be an expression of your preparation.

WEEKLY OVERVIEW

	M	T	W	TH	F	SA	SU	TOTAL
S1	30–45 min.	70 min.	40–50 min.	30–40 min.	40 min.	20 min.	IM 70.3 RACE	4.8–
S2	—	—	20–30 min.	30–60 min.	—	10–20 min.		7.25 hr.

MONDAY

SESSION ONE

SUPPORTING BIKE
TECHNICAL Prep, 30–45 min.

Main
30–45 min. spin recuperation
First and last 10 min. high rpm in a small gear

TRAINER OPTION

Warm-Up 10 min. spin

Pre-Main
3 × 2 min. smooth, with 30 sec. at 75, 85, 95, 105 rpm
30 sec. break between intervals

Main
3 × 2 min., ramp by 30 sec. from easy to strong
2 min. spin very easy between intervals

Add-On 5 min. spin easy at higher rpm

Scale for Time Trim as needed or skip if unable to complete.

Scale for Fatigue If you're sore from last week, convert to a 30–45 min. flush/spin on the bike or very easy 1–2 km swim.

SESSION TWO

PM OFF

TUESDAY

SESSION ONE

KEY BIKE + RUN
TECHNICAL Prep, 70 min.

Warm-Up 10 min. spin

Pre-Main
3 min. ramp Z1 to Z3/Z4
3 min. Z2 build rpm to fast
3 min. ramp Z1 to Z3/Z4
3 min. Z2 build rpm to fast

Main
4 × 2 min. build by 30 sec. to Z4+
90 sec. Z1 spin between intervals
3 × 1 min. build by 20 sec. to Z5
90 sec. Z1 spin between intervals
2 × 30 sec. build by 10 sec. to Z5+
90 sec. Z1 spin between intervals

Then 10 min. smooth Z2

RUN OFF THE BIKE

3 min. ramp to IM 70.3 effort
2 min. Z2 easy
30 sec. build to feel strong
2 min. Z2 easy
30 sec. build to strong
2 min. Z2 easy
30 sec. build to very strong

Scale for Time Cut Pre-Main to 2 × 3 min. Then Main is two rounds of each set.

Scale for Fatigue Remove the Main set but add a 15 min. build by 5 min. to the last 5 min. feeling steady and open.

SESSION TWO

PM OFF

344

WEDNESDAY

KEY **SWIM**
ENDURANCE Building, 1700–2100

This is a recommended session.

Warm-Up 10 min. smooth

Pre-Main
Pull 200, 175, 150, 125, 100, 75, 50, 25; progress to 80–85%.

Main
8 × 100–150 build effort by 2 intervals to the last 2 being above race effort
Always 30 sec. rest

Scale for Time Reduce the Pre-Main set to begin at the 150. Drop to 6 Intervals in Main set as: 1 at 65%, 1 at 70%, 1 at 75%, 1 at 80%, 1 at 85%, 1 at 90%.

Scale for Fatigue Reduce the Pre-Main set to begin at the 150. Drop to 6 Intervals in the Main set and only build to 85%.

SUPPORTING **RUN**
TECHNICAL Prep, 20–30 min.

Warm-Up 10 min. easy
Add dynamic warm-up if possible.

Main
10–20 min. low stress
Every 4th min. or so, check on form, posture, etc. Aim for best MFP. Do not exceed Z2 effort.

Scale for Time Simple scale of duration as needed.

Scale for Fatigue Trim duration or skip if needed.

THURSDAY

SUPPORTING **SWIM**
TECHNICAL Prep, 1250–1500

This is a recommended session.

Warm-Up 10 min. easy

Main
5 × 150–200 progress 1 to 5 to 80%
12 × 25, do as 3 rounds of: easy, build, fast, fast

Then, 200 easy

OPEN WATER

Warm-Up 10 min. smooth

Pre-Main
5 × 90 sec. progress 1 to 5 to 80%

Add-On 4–6 × 30 sec. blasts with 1 min. easy between efforts

Scale for Time Reduce duration as needed.

Scale for Fatigue Skip this swim if fatigued.

SUPPORTING **BIKE**
TECHNICAL Recovery, 30–60 min.

This is a recommended session.

Main
30–60 min. smooth endurance
Nothing hard.

Add-On Do a 20–30 min. very low stress shake-out run after you finish the ride.

Scale for Time Scale as needed, but this may become a walk if time-crunched.

Scale for Fatigue Going for a walk and moving the blood is a good thing.

IRONMAN 70.3

RACE SPECIFIC

FRIDAY

SESSION ONE

SUPPORTING BIKE + RUN
TECHNICAL Prep, 40 min.

This is a recommended session.

Warm-Up 15 min. smooth

Pre-Main
3 × 3 min. build by 1 min. to Z3+/Z4

Main 6 min. as:
2 min. smooth,
2 min. ramping effort,
2 min. at IM 70.3 effort

Smooth home and feel good

RUN OFF THE BIKE

10 min. smooth as:
5 min. ramp to IM 70.3 effort,
5 min. form-based running

Scale for Time Scale duration as needed.

Scale for Fatigue Skip this session.

SESSION TWO

PM OFF

SATURDAY

SESSION ONE

KEY SWIM
TECHNICAL Prep, 20 min.

Open water session at the racecourse.

Main
10 min. to loosen up
4 × 2 min. build by 30 sec. to 90%

Then a few take-out efforts if you need to spark it up a touch.

Scale for Time Scale as needed; you are the boss to make yourself feel good for tomorrow.

Scale for Fatigue Not needed.

SESSION TWO

KEY BIKE
TECHNICAL Activation, 10–20 min.

Main
10–20 min. smooth easy endurance
Include 3 × 30–45 sec. ramp to strong but not deep effort
3-4 min. riding between intervals

Follow the pattern and theme of previous weeks and nail this ride. Note that this is your last chance to check out your equipment prior to the race.

Scale for Time Not needed.

Scale for Fatigue Not needed.

SUNDAY

IRONMAN 70.3 RACE DAY

Workout Glossary

For each discipline, there are four general categories of workouts, and they contain descriptions that further define the intent of individual sessions. You'll want to become familiar with the themes and focus of each workout so that when you scan a week of training, you can quickly understand the focus of the session. Here's an example:

> KEY **BIKE**
> END-OF-RANGE Strength-Endurance, 1.5–2 hr.

- *Priority:* Whatever the discipline, workouts specified as "key" are not to be missed.

- *Category:* End-of-Range is a style of riding that focuses on evolving cadence, usually with a very low or very high rpm at a moderately strong to very strong effort.

- *Intent:* Strength-Endurance means that the session is designed to develop muscular strength and resilience, so you can expect to focus on lower cadences.

Here's a very different bike workout:

SUPPORTING RUN
TECHNICAL Activation, 50–70 min.

- *Priority:* Supporting workouts have a role in your preparation. Get them in if you can, but these workouts are candidates for scaling or skipping altogether if life gets busy or you experience excessive fatigue. (You'll find specific notes on scaling for time management or heavy fatigue in the race-prep training plans.)

- *Category:* Technical workouts entail less physical stress on the body. This is a chance to work on form and skills.

- *Intent:* Here the main goal of the session is recovery—these workouts facilitate recuperation from a previous, challenging session.

You can see how this terminology explains the intent and theme of any session. Let's get studying!

Swim Workouts, Technical

These swims are focused on recovery, technique and form development, or preparation for an upcoming session or race.

Recovery: Recuperation sessions with lower physical stress, which provides a great opportunity to focus on technique and form.

Form: Low-stress sessions that focus on body position, pulling form, and synchronization. Typically include some work with swimming tools, such as fins, paddles, and pull buoy, to help with form.

Speed and Power: "Over-recruitment" best describes this work, which still has a place in technical swims. Some fast swimming is added to ensure the body is working to its full potential.

Prep: Designed as preparation for an upcoming workout or race, these sessions feature some activation and building work, without causing fatigue.

Swim Workouts, Endurance

Open-water races require high levels of cardiovascular and muscular endurance. These sessions develop your ability to maintain specific efforts in open water.

Short Intervals: Focused on maintaining form under fatigue, a key performance criteria. Hit each interval with good form and maintain it through the session.

Over-Distance: Conditions the mind and the body to handle the challenge of race distance and beyond. Use these sessions to convert the endurance of short-interval work into extended swimming.

Building: Lessons in pacing and self-management, these sessions "build" effort across a series of intervals. Increase effort and speed through the progression. Master the art of efficiency and speed change.

Swim Workouts, Intervals

Raises the sustainable ceiling of your performance and develops your resilience to fatigue. Intervals are often executed at maximal sustained pace, but not at the cost of retaining rhythm, supple tempo, and good form. Never fight the water, even in these interval workouts.

High-Intensity: Drives adaptation of synchronization, power, and capacity to your swim stroke and your ability to produce force. Swim toys are used to improve speed or force over-recruitment.

Building: Strong intervals with progressive intensity. Different from the building sets of an endurance focus, these are mostly shorter intervals that progress toward maximal effort, creating a great delta of both effort and speed through the main set.

Swim Workouts, Event-Specific

Designed as preparation for races and specifically for the demands of open-water swimming. Translate these physical and mental skills into your race execution and performance.

Pyramid: Progressive distance with a focus on great form as the distance sets become longer and more challenging. Mimics the feeling of fatigue and the difficulty of maintaining form in a race.

Threshold: Notoriously tough and challenging. Done properly, these sessions can increase tolerance for very strong efforts. Often integrates open-water skills, such as sighting, but retaining form despite fatigue is critical.

Race Simulation: Recreates in the pool the variability that happens in open water, including race starts, swimming in a group, buoy turns, establishing a rhythm, surges of speed, and swim finishes.

Open Water: Many athletes have limited access to open water. For information regarding open-water swim sessions, visit the Purple Patch website.

Bike Workouts, Technical

Lower-stress sessions that focus on technique, skills, preparation, or recovery over physical strain or load. It's common to turn off the mind in these feel-good sessions, but that is a mistake. Build cycling skills, terrain management, and course execution to yield better performance with lower physical cost.

Prep: A chance to physically and mentally get ready for the work to come. Because this ride is rejuvenating, it may precede a race or key session. Learn what makes you feel good and what you enjoy.

Recovery: Pure recuperation with minimal, if any, efforts. Get the blood moving to help address any soreness or fatigue. Take the opportunity to get comfortable on the bike, practice handling skills, and ride well with great form.

Activation: Easier sessions that include some short, intense efforts. These will stimulate the muscles and movement patterns needed in future sessions. These sessions should not create deep fatigue, despite the somewhat higher intensity.

Bike Workouts, Endurance

Fitness and endurance on the bike underpin performance both on the bike and on the run. Smooth, efficient riding demands great focus on form and terrain management. Endurance is the bedrock of your racing preparation.

Over-Distance: Elevates cardiovascular and muscular fitness, improves postural fitness, develops mental focus and resilience, and provides a platform to work on proper fueling and hydration strategies.

General Endurance: Develops a baseline of fitness, form, and good habits and builds resilience. Endurance sessions, executed properly and consistently, make up the backbone of race readiness.

Bike Workouts, End-of-Range

The "special sauce" of Purple Patch training. A high percentage of racing happens in a narrow range of output and cycling cadence (rpm), but there is great value in developing a wide range of intensity and cadence. Consistency in these sessions establishes an awareness of your natural strengths, tools for managing various terrain and conditions, and the chance to vary loads for consistent output and speed. Expect plenty of very low cadence, and very high cadence, in these varying and challenging sessions. Do this work to be better prepared and more aware as a rider.

Strength-Endurance: Focuses on low rpm at moderate to very heavy tension on the chain. Develops resilience, strengthens pedal stroke, and reduces cardiovascular stress at opportune times.

Building: Use these intervals to develop a sense of pacing and progressive effort, especially with uncertainty over past efforts. These intervals often start at low cadence but progress from smooth to maximal effort over a series of intervals or within each interval.

High Cadence: Work the other end of range by pedaling very fast while keeping tension on the chain. Cardiovascular and neurological stress is high, but cadence is an important tool to develop. In the real world of cycling, this work is relevant to maintaining power and speed while riding downhill or in a tailwind.

Bike Workouts, Event-Specific

Focus on specificity for an upcoming race. Find the pace, effort, or power output appropriate for race goals and simulate (train) for the experience and pacing of it. Also work to blend your natural strengths, terrain management, and hydration and fueling strategies.

Building: Rides start with good posture, position, and pedaling and gradually progress effort through the session. Focus on delivering your best effort and form in the final third of the series of intervals or ride as a whole. Ingrain great riding in the final third of every ride.

Intervals: Efforts are just under, at, or perhaps just above, goal race effort. Consistency and smart management of these sessions will help you develop self-management and internal pacing.

Race Simulation: Designed to test effort and fueling strategies for race day. These challenging sessions are some of the most important ways to test and track progress along the journey.

Run Workouts, Technical

Removes physical stress and focuses on run form, technique, or lower stress running for resilience or recovery. Sessions may include focused walking, hopping, bounding, or very easy running, More advanced runners might need to intentionally hold back on some elements of good form, such as leg propulsion and foot speed, to allow easy running. Posture and proper arm carriage remain essential.

Recovery: Make sure these easy runs are truly easy in nature. If necessary, incorporate walking in these sessions to retain the goal of low stress.

Prep: Short runs designed to help you feel good in the days leading up to key run sessions or races. Explore the options provided to develop a sense of what works best.

Activation: Includes strides, over-recruitment running, and similar efforts that will improve the dialogue between brain and muscles, enhancing readiness for upcoming key sessions or racing without leading to fatigue or soreness.

Run Workouts, Endurance

Develops the cardiovascular and muscular conditioning, qualities that make up the backbone of successful run training. Sessions focus on the consistent layering of effort to build a platform of resilience.

Over-Distance: In run training, over-distance entails an extended duration of time, not necessarily running longer than the race distance. Form is key, as is self-management and holding on to form despite fatigue.

General Endurance: Develops resilience while maintaining good form. Sessions typically specify minimal form pace (MFP) running, or retaining as many of the elements of good form as possible for the specified time.

Run Workouts, Intervals

These sessions vary speed and effort in a wide range of intensities depending on the goal of the session. Realize that it isn't just about effort; awareness and form must be retained.

Strength: Runs are executed on hills or a loop that you can repeat to develop strength and form in your legs that will translate to better running on the flats and varying terrain.

Tempo: Sustained efforts at an uncomfortable but sustainable pace or effort. An important tool to evolve pace and overall development.

Speed: Prescribed in small doses, these sessions include some sustained efforts at higher-than-race-pace running. As a stand-alone workout, these are labeled speed work.

Run Workouts, Event-Specific

Practices the style and personality of running specific to an upcoming race. This training is fundamental to race execution. Aim to develop your experience of what you will encounter on race day.

Building: Smooth, progressing effort and tempo extending through the main workout. Other sessions ramp up to race pace quickly, but these sessions are preparation for best performance the last third of the run, in terms of both form and pace.

Intervals: Different from the interval workouts, event-specific intervals always focus on race effort/pace. Expect to see some longer intervals focused on race effort.

Run Off the Bike: Use these brick sessions to add resilience, sneak in running frequency and duration in a block, and train your ability to ramp up to pace quickly off the bike. Also work on the transition piece, which can be a great place to save time on race day.

Race Simulation: Designed to prepare you for the experience of race day. Treat these sessions as mini-races and practice race day breakfast, fueling, equipment choice, and event-specific terrain whenever possible. Practice self-management for your best route to success.

Index

Note: Italicized page numbers indicate a figure.

Acknowledgments

To the athletes: Most coaches will tell you that while our job is to coach, edu-cate, and guide athletes to new levels of performance, every athlete provides the opportunity for learning and growth in the coach. Through that lens, I realize this book has come to fruition via the lessons, observations, and challenges that every athlete I have coached has provided. While I have been immensely lucky and proud to coach many world-class athletes, most of the lessons in this book have emerged through working with athletes who don't compete at that high-est level. With this said, many of them are world-class people. Whether it is the many CEOs and other leading executives, whose sporting aspirations and com-plex lives have forced me to think outside the box to create performance solu-tions, or those who arrived on the back of chronic fatigue and over-training and sought balanced energy and dared to have sporting dreams again, the influence and time-starved methodology described here has emerged from your journeys.

To Paul Buick: I met Paul more than ten years ago, a man who just loved to help people ride their bikes better. Little did I know that he would evolve to become the most trusted and influential partner in the Purple Patch method-ology and approach to coaching. His genius is, in my mind, as unparalleled as his uniqueness a person. He is a massive part of the Purple Patch success and an irreplaceable part of the Purple Patch Team.

To the Purple Patch Team: In addition to the athletes, our coaching couldn't happen if I were not surrounded by a wonderful team at Purple Patch. Beyond the joy and inspiration of building Purple Patch with my wife, Kelli, I am lucky for the trust, belief, effort, and dedication of the entire team who, with an athlete-first mindset and a commitment to constantly aim for the better, I believe are on our own path of excellence.

To the contributors: This book could not have been possible without the people who contributed to framing, building, revising, and filtering the most important elements to cram into these precious pages. Michael Lord DC, Brendon Rearick, Brian Metzler, Renee Jardine, Dr. Chris Winter, and all the other highly gifted and smart people who have influenced and contributed to my coaching mindset, thank you.

To the influencers: Beyond athletics, Kelli and I have been fortunate to have highly influential and helpful advisors and mentors who have helped shape our mindset, path, and approach. These very special people have had a direct and an indirect influence on the pages of this book, and I can never fully express how helpful and important you have all been. There are too many to name all, but some of the key players include Sir Michael Moritz, Derek Robson, Tom Andrews, Gerry Rodrigues, Alan Waxman, Tyler McMaster, Tom Wildhart, Max Levchin, Jesse Thomas, Scott McMullin, Pat Romano, Carmel Galvin, Pete O'Dea, Brian Weaver, Josh Ross, Alex Kaplinsky, and many more.

Sami the Bull: And a special word to Sami Inkinen, who was the first living case study of the clear solutions-based approach to performance within a busy life. A shared journey to an age-group world championship, in parallel to taking a company from concept to IPO, is a rare chance for personal development and joy. Our concepts and theories live on, now tried and trusted, and I hope we can continue to be a positive influence in the pursuit of helping every inspired person to real their own potential of human performance.

Thank you for reading. Onward in the journey of potential and performance.

About the Author

MATT DIXON is an exercise physiologist and an elite coach. He is founder and president of Purple Patch fitness, a fitness and coaching company serving triathletes and endurance enthusiasts of all levels, from world champions to novices. His clients include leading professional triathletes and endurance athletes, executives of global companies, serious amateur triathletes, and fitness aficionados looking to improve both their lives and their performances.

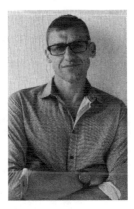

Over the past few years, Purple Patch athletes have laid claim to over 250 professional Ironman- and half-Ironman-distance championships and podium finishes, over 125 of which have been victories. The winning formula is rooted in the Purple Patch pillars of performance. When endurance, strength, nutrition, and recovery are adequately and equally developed, athletes enter into a "purple patch" in which top performances become a reality. Matt has developed numerous athletes from the amateur ranks to have highly successful professional careers. He has also helped more than 150 athletes qualify for and compete in the Hawaii Ironman World Championship, including multiple age-group world champions. Matt's coaching career is steeped in his own experience, first as an elite swimmer and then as a professional triathlete. He was a two-time Olympic trials finalist for Great Britain and an NCAA Division I swimmer. His triathlon career spanned multiple seasons; he competed as a pro at the Hawaii Ironman and won Vineman 70.3.

Starting out as a coach in a national champion swimming program, Matt went on to become an NCAA Division I collegiate swimming coach while completing his master's degree in clinical and exercise physiology. He ultimately landed in triathlon and has been coaching triathletes since 2001. Matt is the author of *The Well-Built Triathlete*, a complete training manual that develops the whole athlete for greater performance. He has been featured in the *Wall Street Journal*, the *New York Times*, *Outside* magazine, *Men's Fitness*, *Men's Health*, *Triathlete* magazine, *Triathlete Europe*, and *Lava Magazine*. Contact Matt through his website, Purple Patchfitness.com.

Matt lives in San Francisco with his wife, Kelli, their son, Baxter, and their naughty dog, Willow.

AS A FAST-TRACK TRIATHLETE

PURPLE PATCH WOULD LIKE TO OFFER YOU

3 FREE MONTHS

OF THE **PURPLE PATCH EDUCATION PROGRAM**

THE PROGRAM INCLUDES:

➡ A comprehensive library of performance videos and education

➡ A weekly educational bulletin written by Matt Dixon

➡ Access to special performance webinars by Matt Dixon

...and more!

Redeem this one-time offer at
purplepatchfitness.com/fast-track-triathlete-offer
and enter the code **IAMFASTTRACK**

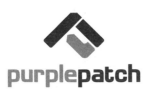

purplepatch